Praise for

Dining Lean

How to Eat Healthy in your Favorite Restaurants

"Dining Lean...offers Lichten's innovative 'Calorimeters,' easy-to-use charts that group foods by type and serving size to help readers estimate the total energy and fat grams in any food item."
- Journal of the American Dietetic Association

"'Rather than give up on restaurant dining, order more wisely', suggests Joanne V. Lichten, a Houston-based registered dietitian...'Dining out healthfully is about choices – not deprivation'. That's the word from...Lichten, who's living proof that you can dine out and maintain a healthful eating style...'[*Dining Lean*] has a different philosophy than diet books that say don't eat this'. ...For Lichten, no food is off limits. It's a matter of priorities."
- Karen Haram, San Antonio Express News

"Eating Out? Watch the Fat...*Dining Lean* has useful diagrams and comparative drawings to help determine serving size...contains information that some may find surprising."
- Ramin Jaleshgari, Newsday

"*Dining Lean* breaks out healthy choices by appetizer, accompaniments, sauces, and entrees in a variety of ethnic and chain restaurants."
- Frequent Flyer Magazine

"If you're on a perpetual diet, a quest to eat healthy, or just curious about the dietary impacts of dining out, then this handy nutritional guide was written just for you. The book also includes information on what to avoid – and what to order – for healthy eating at restaurants varying from Indian to Italian."
- Independent Publisher

"It's easy to control what you eat when you are in control in the kitchen. But, dining out is another challenge altogether. Dr. Joanne Lichten's *Dining Lean* is an exhaustive reference for maintaining your healthy habits in restaurants. Well researched, yet easy to read and friendly, it is filled with tips, nutrition facts, and specific information on the most popular restaurants. Don't leave home without it!"

- Mary Guay, Author of *Don't Diet - Live It!*

"Joanne V. Lichten, a dietitian and PhD, has written a new guide on how to eat healthfully while eating out. It contains listings of hundreds of fast food and other restaurant foods, plus actual-size drawings of portions to help you make dine-out decisions."

- Ann Criswell, Houston Chronicle

"Lichten packs a ton of easy-to-understand nutritional information in this 284 page paperback ...The first two chapters – a sort of crash course in 'Nutrition 101' – are especially useful. *Dining Lean* is an excellent resource to keep handy for answers to your most common nutrition questions."

- Karen Andreas, The Salem Evening News, Salem, MA

"...offers positive, realistic steps toward eating healthfully....Although her chapters are oriented to restaurant dining, they are just as applicable for meals you eat at home.

- The Desert Sun, Palm Springs, CA

"Lichten's book is about making informed decisions."

-Barbara M. Houle, Telegram & Gazette, Worcester, MA

"...in this business it's all too easy to grab a burger on the way to a story, and thus I'd fallen off the 'eating healthy' wagon many, many times...your book will be able to help our entire newsroom."

- Shea Daugherty, KZTV, Corpus Christi

"If you eat, read this book! Dining Lean is full of easy-to-digest facts and suggestions on how to gain the upper hand regarding your dietary decisions. I highly recommend it!"

- Tony Alessandra, PhD, Author of The Platinum Rule & Charisma (Warner Books)

Dining Lean

How to Eat Healthy in your Favorite Restaurants

Joanne V. Lichten, RD, PhD

Nutrifit Publishing

Dining Lean

How to Eat Healthy in Your Favorite Restaurants
2nd Edition

Joanne V. Lichten, RD, PhD

Published by:
Nutrifit Publishing
PO Box 690452
Houston, TX 77269-0452
(281) 955-LEAN
(888) 431-LEAN
Email: DiningLean@aol.com
Web: www.DiningLean.com

Printed in Canada by Hignell Printing

Publisher's Cataloging In Publication data:
Lichten, Joanne V.
Dining Lean: How to eat healthy in your favorite restaurants. Second edition
304p. 22cm. Includes index.
ISBN: 1-880347-00-8: $14.95 (pbk.)
1. Nutrition - Handbooks, manuals, etc. 2. Restaurants - United States - Guide-books. 3. Low-fat diet.

TX907.2   2000
613.2-dc20

Cover design by Pat Packard, Houston

This book is dedicated to the two "sweeties" in my life: Lorin & Alexandra who always knew to peak around my desk to see how my writing was coming along. You always seemed to know when I needed company, a hug or to be left alone in my tears. Thanks for understanding my personal need to write Dining Lean and, now, this new edition.

Many thanks also to my parents, Dr. Mary Ann and Richard Valinski, who spent countless days reading my book and offering suggestions.

Without Denise Vargo's countless hours meticulously checking my numbers, I wouldn't have made the deadline. Thanks.

I'm also grateful for the editing by Christy Craig and the illustrations (and the updated cover) by Teresa Southwell.

HOW TO USE THIS RESTAURANT GUIDE

Many people are under the assumption that it is nearly impossible to "eat right" while "dining out." This book demonstrates that it just isn't so! Many restaurants offer menu items that are low in both calories and fat. In addition, just about every restaurant has menu items that can be modified to meet your healthy eating program.

The information in this book was up-to-date at the time of the printing. All nutritional information from the restaurants was obtained from the restaurant's corporate headquarters or from their web site. All restaurants were given an opportunity to review the information prior to printing.

Before you order foods at these restaurants based on the information in this book, consider the following. Restaurants frequently change menus, recipes, and chefs. In addition, there may be errors in the contents of this book due to typographical mistakes or misunderstandings between myself and my sources. So always verify the information in this book before ordering.

Dining Lean is a guide book that lists menu items including the lowest fat and calorie menu items available at each restaurant. These are not exact prescriptions of what *you* should be eating. As with any book that suggests foods for better health, it is impossible to generalize to the entire population. Always consult with a Registered Dietitian or Medical doctor regarding how to tailor this restaurant guide to your particular health needs. Bon Appetit!

Dr. Joanne Lichten

Table of Contents

PART
1

The Beginning

Introduction

Nearly half of all Americans eat out on a typical day.

Eating out used to be a rare social event. Now, as a result of dual career families, business meetings planned around meals, hectic schedules, and fatigue, we eat out more frequently. According to the National Restaurant Association, nearly half of all adults eat out on a typical day. The USDA reports that 27% of all meals are purchased from restaurants. Of the meals we eat out, half of these meals are take-out or delivered food. And...

Many Americans want to eat healthier.

The average American gains a pound a year after they reach the age of 25, contributing to nearly half of all adults being overweight. Studies reveal that Americans are constantly trying to lose weight. Since heart disease is the number one killer in the United States, many of us are also concerned with our serum cholesterol. For those reasons, about 40% of all restaurant customers are trying to eat healthier food items not only at home, but also when eating out. Dining out can no longer be used as an excuse for unhealthy eating habits. Because...

Restaurants are responding with healthy foods.

A recent survey of table service restaurants confirmed that 40% currently feature healthful menu items. Results from another study indicated that nearly half of the restaurants plan to add more nutritious menu items in the future. Even fast food restaurants (representing one third of all restaurant visits) are serving new, good-tasting, healthy foods. And...

DINING LEAN has made it easier than ever to select the healthiest food at every restaurant.

This book provides you with the following information:

■ Your daily recommendation of calories, fat, and sodium.

■ How much calories, fat, and sodium you actually *consume* each day.

■ Calorie, fat, carbohydrate, and sodium content of thousands of restaurant food items.

■ "Calorimeter" charts and portion size depictions for estimating the calories and fat grams of *any* food (when nutritional information is not available).

■ Exchanges for people with diabetes or on a weight management program.

■ Lists of recommended preparation and serving modifications to request.

Why does DINING LEAN stress low fat menu selections?

In the second chapter, you will discover that it is the excess fat in our diet that is increasing our serum cholesterol and keeping us fatter than we would want to be. Most people don't realize that:

■ Fats have twice as many calories as equal weights of carbohydrates or protein.

■ Fats in the foods we eat are very close in composition to the fat on our body. Whenever we eat more fat than we need, they are just "sucked up" by our fat cells.

■ All fats, whether "healthy" fats (such as tub margarine or vegetable oil) or "unhealthy" fats (like butter or lard), have the same number of calories and make us *equally* fat.

■ "Cholesterol Free" *does not* mean the product is calorie-free, lower in calories, fat-free, or lower in fat.

■ Simply cutting back on dietary cholesterol is not enough to lower your blood cholesterol; cutting back on your total fat intake is also necessary.

Therefore, the bottom line is: if you want to lower your serum cholesterol or lose weight decrease your *fat* intake!

How this Book is Organized

The next two chapters in **Dining Lean** include a discussion of nutritional needs and general guidelines for eating out healthy at *any* restaurant. The remainder of the book is organized into separate chapters based on the type of food served. Each chapter, illustrated with easy-to-read comparison charts and lists, contains recommendations on how to reduce your intake of both calories and fat. In addition, nutritional information (calories, fats, carbohydrates, and sodium) is provided for all commonly served foods. Exchanges are also listed for persons following a diet for diabetes or for weight loss and maintenance. There is no implied comparison of one restaurant against another. The last chapter contains nutritional information of menu items found in many of your favorite restaurants.

Other Important Information

The calories, grams of fat, and sodium listed in the introductory sections of the chapters were obtained from USDA food composition tables, averages from restaurant's nutritional information, food manufacturers, and scientific literature. The nutritional information listed under each restaurant was obtained directly from that restaurant. Prior to publication, each restaurant was given an opportunity to review the written text. Calories were listed exactly as the numbers were provided. Fat grams larger than one were often rounded to the nearest whole number for simplicity. Some exchanges were provided by the restaurant but most were calculated by the author using the restaurant-provided nutritional information.

No Nutritional Information Available? No Problem!

Most restaurants do not provide nutritional information. Even if you could find the food in a calorie book, it is still difficult to know how many calories are in *your* food since portion sizes vary greatly.

For example, if the calorie book lists an *average* roll as having 150 calories, you still don't know how many calories are in *your* roll. What does an *average* size roll look like anyway?

If your calorie guide book states there are 600 calories in a 10 oz serving of lasagna, are you any closer to knowing how many calories you consumed? Is a 10 oz serving of lasagna a small portion or a large one?

It doesn't have to be confusing to accurately calculate the calories in your favorite meals. We just need two pieces of information which **Dining Lean** provides:

❶　Weight or size of the food. Throughout the book you will find size descriptions of many food items (such as *"the size of a deck of cards"*). In addition, there are numerous measurements and actual-size drawings. These measurements, pictures, and descriptors make it easy to determine *your* specific portion.

❷　Calories per ounce for specific food items. **Dining Lean** provides what the author has termed *"Calorimeters"* to assist you in calculating the number of calories *at a glance*. All foods have roughly between zero and 200 calories per ounce. Pure fat, such as butter or oil, has 200 calories per ounce. Water, at the other extreme, has zero. All other foods fall somewhere in between these two numbers.

What is a Calorimeter?

The "Calorimeter" is an easy-to-use chart that illustrates calories in a specific portion. Food items are logically grouped for comparative purposes. The calorimeter, at a glance, will enable you to compare food choices by the ounce and by the serving size. This simple tool enables you to make well-informed food selections. Let's take a look at a calorimeter for a variety of foods.

Calorimeter: Calories per ounce

200	Pure fats - oil, butter, margarine
180	Nuts
150	Chocolate candy
140	Brownie
130	Cookies, plain croissants, cake doughnuts
120	Chocolate cream filled doughnuts
110	Danish, cheesecake, plain & frosted cakes, pasta (plain)
100	Muffins, coffee cake, yeast doughnuts, sausage, fried meats
80	Bagel, custard pies
75	Thin crust cheese pizza, steaks
70	Bread, lowfat muffins, fruit pies
60	Ice cream
50	Fruit cobbler, chicken
40	Soft serve, ice milk
30	Fish
0	Water

As you can see, all foods have between zero and 200 calories per ounce. To find out how many ounces are in each food, calorimeters are often accompanied by pictures depicting the most common portion sizes. For example, knowing that a 3 oz. portion of meat is the size of a deck of cards, you can easily estimate the calories and fat grams of *your* meat portion.

Do You Want to Lose Weight?

In the next chapter you will learn that by eating 100 fewer calories each day, you can lose a pound a month, effortlessly! To help you lose weight, there are numerous suggestions preceded by a check (✓). Frequently, these suggestions are combined with an example of the calorie and fat savings.

Dining Lean Basics:
Facts about Calories, Fat, & Sodium

Did you know that you can begin losing weight or prevent the typical trend of gaining weight as you age by making *very small* changes in how you eat? This chapter explains how to maintain a healthy weight *and* keep your cholesterol level normal.

Why Am I Gaining Weight?

There is only one reason why we gain excess weight. It is simply because we eat more calories than our bodies need. There are two general solutions to treat and prevent excess weight gain: ❶ eat fewer calories and ❷ exercise more to burn more calories.

Some diets promote a specific pattern of foods to eat, when to eat it, and exactly how much to eat of it. These programs often state or imply a mindset of good and bad foods and set strict guidelines making the program difficult to follow. **Dining Lean**, instead, suggests that each of us determine how many calories we need in a day so *we* can decide how to best *spend* our calories. Think of the number of calories we need in a day as our "budget." When you eat more calories than you need, you will gain weight. When you eat fewer calories than you need each day, you will lose weight. It really is that simple.

The options on how to spend your calories are nearly limitless, but no single food is "off" the program. Certainly, eating all fried foods or high sugar foods on a daily basis would not be healthy. But eating these foods on an infrequent basis is still acceptable and can still fit into your daily "budget." According to research conducted by the author, people who have been successful at losing weight are the ones who have made *slow*, healthy changes in their lifestyle and didn't give up all the foods they love. Typically, when you cut out all the foods you love, it becomes difficult to "stick with the program." Have some flexibility - it's a lot more fun and gives you the greatest chance of success in the long run. Before we can be flexible, we need to be informed. So let's start!

How Many Calories Should I Be Eating?

The number of calories we need every day to maintain our present weight can be calculated using the simple formula below.

Estimating Daily Calorie Needs

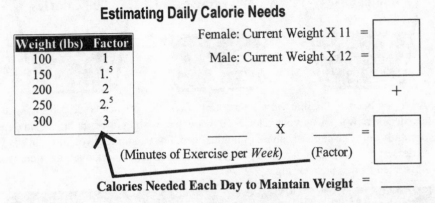

Weight (lbs)	Factor
100	1
150	$1.^5$
200	2
250	$2.^5$
300	3

Female: Current Weight X 11 =

Male: Current Weight X 12 =

+

_____ X _____ =

(Minutes of Exercise per *Week*)   (Factor)

Calories Needed Each Day to Maintain Weight = _____

If you want to lose weight, you will have to either ❶ eat fewer calories or ❷ exercise more to burn more calories. Read on to find out how you can eat fewer calories.

More Food for your Calorie Needs

Calories come from three basic nutrients: carbohydrates, proteins, and fats. Vitamins, minerals, and water (the other three nutrients) have no calories.

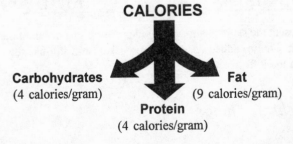

CALORIES

Carbohydrates
(4 calories/gram)

Protein
(4 calories/gram)

Fat
(9 calories/gram)

FACT: Fats are more than twice as caloric (or fattening) as carbohydrates and proteins. While carbohydrates and proteins have only 4 calories per gram, fats have a whopping 9 calories per gram. That translates to approximately 112 calories per ounce of protein or carbohydrates. One ounce of fat has over 250 calories!

That's why you can eat a greater *quantity* of foods that are low in fat than of those that are high in fat. For example, a medium sized apple (high in carbohydrates) has no more calories than two tiny pats of margarine (pure fat).

To illustrate the point further, a cup of white flour has 400 calories and a cup of sugar has 800 calories. In contrast, a cup of oil (pure fat) has 2000 calories!

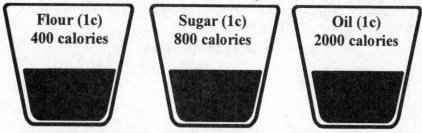

| Flour (1c) | Sugar (1c) | Oil (1c) |
| 400 calories | 800 calories | 2000 calories |

After you become familiar with the amount of calories in your favorite foods, you can decide how to spend your calories so that you are eating fewer calories than you currently eat. The choices can be individualized. For example, if you look forward to dessert you may consider saving calories in your dinner. Check out the difference illustrated in this next example.

A Typical Dinner	Calories	Fat (g)	More Food & Less Calories	Calories	Fat (g)
4 oz. Margarita	240	0	4 oz. Wine	100	0
1 sl. Bread w/1 t. butter	125	5	1 slice Bread – no butter	80	0
Salad w/ 3T. dressing	250	24	Salad w/ 1T. dressing	105	8
Loaded baked potato	400	25	Dry baked potato	160	1
8 oz. Fried fish	600	32	8 oz. Broiled fish w/	250	5
¼ c. Tartar sauce	320	36	lemon		
Broccoli/cheese sauce	125	12	Steamed broccoli	25	0
			Cheesecake (big 6 oz)	600	35
TOTAL:	**2060**	**134**	**TOTAL:**	**1320**	**49**

Both meals represent the same quantity of food prepared in a different manner. The meal on the right side has added dessert (cheesecake!) and still has fewer calories than the meal on the left.

It's Just the Little Things

FACT: There are 3500 calories in each pound of body fat. Eating just 10 calories extra every day could contribute to one pound gained each year.

> ## 10 calories/day X 365 days = 3650 extra calories a year

Ten calories is just 1 hard candy, 1 nibble of a cookie, a sip of soda, *or* a thin smear of butter. Just one of these ten additional calories every day could account for the average one pound many Americans gain each year.

An extra 100 calories consumed each day adds up to nearly a pound a month.

> ## 100 calories X 30 days = 3000 extra calories a month

That extra pound each month could come from eating just a third of a doughnut, 8 oz of beer, 8 oz of soda, an extra tablespoon of salad dressing, $2/3$ oz of chips, *or* just 10 French fries extra each day.

Conversely, if you eat just 100 calories *less* each day, you can lose almost a pound a month or 10 pounds a year with very little effort. This book is loaded with numerous small changes you can undertake to make a *major* impact upon your weight.

A Calorie is a Calorie is a Calorie - or is it?

FACT: The more fat you eat, the fatter you become. Excess fat consumption works against weight control and weight loss efforts in two ways. The first, and more obvious, is the calories per gram as compared to the other two nutrients. The second, and more insidious, is the way our bodies process the fats we eat.

Our bodies change all of the three calorie-containing nutrients (carbohydrates, proteins, and fats) into fuel that our body runs on. Whenever we eat more calories (from any source) than we need each day, our body stores the extra calories as *body fat*.

Eating an extra 100 calories of carbohydrates or an extra 100 calories of protein does not build as much body fat as eating an extra 100 calories of fat. A recent study at the Stanford Center for Research in Disease Prevention demonstrated that dietary fat might be even more caloric than the 4/4/9 ratio indicated.

When we eat more carbohydrates or proteins than we need, twenty three percent (23%) of all the calories is lost in switching the carbohydrates chemically to stored fat. Because the fat that we eat is very much like the fat that we store on our body, very few calories (3%) are needed to convert it. So, nearly all of the fat calories become excess fat on our body. Therefore, fats are probably *three* times more fattening than carbohydrates and proteins.

Simple mathematics makes a demonstrable case for controlling fat consumption. By cutting back on the fats we eat, we can enjoy more real food and lose weight painlessly.

Cut Back on Fats to Decrease Your Cholesterol

FACT: Heart disease is the #1 killer in the United States. Half of all Americans die of heart disease. That's why so many people are concerned about their serum cholesterol level. Levels over 200 mg/dl are considered high for most adults. Research demonstrates that lowering your serum cholesterol level can reduce your risk of developing heart disease.

FACT: Simply cutting back on your dietary cholesterol intake will not lower your serum cholesterol level! Many people think that simply cutting back on the cholesterol content of their food will reduce their serum cholesterol level. While this may have a small effect, it is *far more important* to lose weight and lower your total intake of fat. When you eat *excess fat* your liver simply responds by making *more serum cholesterol.* Cutting back on your cholesterol intake will not necessarily lower your fat intake. However, lowering your fat intake usually lowers your cholesterol intake.

FACT: There are two types of fats. The fats we eat can be categorized into either HEALTHY fats or UNHEALTHY fats. Decades ago, we were told to simply replace the UNHEALTHY fats with the HEALTHY fats. The HEALTHY fats tend to lower the serum cholesterol while the UNHEALTHY fats tend to raise the serum cholesterol.

HEALTHIER FATS (*lowers* cholesterol)	UNHEALTHY FATS (*raises* cholesterol)
Monounsaturated Fats:	**Saturated Fats:**
Avocado	*(Animal)*
Cannola Oil	Bacon, Sausage
Olive Oil	Lard
Peanut Oil	Butter
Polyunsaturated Fats:	*(Vegetable)*
Corn Oil	Coconut Oil
Cottonseed Oil	Palm Oil, Palm Kernel Oil
Soybean Oil	Stick Margarine
Sunflower Oil	
Safflower Oil	**Hydrogenated Fats:**
Soft Tub Margarine	Hydrogenated Vegetable Shortening

Unfortunately, many people believe that HEALTHY fats can be eaten in unlimited quantity. It is not that simple. The *total* fat content of our diets must be lowered.

FACT: All fats have the same number of calories per gram. All fats have 9 calories per gram or about 200 calories per ounce. While soft margarine and oil may be healthier than butter or lard, each contain 100-120 calories per tablespoon - so they're equally fattening!

FACT: Only animals have livers so only animals can produce cholesterol. Cholesterol is manufactured in the liver. Since only animals have livers, only animal products contain cholesterol. That is why cholesterol can be found in animal products such as butter, lard, meat, cheese, and eggs.

FACT: *NO* vegetable products have cholesterol. Vegetables do not have livers so vegetables cannot produce cholesterol. Non-animal products such as wheat, vegetables, fruits, olive oil, margarine, vegetable oils, and tofu (soy bean curd) do not have any cholesterol. A vegetable oil that claims to have "No Cholesterol" may be misleading if you were to conclude that the product has been modified. Vegetables don't have livers; therefore, vegetable oils never had cholesterol and never will.

FACT: Cholesterol Free *does not mean* it is calorie-free or fat-free. "No or low cholesterol" products result from either food that is *naturally* low in cholesterol or from food in which some of the cholesterol has been removed. You can remove the majority of cholesterol from animal products by removing the fat. There is very little cholesterol in skim milk and cheeses made with skim milk. Egg substitutes are made of egg white; the high cholesterol egg yolk has been mostly or completely removed.

Manufacturers of many "no or low cholesterol" foods have just simply changed the type of fat used in a food product. They may have replaced some or all of the animal fat with a vegetable fat in products such as imitation cheese, crackers, or French fries.

In many cases, a "cholesterol-free" product has just as much fat as the original - and therefore, just as many calories. A vegetable oil is pure fat. Lard (animal fat) is pure fat. Vegetable oil may be a little healthier for your heart, but it is just as caloric as lard. Advertising campaigns have successfully misled many consumers into believing that low cholesterol means lowfat or low cholesterol.

FACT: There is no such thing as a no-cholesterol, no-fat oil. You can't remove the fat from oil because vegetable oil is 100% fat - removing the oil would leave you with an empty bottle. Diet margarine has less calories only because some of the fat has been replaced with water and then whipped together. You can't cook well with diet margarine for that reason; the water simply evaporates. Because water has no calories, 100% of all the calories in diet margarine are *still* coming from fat.

Don't believe it if someone tells you that they are frying with a no-cholesterol, *no-fat* oil. There simply is not such a product. There are sprays that have 0 calories per spray (or less than 0.[5] mg by labeling law) but are still made up of fat. These still need to be used sparingly; over spraying can still add on calories.

FACT: Fat-free salad dressings may not really be fat-free. It's true. The Food and Drug Administration allows manufacturers to label foods fat-free if one serving contains less than 0.⁵ gram of fat. If you eat two servings, you've just consumed 1 gram of fat. So clearly, you can see that if you eat salads with a great deal of salad dressing, that fat-free dressing could still add up to a significant number of calories and grams of fat. Comparing the same serving sizes, the fat-free salad dressing is still a better choice over regular salad dressing.

Fat-Free Dressing contains Calories, but Less:	Calories	Fat (g)
Ranch Dressing, 4 Tablespoons	240	20
Fat-Free Ranch Dressing, 4 Tablespoons	120	0-1
Savings:	**120**	**19-20**

FACT: The American Heart Association recommends that Americans eat no more than 30% of their total calories from fat. Simply cutting back on your dietary cholesterol intake *will not* lower your serum cholesterol. That's why the American Heart Association has been recommending for years that we eat less than 30% of all our calories in the form of fat. Simply replacing butter with margarine and frying with vegetable oil instead of lard will not significantly lower your cholesterol (and certainly won't cause a weight loss). You need to cut back on the total amount of fat.

What Foods Are High in Fat?

Most of the fat we eat is not from visible fat such as butter on bread or on a potato. It is hidden from us in the form of egg yolks, meat, cheese, whole milk, fried foods, foods prepared with fat, salad dressing, margarine on vegetables, or sauces.

FACT: Many foods in their natural state are low in fat and calories.

LOWER FAT FOODS	HIGHER FAT FOODS
Vegetable juices, vegetables prepared with little or no added fats, starchy vegetables (corn, potatoes) made with little or no added fats	Fried vegetables such as fried onions, mushrooms, okra, zucchini or French fries; vegetables with added fats such as broccoli with cream sauce or greens prepared with bacon drippings; loaded baked potatoes; potato skins
Most fruits and fruit juices	Avocados, coconuts, olives, nuts, seeds, and peanut butter

LOWER FAT FOODS	HIGHER FAT FOODS
Legumes (beans, peas) prepared with little or no fats	Refried beans
Pasta (plain or with tomato sauce), rice or couscous with little added fats	Pasta with butter or a cream sauce, pasta with a meat sauce, fried rice, "dirty" rice prepared with sausage
Bread and flour products with little added fats (tortillas, yeast rolls, bagels, pancakes)	Cornbread, fried tortillas, biscuits, garlic bread, buttered bread, croissants, waffles, chips, nachos
Most cereals	Granola, cereal with nuts, grits with butter and/or cheese
Desserts such as sorbet, ice milk, lower fat frozen yogurts, low-fat and fat free muffins	Cake, cookies, pies, danish, doughnuts, muffins, ice cream
Skim, nonfat or 1% low fat milk Yogurt, cottage cheese, and aged cheeses made with skim or 1% low fat milk	2% milk, whole milk, yogurt made with whole milk, most cheeses, coffee creamer, non-dairy coffee creamer, sour cream, cream cheese
Egg whites or low fat egg substitute	Egg yolks, fried eggs, scrambled eggs, omelets
Baked or grilled lean protein sources such as fish or shellfish, chicken or turkey without skin, lean beef round, trimmed pork tenderloin, or wild game without skin	Fried shrimp, fried oysters, fried catfish, fried chicken pieces or nuggets, poultry with skin, heavily marbled beef, pork chops, chicken fried steak, hot dogs, prime rib, hamburger, sausage, bacon
Broth-based soups	Cream-based soups, French onion soup with cheese
Fat free salad dressing, flavored vinegar, picante sauce	Regular salad dressings
Cooking with herbs, broth, or water	Butter, margarine, oil, bacon drippings, lard, hydrogenated vegetable shortening

How much Fat Could I Possibly be Eating?

Picture yourself placing an entire stick of butter on a slice of bread. Roll up that slice of bread and take a bite. Do you think that is disgusting? Well, many Americans eat more fat than the equivalent of a stick of butter each day!

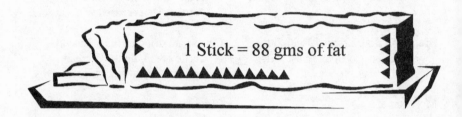

1 Stick = 88 gms of fat

Considering that each stick of butter (or margarine) has 88 gram of fat, let's look at a few typical meals eaten out:

Breakfast	Fat (g)	Italian Lunch	Fat (g)	Mexican Dinner	Fat (g)
2 Scrambled Eggs	15	Salad w/3T. Italian Dressing	26	18 Tortilla Chips	18
3 Slices Bacon	12	Minestrone Soup	5	Mexican Rice	10
1 Spoonful Fried Potatoes	10	2 Buttered Breadsticks	12	3 Cheese Enchiladas	50
Plain Biscuit, 1	8			Refried Beans	10
TOTALS:	**45g**		**43g**		**88g**

These three meals add up to a total of 176 grams of fat or 2 sticks of butter. How much fat do you eat each day? Are you feeling queasy yet?

Calculating the Percentage of Fats in Foods

FACT: The average American eats 35 - 40 percent of all their calories in the form of fat. How do you know if you are hitting the target of "less than 30%?"

Dietary fats such as margarine, butter, oil, or shortening get nearly 100% of all their calories from fat. On the other hand, most of the fruits, vegetables, and starches in their unadulterated state derive less than 10% of all their calories from fat.

FACT: Calculating the percentage of fat in an individual food is easy. To calculate the percentage of fat in a food, use this simple formula:

Calculating the Percentage of Fat in a Food

Step 1➡	Grams of Fat X 9 = Fat Calories
Step 2➡	(Fat Calories ÷ Total Calories) X 100 = % Fat

FACT: Food labels that claim "% *fat-free*" are misleading. Fats have more than twice as many calories as the same amount of carbohydrates or proteins. Therefore, the percentage of calories coming from fat will also be disproportionately higher than it would appear from the numbers on a food label. This is illustrated in the following example.

	½% Milk, 1 c.	Whole Milk, 1 c.
Calories:	90 calories	150 calories
Fat (g):	1 gram fat	8 gram fat
Step 1➡	1 X 9 = 9	8 X 9 = 72
Step 2➡	9 ÷ 90 = .10	72 ÷ 150 = .48
	.10 X 100 = **10% FAT**	.48 X 100 = **48% FAT**

Even lean meats can get a large percentage of calories from fat. As you can see, the labeling of a certain percent fat-free (such as 95% fat-free luncheon meats) has *nothing* to do with the American Heart Association's recommendation of 30% fat. The manufacturer is referring to the percentage of *the weight of the product* that is fat-free and not the percentage of *calories*.

	95% Fat-free Meats, 1 oz	Bologna, 1 oz
Calories:	35	72
Fat (g):	2	7
Step 1➡	2 X 9 = 18	7 X 9 = 63
Step 2➡	18 ÷ 35 = .51	63 ÷ 72 = .88
	.51 X 100 = **51% FAT**	.88 X 100 = **88% FAT**

FACT: Eating just a "dab" of margarine, oil, or dressing can really add up over time. Even though vegetables and starches, as they are found in nature, are fairly low fat, adding fats can make a BIG difference. All you need for sustained health is "a dab" of fat a day, but instead most of us add "just a dab" to everything we eat. And that adds up quickly as you can see in the next two examples.

	Vegetable Salad, without Dressing	Vegetable Salad with 2T Dressing
Calories:	30	190
Fat (g):	$0.^2$	16

Step 1→ | $0.^2 \times 9 = 1.^8$ | $16 \times 9 = 144$

Step 2→ | $1.^8 \div 35 = .05$ | $144 \div 190 = .76$

$.05 \times 100 =$ **5% FAT** | $.76 \times 100 =$ **76% FAT**

	Yeast Roll, no butter or margarine	Yeast Roll with 1 teaspoon margarine
Calories:	110	145
Fat (g):	1	5

Step 1→ | $1 \times 9 = 9$ | $5 \times 9 = 45$

Step 2→ | $9 \div 110 = .08$ | $45 \div 145 = .31$

$.08 \times 100 =$ **8% FAT** | $.31 \times 100 =$ **31% FAT**

As you can see, many foods are more than 30% fat. This does not mean that you should not be eating them nor does it mean that you have to become a mean fat-calculating machine before you put something into your mouth. There is a far simpler way to decrease our fat intake than calculating the fat percentage in each and every food. A easier way involves three steps:

❶ Determine the maximum *grams* of fat you need each day (see the chart on the next page)

❷ Examine the fat grams in the foods you enjoy (using the Calorimeters and nutritional information throughout this book)

❸ Keep your fat intake below that level

How Much Fat Should I Be Eating?

Fats contribute to the texture and taste of foods and our satiety level (feeling of fullness) but cutting our fat intake back to 30% of our total calories is a sensible and achievable level. Getting your fat intake down to 20% of your total calories is also healthy but requires more discipline.

Because Mother Nature provides a small amount of fat in just about every food item (in it's natural state) you can keep your fat intake to 10% of total calories only if you exclude nearly all meat, chicken, fish, eggs, cheese, salad dressing, oil, margarine, avocados, and nuts. In other words, this regimented vegetarian diet would *still* contain 10% of the total calories coming from fat. For most of us, this strict dietary approach is unpalatable, unrealistic, and unnecessary.

Earlier in this chapter, we estimated the number of calories we need to maintain our weight. Now take a look at the chart below - and keep your fat intake between 20 and 30% of your total calories.

What are the *Maximum* Grams of Fat I Should Eat?

Calories	30% Fat (g)	20% Fat (g)
1000	33	22
1200	40	27
1500	50	33
1800	60	40
2000	67	44
2500	83	56
3000	100	67

Should I Restrict my Sodium Intake?

High blood pressure increases your risk of strokes, heart attacks, and other forms of heart disease. For that reason, the Joint National Committee on Detection, Evaluation, and Treatment of High Blood Pressure recommends that individuals with high blood pressure should take off excess weight, cut back on alcohol, increase their physical activity, eat more foods high in potassium, and eat less sodium. Results from the recent DASH studies recommend we also eat more fruits, vegetables, and milk products to lower blood pressure. Notice that to decrease high blood pressure, reducing sodium is not the *only* recommendation - often losing excess weight brings about more dramatic results.

The typical American eats 4000 milligrams (mg) of sodium eat day while the National Academy of Sciences recommends that healthy individuals consume no more than 2400 mg of sodium per day. A teaspoon of salt contains 2100 mg of sodium. However, very little comes directly from the salt shaker on the table; 80% comes from processed foods.

What Foods are High in Sodium?

LOW SODIUM FOODS	HIGHER SODIUM FOODS
Fresh and frozen fruits and vegetables	Canned vegetables, canned tomato sauce, sauerkraut, soups, broth, canned vegetable juices, processed potato products, olives
Fresh & dried herbs and spices such as basil, cinnamon, curry powder, paprika, and sage; vanilla & almond extracts, lemon juice, vinegar	Table salt, cocktail sauce, soy sauce, most gravies, steak sauce, catsup, tartar sauce, teriyaki sauce, meat tenderizer, garlic salt and other herbs & spices made with salt such as garlic salt, MSG, chili con queso
Chicken, beef, turkey, veal, fish (fresh water & salt water), fresh roast beef or sliced turkey	Bacon, ham, bologna, salami, sausage, pastrami, corned beef, hot dogs, pepperoni, canned tuna & other canned fish, pickled herring, anchovies, prepared meat salads such as tuna salad, casseroles
Pasta, rice, fresh beans	Pasta with sauce, rice prepared with sausage or broth, canned beans
Low sodium cheeses	American and aged cheeses, cottage cheese
Unsalted nuts, unsalted chips, puddings made from scratch	Pickles, salted nuts, potato chips, instant pudding
Oil, unsalted butter *or* margarine	Salted butter & margarine, prepared salad dressings
Fresh fruit, gelatin, frozen yogurt	Baked desserts

General Recommendations to Decrease Sodium

■ Request grilled or baked foods rather than fried foods

■ Choose fresh meats rather than cold cuts or sausage. Avoid smoked or pickled foods

■ Order salads, burgers, tacos, omelets, and other foods without cheese

■ Ask that your food be prepared without salt, MSG (monosodium glutamate), or soy sauce

■ Request unsalted butter or margarine

■ Request all sauces to be served on the side and used sparingly

■ Have salad with minimal dressing instead of soup

■ Order your sandwich without pickles

■ Use lemon or oil & vinegar instead of bottled salad dressings

■ Ask for fresh fruit instead of chips with your sandwich.

■ Enjoy yeast breads rather than biscuits, cornbread, or other quick breads prepared with baking soda or baking powder.

■ Order fruit, low fat ice cream, frozen yogurt, or gelatin instead of baked desserts.

Now that you have mastered a basic understanding of your calorie, fat, and sodium needs, the nutritional information in the balance of the book will be more valuable. As an additional reference, read the next chapter on *General Guidelines for Dining Lean*. These are suggestions you can use in any restaurant.

General Guidelines for Dining Lean

If you think you lack the willpower it takes to dine out low fat, read on. There really is no such thing as willpower. What you need to prevent overeating is pre-planning skills. This chapter includes some of the skills that will help you eat right when you are dining out. Each change will deliver significant savings of calories and grams of fat.

Speak to the Manager

It may be difficult to know what to order just by looking at the menu. The wait staff may be too busy (or may not know enough about the food) to really help you with your decisions. Instead, contact the restaurant ahead of time and ask the manager specific questions about serving sizes and preparation methods. Tell the manager about your nutritional concerns and ask what they may be able to prepare for you. The best time to call the manager is between the hours of 9 and 11 in the morning and between 2 and 5 in the afternoon.

Be Assertive

At the restaurant, be assertive about what changes you want emphasizing the key words such as "on the side" or "without butter." Send it back if it doesn't come the way you requested it. Does that make you uncomfortable? Well, think about this: if you went to the store and asked for a size ten blouse and, instead, they gave you a size six, wouldn't you send it back? Ordering food is no different!

Did Mother say "Never Play with your Food"?

If the food delivered to your table does not comply with your special request and you do not want to wait for another dish to be prepared, feel free to play with your food. Using your knife, wipe off the extra sauce, trim away the fat, or remove the skin off your chicken. Pour the sauce off your dinner plate and onto an empty bread plate. Use a paper napkin to blot away the extra fat on your slice of pizza.

Get the "Doggie Bag" with Dinner

Since most restaurants serve twice as much food as you really need, ask for a doggie bag as soon as you get your dinner. Put half of the dinner in the doggie bag for tomorrow's lunch. If you can't take the extra food home in a doggie bag, don't feel you need to "clean your plate." The starving children in Africa will not benefit from your overeating. Remember, you can either "waste it" or "waist it." The choice is yours!

Don't Feel Guilty About Eating

Eating is necessary for sustaining life; eating should be pleasurable. There's no need to feel guilty about enjoying the foods you love. This book was written to educate you on the nutritional value of specific foods available in restaurants. Use this information as a tool to help you decide exactly how you are going to *spend* your calories and grams of fat. A frequent question you should be asking yourself is: "Considering the calories and fat grams in this food, is it worth it?"

This book is not written as a prescription; set your own priorities. One person may order salad *with* dressing and *fried* fish. Another person may eat both the salad and the potato "dry" and order the fish baked, just so they can "splurge" on a rich, creamy dessert. This book is about making informed decisions.

Eating low fat may require some time to get used to - don't make all of the recommended changes at the same time or you might find the food unpalatable. Make these changes slowly and your taste buds will adapt. Yes, it's true! There really may come a time when you actually prefer the low fat versions of some of your favorite foods.

Eat Slowly and Taste Every Bite

Some people eat more than they need simply because they are speed eaters. They are focused on the physical process of eating as opposed to savoring the food. If you don't swallow until all the flavor of the food is gone, you will enjoy the food so much more and you will end up eating less. Logically, this suggestion is more significant when the food contains a lot of calories. If you have decided to spend the extra calories on a dessert, for example, take thin slivers and savor every bite!

Eat Till you "Feel Fine" - Not Stuffed!

Special occasions, in the past, were celebrated by dining out. The infrequency often led to overindulgence. Today, due to the frequency of dining out, the quantity consumed needs to be moderated. Start listening to your body. Remember that it takes 20 minutes for the full stomach to tell the brain that it is full. So eat slowly! Give the brain time to do its job. Stop when you feel comfortable. Don't feel compelled to clean your plate - the restaurant staff will do that for you.

Concentrate on the Atmosphere

Focus on people you are with and the conversation that is going on around you. Then you can concentrate less on the food. Haven't you ever been so caught up in a conversation during a meal only to realize that you didn't finish you food and you were still satisfied?

Proximity can be a Problem

Does just seeing certain foods prompt you to eat? If so, keep food reminders to a minimum. That may sound difficult in a restaurant, but here are some ideas:

- Stay away from all-you-can-eat buffets or at least don't sit next to the buffet.

- Ask for a table away from the steady traffic coming from the kitchen.

- Have the bread, chips, and butter removed from the table or at least moved outside your reach.

- Be assertive with your requests regarding serving sizes; ask for just one piece of bread or just a half serving of a meal or dessert. That's easier than having a full serving and telling yourself to eat just half. You can't eat what isn't there!

- Hand the dessert and liquor menus back to the server.

- Ask the server not to bring the dessert cart to the table.

Have Closure to the Meal

Most of us need a signal that the meal is over. For many of us, it is when the food is gone and the plate is empty. But since restaurants serve more than most of us need to eat using that signal is a prescription for weight gain. Other suggestions for signals include:

- When you've eaten enough and feel *comfortable*, not stuffed, ask for the doggie bag.

- If you will not be taking the leftovers home, ask your server to clear off your plate so you won't have to look at the temptation.

- If the server is nowhere around, make your food unpalatable so you won't continue to nibble. Try salting your food excessively or pouring on the hot sauce. Another method is to get the food out of sight by placing your napkin over the plate.

■ Sip coffee or hot tea; use this activity as your signal that the meal is over.

■ Bring a mint or piece of hard candy to clear your palate

Order the "Luncheon" or "Appetizer" Portion

Some restaurants will allow you to order the "luncheon" portion at dinner for a discounted price. The luncheon portions are generally half of the dinner portions. These restaurants generally do not mention this on the menu - you need to ask.

Studies conducted by University of Pennsylvania marketing professor Brian Wansink, PhD proved that consumers tend to use more of a food product if it comes in a larger package. Is that also true for *you* in restaurants?

Know the Menu Terminology

Knowing how to read and interpret the menu can help you to make wiser decisions. If you don't understand a menu item or the description, *ask* your server.

■ Leaner ways to cook meats and vegetables include broiling, roasting, char-grilling, grilling, poaching, stir-frying, boiling, and steaming.

■ Restaurants may still brush or baste the meats with fats during or after the cooking process. Haven't you noticed how it shines?

■ Some meat may be marinated in oil or a high fat substance, which can add both calories and fat.

■ The term "Prime" often refers to meat that is very high in fat.

■ Many restaurants add margarine, butter, oil, or other sauces before serving boiled or steamed vegetables. Ask that it be left off.

■ Terms that indicate a high fat food:

Fried	Pan-fried	Hollandaise
Crispy	Escalloped	Creamed
Creamy	Stewed	In its own Gravy
Buttery	Casserole	Au Gratin
In a Butter Sauce	Hash	Parmesan
In a Cream Sauce	Pot Pie	In a Cheese Sauce

Think Before You Drink Your Calories!

Always have a calorie-free beverage such as water, mineral water, club soda, unsweetened iced tea, black tea or a diet soda nearby so you can quench your thirst. These fluids also help to fill you up. Watch out for the latest fruit juice sparklers -

most have over 100 calories per 10 oz serving. Nearly all restaurants in this book offer some non-caloric options other than water, coffee, and tea.

Look at the measuring cups in your kitchen to become familiar with fluid ounces. Eight fluid ounces is equivalent to a one cup measuring cup. This is about the size of a small Styrofoam coffee cup. Keep in mind that most of us drink these beverages in portions larger than 8 oz. Most people don't realize how many calories there are in the beverages they drink. Look at the comparisons in the *Beverage* chapter.

Make Appetizers the Meal

Many appetizers are fried; just eating one choice could easily blow your fat allotment for the whole day! But if you are going to eat something fried - at least eat it in an appetizer portion instead of the entree portion.

If you find some leaner appetizers such as shrimp cocktail or beef strips on a skewer - consider making that your entree. Appetizer meat portions are often only 2-4 ounces, rather than the 8-10 oz entrée size.

Pasta, in Italian restaurants, is often offered in both the entree and the appetizer portion. Having two or three appetizers for a meal can be a viable option or an appetizer, salad, and some bread.

Breads Aren't Fattening

Plain bread or yeast rolls are relatively low in fat and calories. It's the butter and oil that is added that does the damage. Most plain, unbuttered breads have only about 70 - 80 calories per ounce (the size of an average slice of bread). Garlic bread can often have twice as many calories!

Cornbread, croissants, buttered breadsticks, and muffins can add on substantially more calories than the plain yeast rolls. These are often 100-125 calories per ounce even before you butter them. For more details, see the discussion in the chapter entitled *Breads & Spreads.*

Salads Aren't Always Low Calorie Fare

Raw vegetables are low in fat. But, the dressing and the mayonnaise-laden salads can really add up the fat and calories. Salad dressings have about 80 calories per level tablespoon and most restaurants are generous! They usually put on 3 or 4 tablespoons (that's about 200 calories of pure fat) on a *small* garden salad. Oil and vinegar isn't much better - remember oil has 125 calories per tablespoon. Read the *Salads* chapter to discover why a salad can sometimes have more calories and fat than a hamburger and fries.

Beware of "Reduced Calorie" Salad Dressings

Don't rely on restaurants to carry very low-calorie dressings. Even if they do have lower calorie dressings, they may not be as low as you had hoped. While regular salad dressings have about 80 calories and 9 grams of fat per tablespoon, lower calorie salad dressings may range anywhere from 6-50 calories and 0-5 grams fat. Generally, salad bars have the lower calorie dressings while the more upscale restaurants select those in the higher calorie range.

Always Ask for Your Dressing on the Side

Don't let the person in the kitchen determine how much salad dressing you like and how many calories you need. Always ask for your salad dressing on the side so *you* can control how much to add. A good way to get a taste with every bite is to dip your fork into the salad dressing and then into your salad.

There are other Low Calorie Dressings Available

Vinegar is almost always available although rarely mentioned as a dressing option. Many of them are flavorful such as red wine vinegar, balsamic vinegar, and tarragon vinegar. A squirt of lemon on your salad may satisfy your palate. Picante sauce (at 10 calories per tablespoon) also makes a great low calorie dressing or a topping for your baked potato.

Bring Your Own Dressing

Some food companies such as Estee, Dieter's Gourmet, Weight Watchers, Skinny Havens, and Pritikin sell dressings in individual, one-serving packets. If you are going to a restaurant that doesn't serve a lower calorie dressing, bring your own!

Stay Away from Fried Foods

Frying generally doubles in the calories in a given food. Appetizers are notoriously the worst because almost everything is fried. Reviewing the examples below, you may begin to realize that fried foods just may not be worth it!

Order Baked or Grilled rather than Fried:		Calories	Fat (g)
Fried Fish, 8 oz		550	25
Baked Fish, 8 oz		240	3
	Savings:	310	22
French Fries, 10		160	8
Plain Potato, ½ c		100	<1
	Savings:	60	8

If it says "Low Fat" is it Really?

Some restaurants use small red hearts or the terms "heart healthy," "low fat," or "light" to designate menu items that are lower in cholesterol and/or fat. According to new regulations by the Food and Drug Administration, the restaurant must now be able to back up the claim. Typically, that information is not on the menu but can be requested from the server. But keep in mind that there is still the possibility that the cook may not follow the preparation instructions exactly.

Request Healthier Fats

Even if butter is served at the table or used in the cooking, margarine or vegetable oil is almost always available. Request this when ordering. Margarine and oil still has the same number of calories, but it's healthier!

Limit the Animal Protein Portions

Beef, chicken, and turkey are good sources of protein but, unfortunately, they also contain fat - especially saturated fats. Chicken, turkey, and fish are generally leaner than beef but the American Heart Association recommends that we eat no more than 6-8 ounces of animal protein *each day*. That's comparable to eating a piece of meat the size and thickness of a deck of cards for lunch and another piece the same size for dinner.

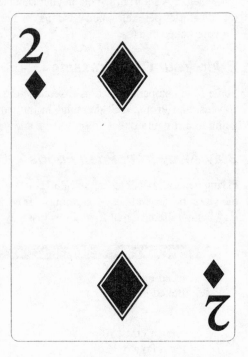

Unfortunately, meat portions served in restaurants are often 6-8 oz at lunch and 8-10 oz at dinner. Occasionally, you will find luncheon portions closer to 3-4 ounces. Ordering appetizers that have 2 or 3 ounces of meat instead of an entree is an excellent way to keep your meat protein to a minimum.

Split an Entree and have an Extra Salad

Again, since entrees are much larger than most people should be eating, consider splitting an entree. Then order an extra salad, a plate of steamed vegetables, or a baked potato.

Simplicity is Best in Entrees

Simply prepared foods are usually the lowest in fats and calories. Butter or oil is often added while cooking the individual servings and can often be omitted if you request. Ask that the vegetables, potatoes, and meats be prepared without added fats.

Broiled foods can be prepared with wine or lemon juice instead of butter. Fish, even with the added fats used when broiling, is usually a better choice than beef. Grilled chicken is almost always offered as well.

Those Little Extras can Really Add Up

Always ask what is added to the menu items that you want to order. Sometimes you'll find it "no big deal" to ask for your dish to be prepared without a few of these extras. In the *Salads* chapter you'll find out that salad dressing, croutons, and sunflower seeds can add up to the calories in a burger! Sauces, listed in the *Entrees & Sauces* chapter, can easily *double* the calories of your dish. When you read the *Mexican Restaurants* chapter, you'll be shocked by the calories in avocados, sour cream, and shredded cheese.

Just a few croutons and a sprinkle of cheese can add an extra hundred calories. Is that how you want to spend your calories and fat? Or would you rather have some dessert? It's up to you!

Order all Sauces on the Side

Most sauces are very high in fat. Unless you know that they are lowfat, it is best to order *all* sauces on the side. That way you can control how much you really want. Dip your fork into the sauce and then into the food for a taste with every bite. This is true for the lemon butter sauce that comes on the fish, the gravy added to the chicken fried steak, the dressing on the salad, and the Alfredo sauce on the fettuccine.

Fill up on Fat-Free Fare

Pure unadulterated starches, vegetables, and fruit are often very low in fat. Plain bread, noodles, potatoes, beans, corn, broccoli, strawberries and melons are all low in fat. It's the toppings that add up the calories and fat grams. So plan your healthy meal with a small portion of meat and larger amounts of these fat-free fare.

Split Dessert, if You Must

Fruit makes a low calorie and sweet ending to a meal. Even if fresh fruit is not listed on the menu, it is often available. Just make sure it is not covered with cream or liquor or served with cheese.

Calories for most other desserts are in the range of 400 to 1000 calories per portion. So if you must have dessert, split one with another person or with the whole table. Our taste buds are mostly sensitized to those first few bites anyway. So take small bites and really enjoy it.

Know the Abbreviations and Measurements

Throughout this book, calories and grams of fat are given for a specific measure of a food item. Measurements such as teaspoon or tablespoon refer to level portions not *heaping* spoons!

Take out the measuring spoons and cups out of your kitchen cupboard and use them when serving yourself at home so you can become familiar with how much is served in a restaurant. Use a postage scale to weigh your food portions at home so you can easily estimate the portions served at the restaurants.

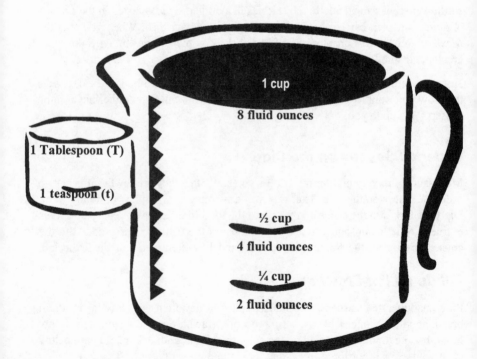

Common Measurements:

$$3 \text{ t (teaspoons)} = 1 \text{ T (tablespoon)}$$
$$4 \text{ T} = \tfrac{1}{4} \text{ cup}$$
$$8 \text{ T} = \tfrac{1}{2} \text{ cup}$$
$$16 \text{ T} = 1 \text{ cup}$$

Abbreviations:

c	= cup	med	= medium
cal	= calories	mg	= milligrams
CB	= cheeseburger	na	= not available
ch	= cheese	oz	= ounce (s)
choc	= chocolate	pkg	= package
chol	= cholesterol	pkt	= packet
ea	= each	#	= pound
fl oz	= fluid oz	SW	= sandwich
gm	= gram(s)	sl	= slice
HB	= hamburger	sm	= small
"	= inch	T	= tablespoon
lg	= large	t	= teaspoon
<1	= less than 1	w/	= with
mayo	= mayonnaise	w/out	= without

Exchange Abbreviations

People with diabetes and those on a variety of weight loss programs are often instructed to use "exchanges" as a simplified way of keeping track of what to eat and how much. Exchanges are lists of foods that are grouped together because they share similar amounts of calories, carbohydrates, proteins, and fats.

Exchanges were provided by some of the restaurants. Whenever possible, exchanges were calculated for the remaining foods listed in this book according to the 1995 edition of Exchange Lists for Meal Planning (American Diabetes Association & American Dietetic Association). For more information or to locate a Registered Dietitian to plan an exchange program for you, call the American Dietetic Association/National Center for Nutrition and Dietetics Hot Line at (800) 366-1655.

Carbohydrate Group:
ST = Starch
FR = Fruit
Mlk = Milk (skim)
CHO = Other Carbohydrates
V = Vegetables

Meat and Meat Substitute Group:
MT = Medium Fat Meat
(leaner meats are noted)

Fat Group:
FAT = Fat

Recommended Exchanges For Healthy Living

So far, we've discussed keeping to your calorie and fat "budget" for health and optimal weight. Based on your calorie budget calculated on page 15, here are some guidelines on how to divide up your calories using exchanges. Each plan is based on approximately 50% of the calories coming from carbohydrates, 30% from fat, and 20% from protein. Although it is not specified how to select your allottment of carbohydrate exchanges, work on eating at least five servings of fruits & vegetables and two servings of milk products every day.

1200 calories/day
6 Meats (MT)
6 Carbohydrates (ST, FR, Mlk, or CHO)
2+ Vegetables (V)
2 Fats (FAT)
(or 5 fats if very lean or lean meats are chosen)

1500 calories/day
6 Meats (MT)
10 Carbohydrates (ST, FR, Mlk, or CHO)
4+ Vegetables (V)
3 Fats (FAT)
(or 6 fats if very lean or lean meats are chosen)

1800 calories/day
6 Meats (MT)
13 Carbohydrates (ST, FR, Mlk, or CHO)
4+ Vegetables (V)
5 Fats (FAT)
(or 8 fats if very lean or lean meats are chosen)

2000 calories/day
6 Meats (MT)
15 Carbohydrates (ST, FR, Mlk, or CHO)
4+ Vegetables (V)
6 Fats (FAT)
(or 9 fats if very lean or lean meats are chosen)

2500 calories/day
6 Meats (MT)
20 Carbohydrates (ST, FR, Mlk, or CHO)
4+ Vegetables (V)
9 Fats (FAT)
(or 12 fats if very lean or lean meats are chosen)

PART
2

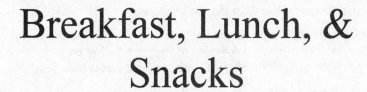

Breakfast, Lunch, & Snacks

Breakfast

Chapter Contents:

- Fresh Fruits, Dried Fruits, & Fruit Juices
- Cereal & Milk
- Eggs & Egg Substitutes
- Breakfast Meats & Potatoes
- Pancakes, Waffles, & French Toast

Most of us are off and running in the morning. Often that means no time for breakfast. No problem, you say, "If I don't eat in the morning I'll have more calories to *spend* later in the day, right"?

WRONG! Research evidence indicates that people who skip breakfast eat larger meals later in the day when their bodies are the least active. Breakfast skippers tend to be more overweight than those that eat breakfast.

When you skip breakfast, you are telling your body that you are still fasting from the night before. That signals a lowering of your metabolism throughout the day. Breakfast literally means "**Break Fast**"- the meal that breaks your fast.

Our weekends can be equally disastrous if we sit down to a more leisurely BIG breakfast or brunch. Often these meals are loaded in both fat and calories. This might be all right if we were to "eat breakfast like a king, lunch like a prince, and dinner like a pauper." But how many of us eat dinner like a pauper? Most of us do not!

Even if eaten just once a week, the traditional bacon, eggs, and biscuit meal can put on excessive unwanted pounds. Check out the calories and fat grams!

A High Fat Breakfast:

	Calories	Fat (g)
Orange Juice, 1c	110	0
Bacon & Cheese Omelet	512	42
Hashbrowns, ¾ c	250	15
Biscuit, 3 oz	375	22
Margarine, 2t	70	8
TOTAL:	**1317**	**87**

What should you eat? If you like a big breakfast, consider making some of the changes noted in this example.

A Large Healthy Breakfast:

	Calories	Fat (g)
Fresh Orange, 1	65	0
Vegetable Omelet made with Egg Beaters	100	5
Grits, ¾ c unbuttered	110	1
Bagel, 3 oz	240	3
Margarine, 1t	35	4
Jam, 1T	54	0
TOTAL:	**604**	**13**

The healthiest breakfast is a low fat, high fiber, high carbohydrate meal. This would consist of fresh fruits and juices, low fat cereals and skim milk, low fat breads, and spreads within your fat limit.

A Smaller Healthy Breakfast:

	Calories	Fat (g)
Fresh Orange	65	0
Wheat Flake Cereal & Skim Milk, 1 c each	190	1
English Muffin, 2 oz	130	1
Jam, 1T	54	0
TOTAL:	**439**	**2**

Next time you think you have no time for breakfast - grab a piece of fruit and a toasted bagel or English muffin with minimal margarine. It's not only fast, it's a healthy choice!

One question to ask yourself is "How do I want to spend my calories"? Secondly, and perhaps more importantly, "What breakfast provides me with the energy that I need for my busy day ahead?"

Fresh Fruits, Dried Fruits, & Fruit Juices

✔ **Fresh fruits, dried fruits, and fruit juices are high in vitamins and minerals and have virtually no fat**; they're great ideas for breakfast. Fresh fruits are also high in fiber and will fill you up quickly. Fresh fruit also makes an excellent topping for pancakes, instead of the usual butter and syrup.

✔ **Dried fruits are considered high in calories** even though they are just as caloric as the fresh fruit they are derived from. A raisin has just as many calories as the grape from which it came from. Only the water was removed. Unfortunately, many people have a tendency to eat far more raisins than they would of the fresh grape.

Select Fresh Fruit Instead of Dried Fruit:		
	Calories	Fat (g)
36 Raisins or 2T	60	0
36 Small Grapes or 1c	60	0
Savings:	**0**	**0**

✔ **Fruit juices are concentrated in calories**. Did you know that ounce for ounce fruit juice has the same calories as most sugar-sweetened sodas? If you are watching your weight, you may want to order the *small* glass of juice. Or better yet, enjoy the high fiber benefits of fresh fruit instead.

Select Fresh Fruit Instead of Fruit Juice:		
	Calories	Fat (g)
½ c Orange Juice	54	0
½ c Diced Cantaloupe	28	0
Savings:	**26**	**0**

Fruits, Fruit Juices, & Dried Fruit

	Calories	Fat (g)	Sodium (mg)	Carbs* (g)	Exchanges**
Fresh Fruit:					
Apple Ring, ea	15	0	3	4	¼FR
Apple, whole medium	80	0.5	1	20	1½FR
Apple, ⅙ slice	15	0	0	4	¼FR
Applesauce, 2T	25	0	1	7	½FR, ¼c=1FR
Applesauce, ½ c	100	0	4	20	1½FR
Banana, 1	110	0	0	22	1½FR
Banana/Strawberry Medley	108	1	6	22	1½FR
Blueberries, ¼ c	20	0	2	5	¼FR, ¾c=1FR
Cantaloupe, diced, ½ c	30	0	7	8	½FR
Cantaloupe, slice	10	0	2	3	6 slices=1FR
Fig, 1 raw	40	0	1	10	½FR, 2 figs=1 FR
Figs canned in heavy syrup, 3	80	0	1	20	1½FR
Fresh Fruit Chunks, ½ c	60	0	2	15	1FR

*Carbs=Carbohydrate, na=not available   **Exchanges:** ST=Starch, Mlk=Milk (skim)
FR=Fruit, CHO=Other Carbohydrates, V=Vegetable, MT=Meat (medium fat), FAT=Fat

Fruits, Fruit Juices, & Dried Fruit (continued)

	Calories	Fat (g)	Sodium (mg)	Carbs* (g)	Exchanges**
Glacéd Fruit, ¼c	50	0	5	12	1FR
Grapes, 25	60	0.5	2	15	1FR
Grapefruit, ½	60	0	0	15	1FR
Grapefruit, canned, ¼ c	25	0	5	6	½FR
Honeydew, slice	15	0	4	4	4 slices=1FR
Kiwi, slice	10	0	1	3	6 slices=1FR
Orange, whole medium, ea	65	0	2	16	1FR
Orange Sections, slice	7	0	0	2	8 slices=1FR
Peaches, sliced & drained, 1 pc	20	0	0	5	3 pc=1FR
Pears, ea	100	0.7	1	25	1½FR
Pineapple, slice	20	0	1	5	3 sl=1FR
Pineapple, chunked, 4 pc	20	0	0	5	12 pc=1FR
Pineapple Bits, 1T	10	0	2	2	1/3 cup=1FR
Prunes, canned, 1	20	0	0	5	3=1FR
Strawberries, 1 ea	10	0	0	3	6=1FR
Tangerine, ea	40	0	1	10	1½=1FR
Watermelon, diced, 1c	50	0.7	3	12	¾c=1FR
Watermelon, sliced, ea	10	0	1	3	3=½FR
Dried Fruit:					
Apricots, dried, 7	60	0	1	15	1FR
Dates, dried, 3	68	0	0	17	1FR
Figs, dried, 2	95	0.4	4	24	1½FR
Peaches, dried, 2	62	0.2	2	15	1FR
Pears, dried,	92	0	2	23	1½FR
Prunes, dried, 3	60	0	0	15	1FR
Raisins, 2T	60	0	0	15	1FR
Fruit Juice:					
Tomato Juice, 6 oz	40	0	0	10	1FR
Apple Juice, 6 oz	85	0	13	21	1½FR
Cranberry Juice, 6 oz	110	0	8	28	2FR
Grape Juice, 6 oz	120	0	5	30	2FR
Grapefruit Juice, 6 oz	70	0	2	17	1FR
Orange Juice, 6 oz	85	0	1	21	1½FR
Prune Juice, 6 oz	130	0	8	32	2FR

Cereal & Milk

✓ **Select skim or low fat milk** instead of whole milk at breakfast. This substitution will save you a substantial amount of calories and fat.

✓ **Grits and oatmeal, prepared plain, are very low in fat,** but the calories go up when fats are added. Ask if the grits can be prepared without butter or margarine. Oatmeal usually is served with milk on the side - request skim or low fat.

---

*Carbs=Carbohydrate, na=not available   ****Exchanges:** ST=Starch, Mlk=Milk (skim)
FR=Fruit, CHO=Other Carbohydrates, V=Vegetable, MT=Meat (medium fat), FAT=Fat

✔ **Most cold cereals are low in fat** provided you select skim milk to go with it. Granola-type cereals or those with added nuts will have substantially more calories and fat.

Healthy Sounding isn't Always Healthy:		
	Calories	Fat (g)
1 c Granola	490	20
1 c Wheat Flakes	100	1
Savings:	390	19

✔ **Birchermuesli, is a cold cereal prepared with oats, fruits, nuts, and cream.** Some restaurants use nonfat plain yogurt in its preparation so it is healthy, but most restaurants still prepare it in the traditional high fat Swiss manner using heavy cream or half & half. Ask before ordering this item.

✔ **Sugar has 16 calories per teaspoon.** Doesn't sound like too much you say? One teaspoon a day translates to extra pound and a half of fat each year! Try artificial sweeteners on your cereal or eat it plain. Your taste buds will adjust to the taste difference within a couple of weeks.

> 16 calories X 365 days in a year = 5,840 calories
>
> 5840 calories / 3500 calories = **1.[7] pounds of fat on your body!**

Cereal & Milk

	Calories	Fat (g)	Sodium (mg)	Carbs* (g)	Exchanges**
Cold Cereals:					
Birchermuesli, ½ c	173	13	212	13	1ST+2½FAT
Flake Cereal, ½ c	75	1	200	15	1ST
Granola, ½ c	245	10	45	30	1ST+1CHO+2FAT
High Fiber Cereal, ½ c	105	0	470	23	1½ST
Raisin Bran Cereal, 1 c	170	1	370	38	1½ST+½FR
Shredded Wheat, 1 c	170	1	0	35	2ST
Sweet Puff Cereal, 1 c	120	1	200	28	1½CHO
Wheat or Corn Flakes, 1 c	100	1	290	26	1½ST
Hot Cereals:					
Oatmeal, ½ c	75	1	300	17	1ST
Grits, unbuttered, ½ c	75	0.[5]	300	18	1ST
Grits, ½ c w/ 1 t margarine	120	6	420	17	1ST+1FAT
Toppings:					
Sugar, 1 teaspoon	16	0	0	4	¼CHO
Brown Sugar, 1 Tablespoon	32	0	6	8	½CHO
Milk (1c):					
Whole Milk	150	8	120	11	1Mlk+1½FAT
2% Low Fat Milk	120	5	120	13	1Mlk+1FAT
Skim Milk	90	0	120	12	1Mlk

> ***Carbs**=Carbohydrate, na=not available   **Exchanges:** ST=Starch, Mlk=Milk (skim)
> FR=Fruit, CHO=Other Carbohydrates, V=Vegetable, MT=Meat (medium fat), FAT=Fat

Eggs & Egg Substitutes

✓ **Eggs are a good source of protein**; one egg has as much protein as an ounce of meat. While egg whites have no fat or cholesterol, one egg *yolk* contains 5 grams of fat and 270 mg cholesterol. For this reason, the American Heart Association recommends no more than 3 egg yolks per week.

✓ **Order egg substitutes** instead of eggs. Egg substitutes are basically colored and flavored egg whites. Their taste has greatly improved over the years.

Egg Substitutes are Low Calorie:	Calories	Fat (g)
Two eggs scrambled in 1 t margarine	200	15
Egg substitutes scrambled in 1 t margarine	60	4
Savings:	**140**	**11**

✓ **Many restaurants will prepare your order with "egg whites only" or with egg substitutes, even if it is not on the menu!** This includes omelets, frittatas, and even French toast.

✓ **Request that your eggs or egg substitutes be prepared with a non-stick spray.** Otherwise, cooks may use generous amounts of butter or oil to prepare these products.

Eggs

	Calories	Fat (g)	Sodium (mg)	Carbs* (g)	Exchanges**
Egg, poached or boiled, 1	75	5	70	0	1MT
Egg, scrambled or fried, 1	100	8	150	0	1MT+½FAT
Egg whites, 2	32	0	100	0	1MT(very lean)
Scrambled Eggs, ¼ c	100	8	150	0	1MT+½FAT
Egg substitutes, ¼ c	25	0	80	1	1MT(very lean)
Egg Dishes:					
Eggs Benedict 2 eggs w/1 muffin	535	36	1280	10	1½ST+3MT+4FAT
Vegetable Frittata w/2 eggs	230	15	250	5	1V+2MT+1FAT
Meat Frittata w/2 eggs	320	23	600	0	3MT+1½FAT
Quiche Lorraine, 1/6 pie	500	37	460	33	2ST+2MT+5FAT
Quiche Florentine, 1/6 pie	450	25	650	32	2ST+3MT+2FAT
Quiche, w/ham & cheese, 1/6 pie	460	27	500	33	2ST+3MT+2FAT
Omelets:					
Plain, 3 egg	325	26	520	0	3MT+2FAT
Cheese, 3 egg	440	36	695	0	4MT+3FAT
Ham & Cheese, 3 egg	470	37	850	0	4MT+3½FAT
Mushroom, 3 egg	435	37	615	5	1V+3MT+4FAT
Mushroom & Cheese, 3 egg	550	47	790	5	1V+4MT+5FAT

*Carbs=Carbohydrate, na=not available   **Exchanges:** ST=Starch, Mlk=Milk (skim)
FR=Fruit, CHO=Other Carbohydrates, V=Vegetable, MT=Meat (medium fat), FAT=Fat

Breakfast Meats & Potatoes

✓ **Order ham or Canadian bacon instead of bacon or sausage.** Ounce for ounce ham and Canadian bacon are higher in protein and lower in fat. Some people add bacon and sausage to their breakfast thinking they are high in protein. Yet more than 70% of their calories comes from *fat!*

	Bacon, 1 slice	Sausage, 1 oz patty
Calories:	36	100
Fat (g):	3	8
Step 1 →	$3 \times 9 = 27$	$8 \times 9 = 72$
Step 2 →	$27 \div 36 = .75$	$72 \div 100 = .72$
	$.75 \times 100 =$ **75% FAT**	$.72 \times 100 =$ **72% FAT**

✓ **All we need is just six ounces of protein a day** or meat the size of two decks of playing cards. Each egg or serving of egg substitutes counts as an ounce of meat. What meal and source of protein would best satisfy your needs? It's up to you.

✓ **Bacon, ham, sausage, and smoked salmon are all high in sodium** that is added during the processing.

✓ **Hash browns, home fries, or any other fried potato products are high in fat.** Most have more than 50% of their calories coming from fat.

✓ **Ask for a substitute of tomato slices, fresh fruit, or unbuttered grits instead.** Most restaurants will comply.

Accompaniments

	Calories	Fat (g)	Sodium (mg)	Carbs* (g)	Exchanges**
Breakfast Meats:					
Bacon, 1 slice	36	3	101	0	1FAT
Breakfast Ham, 1 slice	25	1	295	1	½MT(very lean)
Canadian-style Bacon, 1 slice	42	2	360	1	¾MT(lean)
Country Ham, 1 oz	60	4	400	0	1MT
Smoked Salmon, 1 oz	35	1.[2]	333	0	1MT(very lean)
Sausage, 1 oz patty	100	8	350	1	1MT+½FAT
Sausage, link	52	5	105	1	1MT

For breakfast steaks and other meats, see the *Entrée & Sauces* chapter.

	Calories	Fat (g)	Sodium (mg)	Carbs* (g)	Exchanges**
Breakfast Potatoes:					
Hashbrowns & Home Fries, ½ c	165	10	50	15	1ST+2FAT
Potato Puffs, ½ c	140	7	460	16	1ST+1½FAT

***Carbs**=Carbohydrate, na=not available   **Exchanges:** ST=Starch, Mlk=Milk (skim) FR=Fruit, CHO=Other Carbohydrates, V=Vegetable, MT=Meat (medium fat), FAT=Fat*

Pancakes, Waffles, & French Toast

✓ **Buttermilk pancakes have just 55 calories per ounce**. Here's a drawing of a 1 and 2 ounce pancake. If your pancakes are 6½" across (an inch wider than this book), you can safely estimate that they are at least 220 calories each! Whole grain pancakes are heavier and have a bit more calories and fat as you can see on the next page.

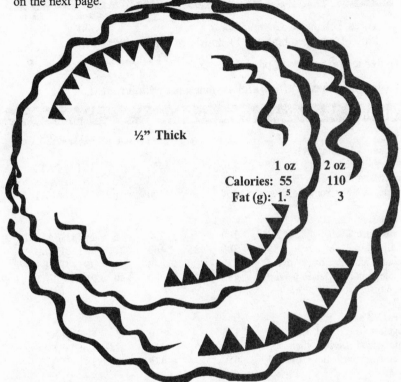

½" Thick

	1 oz	2 oz
Calories:	55	110
Fat (g):	1.5	3

✓ **Waffles are higher in fat and calories than pancakes**. Think about sharing the Belgium waffle with a friend.

✓ **Ask for the non-stick spray**. Waffles are usually prepared with a non-stick spray. Request the spray for the pancakes and French toast as well.

✓ **Request the French toast to be prepared with egg substitute**. This substitution is not available for pancakes since the batter is usually prepared in advance.

✓ **Stay away from deep-fried French toast** unless you can afford the calories.

✓ **Use a minimal amount of syrup**. At approximately 50 calories a tablespoon, the calories in the syrup can be damaging to your waistline. Most restaurants have *diet* syrup (about 10 calories/tablespoon). If your taste buds are not yet ready for the diet syrup, try mixing the regular and the diet together in a small bowl.

✓ **Applesauce, sprinkled cinnamon, and fresh fruit also make delicious, lower calorie toppings.**

✓ **Specify "no butter, powdered sugar, fruit toppings, whipped cream, or other toppings on top."** Request for these toppings on the side; these additions are what converts pancakes and waffles into nutritional disasters.

Get It Plain:	Calories	Fat (g)
Three 2 oz pancakes, plain	330	9
Plus 1T whipped butter & 1T powdered sugar	110	9
Total:	**440**	**18**

✓ **Order a short stack of pancakes.**

✓ **Order pancakes, waffles, and French toast without meat.**

Pancakes, Waffles, & French Toast

	Calories	Fat (g)	Sodium (mg)	Carbs* (g)	Exchanges**
Pancakes (4" diameter):					
Buttermilk Pancakes, 2 oz	110	3	460	16	1ST+½FAT
Buckwheat Pancakes, 2½ oz	135	5	370	18	1ST+1FAT
Wholegrain Nut Pancake, 2½ oz	160	6	390	18	1ST+1½FAT
Waffles:					
Toaster-size Waffle, 4" X 4" X ½"	100	3	230	15	1ST+½FAT
Waffle, 4 oz	300	15	460	31	2ST+3FAT
Belgian Waffle, 6 oz (7" round)	420	20	880	45	3ST+4FAT
Wholegrain Nut Belgium Waffle, 6 oz (7" round)	450	28	880	40	2½ST+5FAT
French Toast:					
Regular-sized Bread, 1 slice	125	4	210	15	1ST+1FAT
Thick-sized Bread, 1 slice	188	6	315	22	1½ST+1FAT
Deep-fried toast sticks, order	450	24	475	47	3ST+5FAT
Sauces & Toppings (1T unless noted):					
Applesauce, ¼ c	50	0	2	3	1FR
Butter	108	12	123	0	2½FAT
Diet Syrup	9	0	6	2	FREE
Fruit Flavored Syrup	55	0	0	14	1CHO
Fruit Topping	24	0	3	6	½FR
Fruit Topping, ¼ c	100	0	11	25	1CHO+½FR
Jelly, Jam, or Marmalade	50	0	3	14	1CHO
Maple Syrup	50	0	20	14	1CHO
Margarine	100	11	100	0	2½FAT
Powdered Sugar	29	0	0	8	½CHO
Whipped Butter	81	9	80	0	2FAT
Whipped Margarine	70	7	70	0	1½FAT
Whipped Topping	12	1	2	0	¼FAT

*Carbs=Carbohydrate, na=not available **Exchanges:** ST=Starch, Mlk=Milk (skim)
FR=Fruit, CHO=Other Carbohydrates, V=Vegetable, MT=Meat (medium fat), FAT=Fat

Burgers & Fast Food

Chapter Contents:

■ General Guidelines for Burgers & Other Hot Sandwiches
■ Other Foods: Salads, Pitas, Wraps, Potatoes, Chili, & Teriyaki Bowls
■ French Fries & Onion Rings
■ Calculating the Calories and Fat grams in your Fast Food Meal

Yes, you really can dine lean at a fast food restaurant - and grilled chicken sandwiches are not your only option. Other lean choices include veggie burgers, fajitas, and roast beef, turkey, chicken, BBQ, and ham sandwiches. And of course, there's always salad with low fat dressing. Stuffed baked potatoes with minimal toppings, teriyaki bowls, low fat soups, and even chili are a nice healthy break from a sandwich. Or you can get a complete meal of roasted chicken, mashed potatoes, and veggies. If you select wisely, you can even have a hamburger every now and then.

Almost anything is acceptable on a lower fat eating program. If you order high fat, high calorie foods, simply balance it by choosing low fat foods throughout the rest of the day so as not to exceed your maximum fat intake as discussed in the *Dining Lean Basics* chapter. Here are some suggestions:

Burgers & Other Hot Sandwiches

✓ **Request the hamburger buns to be grilled "without butter or oil."** Many restaurants brush the buns with butter or oil before grilling them - but it's not necessary. And you probably won't even taste the difference!

Request the Buns to be Grilled without Butter:		
	Calories	Fat (g)
Bun with butter	260	12
Bun without butter	160	1
Savings:	**100**	**11**

✓ **Order the smallest burger available.**

Compare these Burgers:

	Calories	Fat (g)
Half Pound (6 oz cooked weight)	490	35
Third Pound (4 oz cooked weight)	330	24
Quarter Pound (3 oz cooked weight)	245	18

Avoid Double Meat Sandwiches:

	Calories	Fat (g)
Burger King® Double Whopper® Sandwich	920	59
Burger King® Whopper® Sandwich	660	40
Savings:	**260**	**19**

✓ **Ask for the burger to be cooked well done.** The more you cook the burger, the less fat remains.

Well Done = Less Fat:

	Calories	Fat (g)
Third Pound Burger, broiled medium	330	24
Third Pound Burger, broiled well-done	315	22
Savings:	**15**	**2**

✓ **Eliminate the cheese.** Each slice of cheese contains approximately 100 calories. Some sandwiches have more than one slice. Is it worth the calories?

Say "No" to Cheese:

	Calories	Fat (g)
Jumbo Jack® with Cheese	680	45
Jumbo Jack®	590	37
Savings:	**90**	**8**

✓ **Limit the toppings.** Sure they all add flavor, but all these toppings could double the fat grams of your sandwich. So be selective.

Forget the Extras (or at least some of them):

	Calories	Fat (g)
Avocado, ¼	80	8
Bacon, 2 crisp slices	70	6
Cheese, 1 oz slice	90	9
Mushrooms, ¼c sautéed in 1T butter	110	11
Savings:	**350**	**34**

✓ **Use mustard instead of mayonnaise.** While some restaurants are now offering low fat mayonnaise, few restaurants are offering the fat-free version. Choose mustard instead of mayonnaise for a flavorful, low calorie option. Other low fat dressings include salsa, barbecue sauce, and fat-free salad dressings.

Get Used to the Taste of Mustard:

	Calories	Fat (g)
1T Mayonnaise	100	11
1T Mustard	<u>15</u>	<u>1</u>
Savings:	**85**	**10**

Get your Grilled Chicken Sandwich plain or with low fat Dressing:

	Calories	Fat (g)
BK Broiler® Sandwich	530	26
BK Broiler® Sandwich w/out mayo	<u>370</u>	<u>9</u>
Savings:	**160**	**17**

✓ **Order a small roast beef sandwich** and keep condiments to mustard or low fat dressing.

Select Small Roast Beef Sandwiches with Low Fat Condiments:

	Calories	Fat (g)
Arby's® Giant Roast Beef Sandwich	550	28
Arby's® Regular Roast Beef Sandwich	<u>400</u>	<u>20</u>
Savings:	**150**	**8**

✓ **Ham & Cheese Sandwiches are another remarkably low fat option.** Other submarine sandwiches (such as roast chicken and turkey) offered in fast food restaurants may be low in fat and calories also, check out the nutritional information.

✓ **Avoid the fried chicken or fried fish sandwiches.** Are you choosing chicken or fish because you think they are healthier than beef? Not if they are fried! Unless it says "grilled or broiled" assume they are fried.

Ham & Cheese has less Calories than a Fried Fish Sandwich:

	Calories	Fat (g)
Hardee's® Fisherman's Fillet™	530	28
Hardee's® Hot Ham'N'Cheese™	<u>300</u>	<u>12</u>
Savings:	**230**	**16**

Fried Chicken are not leaner than Hamburgers:

	Calories	Fat (g)
DQ® Homestyle Hamburger	290	12
DQ® Chicken Breast Fillet Sandwich (fried)	430	20

Order a *Grilled* Fish Sandwich instead of Fried:

	Calories	Fat (g)
Fried Fish Sandwich, average	460	25
Grilled Fish Sandwich w/lettuce, tomato, onion	<u>410</u>	<u>12</u>
Savings:	**50**	**13**

Other Fast Foods

✓ **Skinless, roasted chicken has less than half the fat and calories of fried chicken.** Your fried chicken contains more fat than it appears. Many fats, especially the saturated fats, solidify after cooking and don't look greasy. A wiser choice is to select roasted chicken and remove the skin.

Select Roasted Chicken rather than Fried Chicken:	Calories	Fat (g)
KFC® Original Recipe® Drumstick & Thigh	390	27
KFC® Tender Roast® Drumstick & Thigh,no skin	173	8
Savings:	**217**	**19**

Order Grilled Chicken rather than Fried Chicken:	Calories	Fat (g)
Chick-fil-A Nuggets®, 8 pack	290	14
Chick-fil-A® Chick-n-Strips®, 4	230	8
Savings:	**60**	**6**

✓ **Select a grilled chicken salad with low fat dressing.** Many restaurants offer grilled chicken salad. The salad vegetables and grilled chicken make for a low calorie, low fat meal. If bacon, cheese, avocado, and salad dressing are added they can more than double the calories.

Request Low Fat Dressing for your Salad:	Calories	Fat (g)
McDonald's® Grilled Chicken Salad Deluxe w/1 pkg Ranch Dressing	350	22.[5]
McDonald's® Grilled Chicken Salad Deluxe w/1 pkg Fat Free Herb Vinaigrette	170	1.[5]
Savings:	**180**	**21**

✓ **Broiled Fish Lunches are both low fat and filling.** As an alternative to a sandwich, consider a broiled chicken or fish plate which often includes rice, vegetables, bread, and more.

Order a *Broiled* Fish Lunch or Platter such as:	Calories	Fat (g)
Captain D's® Broiled Fish Lunch *or*	435	7
Captain D's® Broiled Fish Platter	734	7

✓ **Pitas and wraps can be lean option** if lean meats are chosen and little or no dressing is used.

Order Pitas without Dressing:	Calories	Fat (g)
Chicken Caesar Pita	500	20
Chicken Caesar Pita w/out dressing	420	11
Savings:	**80**	**9**

✓ **Ask for the stuffed potatoes to be prepared without butter**. Potatoes, by themselves, contain only negligible amounts of fat but are rich in vitamins, minerals, and fiber. Keep the meal healthy by adding only lean meats, vegetables, and low fat toppings to your plain potato. Specialty potato restaurants offer broth as an alternative to butter; they may also offer fat-free sour cream and cheese.

Request the "Lite Potatoes with Broth" instead of Butter:		
	Calories	Fat (g)
1 Potato 2® Chicken, Broccoli, & Cheddar	591	37
1 Potato 2® Chicken Fajita Lite (w/broth)	272	2
Savings:	**319**	**35**

✓ **Chicken Teriyaki Bowls are low in fat**. They have more calories than a plain grilled chicken sandwich, which makes it an ideal alternative for people who

Order a Teriyaki Bowl (without the Egg Roll) such as:		
	Calories	Fat (g)
Jack in the Box® Chicken Teriyaki Bowl	670	4

✓ **Chili can be a low calorie meal** by itself or an adjunct to a low fat sandwich or potato.

Try This for a Change:		
	Calories	Fat (g)
Wendy's® Large Chili	310	10

French Fries & Onion Rings

French fries and onion rings contain more than 50% of their calories from fat. Many people, focusing more on their wallet than their waist line, order a combination meal that includes a sandwich, medium or large fries, and a drink. Ways to address this less than ideal combination include:

❶ ask them to substitute a *small* bag of fries instead or

❷ on the way to the table, dump half the fries into the trash can. Remember, you can't eat what isn't there to tempt you.

Select Small rather than Large:		
	Calories	Fat (g)
Whataburger® *Large* French Fries	442	24
Whataburger® *Junior* French Fries	221	12
Savings:	**221**	**12**

Have it Without Cheese:		
	Calories	Fat (g)
Krystal® Chili Cheese Fries	540	28
Krystal® Regular Fries	370	18
Savings:	**170**	**10**

Calculating Calories & Fat grams in your Fast Food Meal

As a group, fast food restaurants are more likely to provide the consumer with nutritional information than any other type of restaurant. The last part of this chapter provides the most current nutritional information from most fast food restaurants. If your favorite burger or fast food restaurant does not provide nutritional information, use the generic information below.

Burgers & Fast Food

	Calories	Fat (g)	Sodium (mg)	Carbs* (g)	Exchanges**
Burgers on Buns (w/mustard, ketchup/pickles unless noted):					
Hamburger, 2 oz, small/kid's	286	12	636	23	1½ST+1½MT+1FAT
Cheeseburger, small/kid's	342	16	895	23	1½ST+2MT+1FAT
Quarter Pound Burger on small bun	452	22	912	32	2ST+3MT+1½FAT
with cheese	505	29	1304	32	2ST+3½MT+2FAT
with bacon & cheese	540	33	1620	32	2ST+3½MT+2½FAT
with mayo	595	35	967	32	2ST+3MT+4FAT
with cheese & mayo	660	44	1015	32	2ST+3½MT+5FAT
Third Pound Burger on medium bun, no toppings	640	34	575	47	3ST+4MT+3FAT
Half Pound Burger on large bun, no toppings	910	49	845	62	4ST+6MT+3FAT

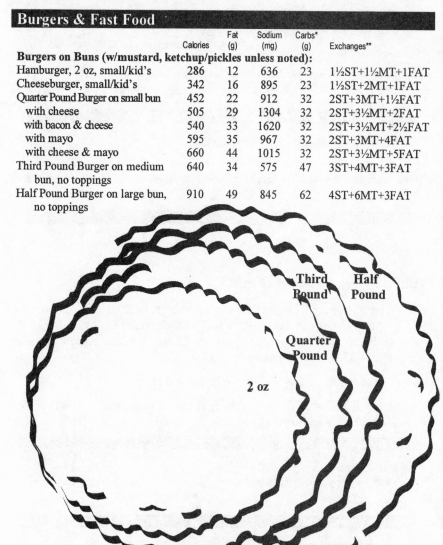

Third Pound   Half Pound

Quarter Pound

2 oz

*Carbs=Carbohydrate, na=not available   **Exchanges: ST=Starch, Mlk=Milk (skim) FR=Fruit, CHO=Other Carbohydrates, V=Vegetable, MT=Meat (medium fat), FAT=Fat

Burgers & Fast Food (continued)

	Calories	Fat (g)	Sodium (mg)	Carbs* (g)	Exchanges**
Grilled Chicken & Fish Sandwiches on Buns:					
Grilled Chicken Sandwich, regular	335	9	900	38	2½ST+3MT(lean)
without dressing	300	5	850	38	2½ST+3MT(lean)
Grilled Chicken Sandwich, large	475	21	930	45	3ST+3½MT
without dressing	385	11	890	45	3ST+3½MT(lean)
BBQ Grilled Chicken SW on bun	395	9	915	40	3ST+3MT(lean)
Grilled Fish Fillet , "no butter on bun"	410	12	na	45	3ST+3MT
Fried Chicken & Fish Sandwiches on Buns:					
Fried Chicken Sandwich	485	24	1047	45	3ST+2MT+2FAT
Fried Fish Fillet Sandwich	460	25	900	44	3ST+1MT+3½FAT
with cheese	552	32	1367	44	3ST+1½MT+4½FAT
Fried Fish Fillet Sandwich w/out cheese, w/out tartar sauce	390	18	750	44	3ST+1MT+2FAT
Fried Fish Fillet Sandwich, large	675	31	1091	59	4ST+2MT+5FAT
Other Fast Food Sandwiches on Buns:					
Hot Dog, regular	250	14	600	23	1½ST+1MT+1½FAT
Cheese Dog, regular	290	18	950	23	1½ST+1MT+2FAT
Chili Dog, regular	280	16	875	25	1½ST+1MT+2FAT
Chili & Cheese Dog, regular	350	22	1050	25	1½ST+1½MT+2FAT
Hot Dog or Sausage, ¼#	460	37	1360	30	2ST+3MT+4FAT
Corn Dog, regular 2½ oz	200	10	620	18	1¼ST+½MT+1FAT
Corn Dog, ¼#	330	17	990	27	1¾ST+1MT+2FAT
Roast Beef Sandwich, small	325	12	875	31	2ST+1½MT+1FAT
regular	375	17	915	39	2½ST+2½MT+1FAT
Gardenburger® on Bun, small	350	4	480	48	3ST+½V+½MT
medium	430	7	765	69	4ST+1V+1MT
steaksize	590	9	1070	98	5ST+1V+1½MT
Other Fast Foods:					
Chicken Pieces, regular order	290	16	697	14	1ST+2MT+1FAT
Chili, Small/regular	220	8	830	20	1ST+1V+1MT+½FAT
large	320	11	1237	30	1½ST+2V+1½MT+½FAT
Buffalo Wing, 1	75	5	500	0	1MT

*Carbs=Carbohydrate, na=not available   **Exchanges:** ST=Starch, Mlk=Milk (skim)
FR=Fruit, CHO=Other Carbohydrates, V=Vegetable, MT=Meat (medium fat), FAT=Fat

Burgers & Fast Food (continued)

	Calories	Fat (g)	Sodium (mg)	Carbs* (g)	Exchanges**
Individual Components:					
Half Pound Burger	490	35	350	0	6MT+1FAT
Third Pound Burger	330	24	232	0	4MT+1FAT
Quarter Pound Burger	245	18	175	0	3MT+½FAT
Small Burger, 2 oz	155	11	90	0	1½MT+1FAT
Turkey Burger, 4 oz	210	15	30	0	3MT
Grilled Chicken Breast, 4 oz	200	8	70	0	3MT(lean)
Grilled Fish Fillet	220	10	na	0	3MT
Hot Dog, ¼#	360	36	1170	2	3MT+4FAT
Hot Dog, 2 oz	180	16	585	1	1MT+1½FAT
Sausage, ¼#	360	32	1100	3	2½MT+2½FAT
Gardenburger® (small, 2.5 oz)	130	3	290	18	1ST+½MT
Gardenburger® (medium, 3.4 oz)	190	4	390	24	1ST+1MT
Gardenburger® (steaksize, 5 oz)	270	6	570	38	2ST+1½MT
4 oz Bun (for ½# burger)	320	3	500	60	4ST+½FAT
3 oz Bun (for 1/3# burger)	240	2.5	375	45	3ST+½FAT
2¼ oz Bun (for ¼# burger)	190	2	270	30	2ST+½FAT
1½ oz Bun (for 2 oz burger)	120	1	190	22	1½ST+¼FAT
Hot Dog Bun, regular	100	1	190	21	1½ST+¼FAT
Butter/Oil on buns, 1T	100	11	0	0	2FAT

Hamburger Bun Sizes:

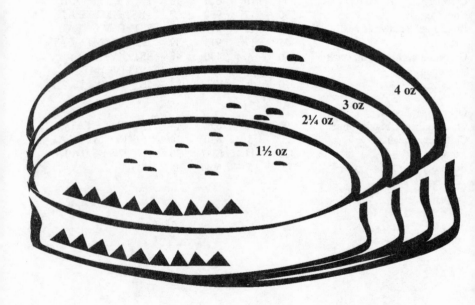

---

*Carbs=Carbohydrate, na=not available   **Exchanges:** ST=Starch, Mlk=Milk (skim)
FR=Fruit, CHO=Other Carbohydrates, V=Vegetable, MT=Meat (medium fat), FAT=Fat

Burgers & Fast Food (continued)

	Calories	Fat (g)	Sodium (mg)	Carbs* (g)	Exchanges**
Toppings:					
Avocado, ¼	78	8	5	3	1½FAT
Bacon, 2 slices crisp	72	6	202	0	1½FAT
Cheese, American 1 oz	90	9	420	<1	1MT+1FAT
Cheddar Cheese, 1 oz	114	9	175	0	1MT+1FAT
Swiss Cheese, 1 oz	107	8	75	0	1MT+1FAT
Lettuce	0	0	0	0	FREE
Mushrooms, sautéed in 1T butter	110	11	125	2	2FAT
Onion, 1 slice	5	0	0	1	FREE
Pickles, 2 slices	1	0	140	0	FREE
Tomato, 2 slices	5	0	0	1	FREE
Condiments (1T) *your sandwich may have more or less*:					
Barbecue Sauce	15	0	250	2	1T=FREE *or* ¼CHO
Chili Hot Dog Sauce	17	1	75	2	1T=FREE *or* ¼CHO
Honey Mustard Sauce	45	4.^{2}	15	1	1FAT
Ketchup	15	0	180	4	1T=FREE *or* ¼CHO
Mayonnaise	110	11	80	2	2FAT
Mustard	15	1	190	1	FREE
Sweet N'Sour Sauce	30	0	35	8	½CHO
Tartar Sauce	70	8	220	0	1½FAT
Accompaniments:					
Onion Rings, regular	297	16	438	31	2ST+3FAT
Large	441	27	838	45	3ST+5FAT
Onion Rings, each	82	6	150	8	½ST+1FAT
Potato Puffs, each	14	0.^{7}	30	1	10=1ST+1½FAT
French Fries, small/junior	232	12	204	25	1½ST+2FAT
Medium/regular	352	18	254	55	2½ST+3FAT
Large	434	21	333	65	3¼ST+4FAT
Extra Large	540	28	758	75	4ST+5FAT
French Fries, 1 c	155	8	170	15	1ST+1½FAT
Skinny French Fries, 1 @ 2½" long	5	0.^{25}	na	na	na
20 @ 2½" long	100	5	75	14	¾ST+1FAT
Regular French Fries, 1@ 2½" long	10	0.^{5}	na	na	na
10 @ 2½" long	100	4.^{1}	na	16	1ST+1FAT
Battered French Fries, 1 @ 2½"	14	0.^{8}	na	na	na
7 @ 2½" long	100	5.^{3}	na	15	1ST+1FAT
Steak Fries, 1 @ 2½" long	17	0.^{9}	na	na	na
6 @ 2½" long	100	5.^{2}	na	15	1ST+1FAT

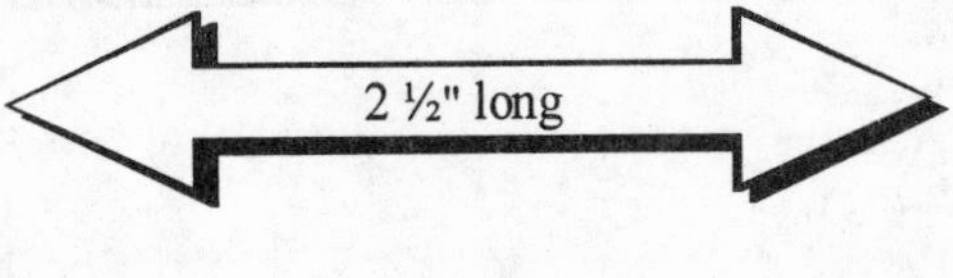

2 ½" long

---

*Carbs=Carbohydrate, na=not available   **Exchanges:** ST=Starch, Mlk=Milk (skim)
FR=Fruit, CHO=Other Carbohydrates, V=Vegetable, MT=Meat (medium fat), FAT=Fat

Deli & Sandwich Shops

Chapter Contents:

- Bread
- Meat, Cheese, and other Fillings
- Condiments
- Accompaniments

Cafes and delicatessens are generally smaller restaurants serving a variety of foods including sandwiches, salads, and soups. Soups and salads are discussed in their own respective chapters in Part 3 of this book. This chapter will focus on the wide variety of sandwiches and typical accompaniments.

Deli sandwiches can be healthy or disastrous depending on how you choose your bread; meat, cheese, or other filling; condiments; and other accompaniments. Take a look at the following example.

A Deli Sandwich Meal Can Be Lean:	Calories	Fat (g)
3 oz Bagel	240	3
2 oz Turkey	60	1
Mustard, 1T	15	1
Baked Potato Chips, 12	110	1
TOTAL:	**425**	**6**

Or It Can Be a Disaster:	Calories	Fat (g)
Tuna Salad, ½ c	380	20
Croissant, 3 oz	360	20
Mayonnaise, 1T	100	11
Cheese, 1 oz	100	8
Potato Chips, 1 oz	150	10
TOTAL:	**1090**	**69**

Bread

There are many people that, when *dieting*, skimp on the bread and eat just the meat. If anything, they should be doing the opposite. Most types of breads are very low in fat. Meat and cheese are much higher in both calories and fat.

✓ **Choose a sandwich made with a low fat bread** such as sliced sandwich bread, French or Italian bread, bagels, pita bread, or rolls. Avoid breads made with eggs and additional fat such as croissants. Check out the difference below:

Bread Calorimeter: Calories & fat per serving

Calories per oz	Bread	Calories & Fat grams (g)				
		1 oz	2 oz	3 oz	4 oz	5 oz
120	Croissants, plain	120	240	360	480	600
		7g	13g	20g	26g	33g
90	Focaccio	90	180	270	360	450
		3g	6g	9g	12g	15g
80	Bagel English Muffin Italian Bread Pita Bread Submarine Roll	80	160	240	320	400
		1g	1g	2g	2g	3g
70	French Roll & Baguette Sandwich Bread Slices	70	140	210	280	350
		1g	2g	3g	4g	5g

How many ounces of bread are you eating? Simply compare the bread in your favorite sandwich with a slice of store-bought sandwich bread which weighs approximately 1 oz. Most deli sandwiches contain at least 2 ounces of bread and as much as 5 ounces! For ease in calculation, various sizes of bagels, croissants, English muffins, focaccio, French & Italian bread, and French rolls are described and/ or illustrated in the *Breads & Spreads* chapter. Pita bread, soft buns, rolls, and Submarine rolls are described below.

Pita Bread

Pita bread is a flat, circular bread that is hollow in the middle. It can be served whole or cut in half. When served whole as a gyro, about 4 ounces of high fat meat is wrapped inside the pita bread and served with a high fat cucumber/sour cream sauce. Pita bread can also be cut in half, opened up and stuffed with a variety of meats, cheese, and sauces. One 6½-7" (approximately 1" larger than the width of this page) round pita is about 2½ oz and contains approximately 190 calories.

Soft Bun

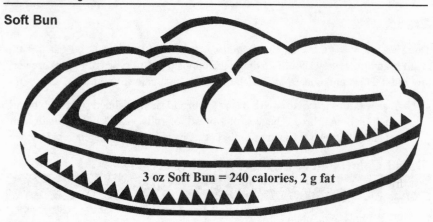

3 oz Soft Bun = 240 calories, 2 g fat

Rolls

A 3¾" crusty French roll weighs about 3 oz. Submarine rolls are fluffier so the portion size is bigger. A 6" submarine roll (slightly longer than the width of this book) will weigh about 2½ - 3 oz.

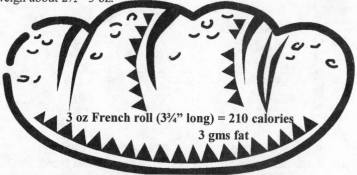

3 oz French roll (3¾" long) = 210 calories, 3 gms fat

3 oz submarine roll (6" long) = 210 calories, 3 gms fat

Sandwich Breads

	Calories	Fat (g)	Sodium (mg)	Carbs* (g)	Exchanges**
Bagel, 3 oz, 3½" diameter	240	1	400	47	3ST
4 oz, 4¼" diameter	320	2	540	65	4ST
5 oz, 5" diameter	400	3	675	81	5ST
Bread, 1 slice ½" thick	70	1	150	15	1ST
Croissant, 3 oz	360	20	400	34	2¼ST+4FAT
English muffin, 3 oz sandwich size	220	2	420	39	2½ST+½FAT
Focaccio bread, ½ of 9" round loaf	450	10	1000	79	5ST+1FAT
French roll, 3 oz	210	3	330	47	3ST
Italian bread, 1 oz slice	75	1	150	15	1ST
Pita bread, 7" round	190	1.⁵	410	37	2½ST
Soft bun, 3 oz	240	2	450	46	3ST
Submarine roll, 3 oz	240	2	450	46	3ST

*Carbs=Carbohydrate, na=not available **Exchanges: ST=Starch, Mlk=Milk (skim)
FR=Fruit, CHO=Other Carbohydrates, V=Vegetable, MT=Meat (medium fat), FAT=Fat

Meat, Cheese, & Other Fillings

Deli meat and cheese range from 30-130 calories/ounce with most sandwiches containing anywhere from 2-8 ounces.

✓ **Choose sliced turkey, chicken, ham, or roast beef**. Cheeses, specialty deli meats such as salami and pastrami, and prepared tuna or chicken salad are at least twice as high in fat and calories.

✓ **Keep meat portions at 3 oz or less**. Three ounces is the size of a deck of cards. If your sandwich contains more than that, consider splitting a sandwich with a friend and having an extra salad, cup of broth-based soup, or some fruit. In a restaurant that really piles on the meat, ask them to go light on the meat or order just a half of a sandwich along with an extra slice of bread. Split the meat between the two slices of bread to make a whole sandwich.

Deli Meat & Cheese Calorimeter: Calories & fat per serving

Calories per oz	Deli Meat & Cheese	Calories & Fat grams (g)				
		1 oz	2 oz	3 oz	4 oz	5 oz
130	Goose Liver Pate	**130**	**260**	**390**	**520**	**650**
		12g	24g	36g	48g	60g
120	Salami	**120**	**180**	**270**	**360**	**450**
		10g	20g	30g	40g	50g
110	Blood Sausage	**110**	**220**	**330**	**440**	**550**
	American, Cheddar, & Swiss Cheese	9g	18g	27g	36g	45g
100	Meatloaf, Braunschweiger	**100**	**200**	**300**	**400**	**500**
	Provolone Cheese	8g	16g	24g	32g	40g
	Pastrami					
90	Bologna, Bratwurst, Brotwurst, Knockwurst, Italian Sausage, Mortadella, Summer Sausage	**90**	**180**	**270**	**360**	**450**
		8g	15g	23g	30g	38g
	Mozzarella Cheese					
60	Headcheese	**60**	**120**	**180**	**240**	**300**
	Chicken Liver Pate	4g	8g	12g	16g	20g
	Lean Corned Beef & Roast Beef					
50	Chicken Breast	**50**	**100**	**150**	**200**	**250**
	Ham, lean	2g	4g	6g	8g	10g
30	Turkey	**30**	**60**	**90**	**120**	**150**
		$0.^5$g	1g	2g	2g	3g

Sandwich Meats & Cheeses

Per 1 oz unless specified:	Calories	Fat (g)	Sodium (mg)	Carbs* (g)	Exchanges**
Blood Sausage	108	10	na	0	1MT+1FAT
Bologna	89	8	280	0	1MT+½FAT
Bratwurst	85	7	158	2	1MT+½FAT
Braunschweiger	102	9	325	1	1MT+1FAT
Brotwurst	92	8	315	2	1MT+½FAT
Chicken Breast	50	1.5	35	0	1MT(very lean)
Chicken Salad, ¼ c	125	9	350	1	1½MT
Corned Beef	72	5.4	325	0	1MT
Corned Beef, lean	60	4	270	0	1MT
Egg Salad, ¼ c	123	11	170	0	1MT+1FAT
Ham	52	3	375	0	1MT(lean)
Headcheese	60	5	355	0	1MT
Italian Sausage	92	7	262	1	1MT+½FAT
Knockwurst	87	8	285	1	1MT+½FAT
Liver Pate, chicken	60	4	na	2	1MT
Liver Pate, goose	131	12	na	1	1MT+1½FAT
Meatloaf	100	8	na	2	1MT+½FAT
Mortadella	89	7	355	0	1MT+½FAT
Pastrami	99	8	348	1	1MT+½FAT
Roast Beef, lean	60	3	10	0	1MT(lean)
Salami	116	10	641	1	1MT+1FAT
Summer Sausage	94	8	375	2	1MT+½FAT
Tuna Salad, ¼ c	190	10	410	2	½CHO+2MT
Turkey	31	0.5	407	0	1MT(very lean)
Cheeses (1 oz):					
American	106	9	406	0	1MT+1FAT
Cheddar	114	9	176	0	1MT+1FAT
Mozzarella	90	7	106	0	1MT+½FAT
Provolone	100	8	248	0	1MT+½FAT
Swiss	107	8	74	0	1MT+½FAT

Condiments

✔ **Have the condiments served to you on the side** except for mustard, fat-free mayonnaise, vinegar, and horseradish. The other condiments are high calorie so use them sparingly.

High Fat Condiments can more than Triple the Fat Grams:	Calories	Fat (g)
6" Sub with turkey, cheese, mayonnaise, & oil	490	25
6" Sub with turkey, cheese, & mustard	300	7
TOTAL:	**190**	**18**

---

*Carbs=Carbohydrate, na=not available   **Exchanges: ST=Starch, Mlk=Milk (skim) FR=Fruit, CHO=Other Carbohydrates, V=Vegetable, MT=Meat (medium fat), FAT=Fat

Condiments

Per 1 Tablespoon:	Calories	Fat (g)	Sodium (mg)	Carbs* (g)	Exchanges**
Aioli Sauce, garlic oil	100	10	3	0	2FAT
Butter	108	12	123	0	2½FAT
Dijonnaise	15	0	210	0	FREE
Guacamole	30	3	105	1	½FAT
Horseradish	6	0	14	0	FREE
Ketchup	18	0	180	4	¼CHO
Margarine	100	11	100	0	2FAT
Mayonnaise	100	11	80	0	2FAT
Reduced Calorie Mayonnaise	50	5	80	1	1FAT
Fat Free Mayonnaise	10	0	130	1	FREE
Mustard	15	1	190	0	FREE
Oil & Vinegar	70	8	0	0	1½FAT
Picante Sauce	5	0	110	1	FREE
Remoulade Sauce	100	11	105	0	2FAT
Sour Cream/Cucumber Sauce	45	3.⁵	na	2	½FAT
Thousand Island Dressing	60	5	110	0	1FAT
Vinegar	2	0	0	0	FREE

Accompaniments

✓ **Request a low calorie accompaniment**. If the meal is typically served with high fat accompaniments (fries, chips) ask for a substitute such as a tossed salad with fat-free dressing, sliced tomatoes, pretzels, fresh fruit, or a big pickle. For more details about ordering a salad, see the *Salads* chapter.

Accompaniments

	Calories	Fat (g)	Sodium (mg)	Carbs* (g)	Exchanges**
Salads (½ c unless specified):					
Cole Slaw	170	12	200	9	2V+2½FAT
Fresh Fruit Salad	60	0	2	15	1FR
Garden Salad	25	1	25	6	1V
2T Salad Dressing	160	16	300	0	3FAT
2T Fat-Free Salad Dressing	20	0	270	4	¼CHO
Macaroni Salad	200	14	360	18	1ST+3FAT
Potato Salad	200	14	660	19	1ST+3FAT
Crunchies:					
Baked Potato Chips, 1oz (12 chips)	110	1.⁵	150	20	1¼ST
Baked Tortilla Chips, 10	120	1	80	22	1½ST
Pickles, 3¾" long	7	0	930	0	FREE
Popcorn, 1 c	55	4	40	6	¼ST+¾FAT
Potato Chips, 1oz (20 reg/12 ripple)	160	10	180	15	1ST+2FAT
Pretzels, 1 oz (48 Sticks)	110	0	530	23	1½ST
Tiny Twists (18) or Regular (8)	100	0	420	19	1¼ST
Thick Twists (4)	110	1	620	24	1½ST
Tortilla Chips, 10	180	8	80	26	1½ST+1½FAT

*Carbs=Carbohydrate, na=not available   **Exchanges:** ST=Starch, Mlk=Milk (skim) FR=Fruit, CHO=Other Carbohydrates, V=Vegetable, MT=Meat (medium fat), FAT=Fat

Pizza

Chapter Contents

- Crust
- Sauce
- Cheese
- Toppings
- Estimating the Calories & Fat in your Pizza

Many people think of pizzas as a high fat dish that one should not eat if they are trying to lose weight or lower their cholesterol. That simply is not true. Pizza can easily fit into a low fat eating program provided you make informed choices.

For the leanest meal, fill yourself up with a green salad and fat-free dressing before eating pizza. Then eat just a few slices of pizza with lower fat toppings such as fresh fruits and vegetables. If you have a hard time stopping at just 2 or 3 slices, buy a small enough pizza so there are no extra slices to tempt you.

Crust

✔ **Pizza crust is generally low in fat and calories.** The pizza crust consists of mostly of flour, yeast, and water so it is very low in fat and has approximately the same amount of calories as bread (ounce for ounce).

✔ **Choose pizzas cooked in the old fashioned pizza ovens.** When using the old fashioned pizza ovens, the pizza is simply placed on the floor of the oven and baked. On the other hand, the newer conveyor belt ovens use a higher tempera-ture which requires extra fat in the dough to allow quick cooking without burning. Thus, pizzas cooked in the conveyor belt ovens are generally higher in calories and fat than those made in the old-fashioned pizza ovens.

✓ **Go with thin or regular crust pizza** rather than pan pizza or thick crust. The calorie difference is even greater with pizza prepared in a conveyor belt oven. In addition to extra oil added to the crust itself, pan or thick crust pizzas cooked in the conveyor belt ovens usually require well-greased pans to prevent sticking. Generally, the thin or regular crust pizzas are placed on a perforated pizza pan without any additional oil.

If you Want more Slices, Order Thin Crust:	Calories	Fat (g)
Round Table® Gourmet Veggie Pan Pizza, 2 sl.	440	15
Round Table® Gourmet Veggie Thin Crust, 2 sl.	320	13
Savings:	**120**	**2**

✓ **Avoid Filled or Stuffed Crusts.** The double crusts and the high fat fillings result in a very high fat and calorie content.

Avoid Stuffed Crust:	Calories	Fat (g)
Pizza Hut® Pepperoni Lover's® Stuffed Pizza, 2 slices	1050	52
Pizza Hut® Pepperoni Lover's® Thin'n Crispy Pizza, 2 slices	578	28
Savings:	**472**	**24**

Sauce

✓ **Tomato or pizza sauce is low in fat; the white sauce is higher.**

✓ **Ask for "no oil on the crust."** Although not common in pizza parlors, some of the upscale restaurants brush the crust with oil before adding the sauce or *instead of* the tomato sauce. Request that oil not be added.

Cheese

✓ **Cheese is high fat**. Mozzarella cheese is the most frequently used cheese, but Provolone and Feta cheese are also seen. Each of these cheeses contain about 6-8 grams of fat per ounce; each pizza slice has roughly 1 oz of cheese.

✓ **Do not order extra cheese**. Extra cheese increases the fat content of each slice of pizza by another 50%!

Don't Do "Extra" Cheese:	Calories	Fat (g)
Pizza w/ Extra Cheese, 2 slices large pizza	370	16
Pizza, 2 slices large pizza	320	11
Savings:	**50**	**5**

✔ **Try pizza with "half the cheese" or even without cheese.** If your favorite part of the pizza is the crust, consider requesting that the pizza parlor add only *half* of the usual amount of cheese on top or request the pizza to be prepared "*light* on the cheese." Ask the manager of your favorite pizza restaurant which term is more understandable to their cooking staff. Managers say that requesting less cheese has become a frequent request from people watching their weight or cholesterol or those with a lactose-intolerance.

"Light" is Better:	Calories	Fat (g)
Thin Crust Vegetable Pizza, 2 slices 14" pizza	265	11
Thin Crust Vegetable Pizza, "light on the cheese," 2 slices 14" pizza	<u>215</u>	<u>6</u>
Savings:	**50**	**5**

Toppings

✔ **Choose the leanest toppings of fresh fruits & vegetables:** onions, mushrooms, green & red peppers, broccoli, tomatoes, roasted pepper, spinach, and pineapple.

✔ **Olives are just about pure fat;** a sprinkling of black and green olives will add another 30 calories and 3 grams of fat per 2 slices. If you don't really care much for them, leave them off your Vegetarian Pizza.

✔ **The leanest meats are: grilled chicken, ham, Canadian bacon, tuna, crabmeat, and shrimp.** Each will add only a couple of grams of fat per slice. Hamburger meat will add a bit more. The high fat toppings such as pepperoni, bacon, and sausage can more than double the fat in each slice.

Choose Leaner Toppings:	Calories	Fat (g)
(For 2 slices of 12" medium Pizza)		
Domino's Pizza®, thin crust, 2 slices, sausage & extra cheese	373	20
Domino's Pizza®, thin crust, 2 slices, w/green pepper, onion, mushrooms, banana peppers, pineapple, and ham	<u>312</u>	<u>13</u>
Savings:	**61**	**7**

Estimating the Calories & Fat in Your Pizza Slices

If no nutritional information is available for your favorite pizza restaurant, use these pictures to estimate the size of your slice. Then check out the chart on the following page.

Extra Large Slice = 10 ½" long
(often sold by-the-slice)

Large Slice = 7" long
(14" pizza pie)

Medium Slice

Buffet-sized

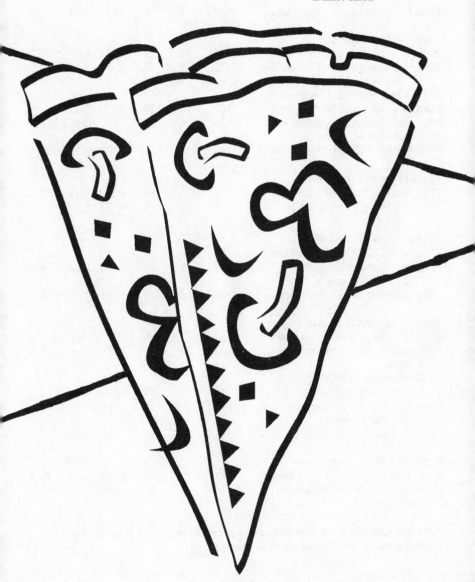

Pizza Calorimeter (per slice):

	Calories	Fat (g)	Carbs* (g)	Exchanges**
Large Slice (thin crust):				
Plain, w/no fat Vegetables*, or Ham	260	8	30	2ST+1MT
Pepperoni, Sausage, Vegetarian, or Lightly Piled Combo	375	15	30	2ST+2MT+½FAT
Extra Cheese or Heavily Piled Combo	420	21	30	2ST+2½MT+1FAT
Large Size (thick crust):				
Plain, w/no fat Vegetables*, or Ham	375	15	38	2½ST+2MT+½FAT
Pepperoni, Sausage, Vegetarian, or Combo	450	21	38	2½ST+2½MT+1FAT
Extra Large Slice (thin crust):				
Plain, w/no fat Vegetables*, or Ham	500	14	53	3½ST+2MT
Pepperoni, Sausage, Vegetarian, or Lightly Piled Combo	655	26	53	3½ST+3½MT+1FAT
Extra Cheese or Heavily Piled Combo	790	36	53	3½ST+4½MT+2FAT
Extra Large Size (thick crust):				
Plain, w/no fat Vegetables*, or Ham	655	25	68	4½ST+3MT+1½FAT
Pepperoni, Sausage, Vegetarian, or Combo	810	37	68	4½ST+4½MT+2FAT
Medium Slice (thin crust):				
Plain, w/no fat Vegetables*, or Ham	200	6	23	1½ST+¾MT+½FAT
Pepperoni, Sausage, Vegetarian, or Lightly Piled Combo	280	11	23	1½ST+1½MT+1FAT
Extra Cheese or Heavily Piled Combo	360	18	23	1½ST+2¼MT+1½FAT
Medium Size (thick crust):				
Plain, w/no fat Vegetables*, or Ham	280	10	30	2ST+1¼MT+½FAT
Pepperoni, Sausage, Vegetarian, or Combo	360	18	30	2ST+2MT+1½FAT
Buffet Size (thin crust):				
Plain, w/no fat Vegetables*, or Ham	140	4	15	1ST+½MT
Pepperoni, Sausage, Vegetarian, or Lightly Piled Combo	190	7	15	1ST+¾MT+½FAT
Extra Cheese or Heavily Piled Combo	240	11	15	1ST+1½MT+1FAT
Buffet Size (thick crust):				
Plain, w/no fat Vegetables*, or Ham	190	6	23	1½ST+¾MT+½FAT
Pepperoni, Sausage, Vegetarian, or Combo	240	11	23	1½ST+1¼MT+½FAT

* No fat vegetables include: onions, green peppers, onions, tomatoes, broccoli, roasted pepper, spinach, and the fruit pineapple.

Snacks

Chapter Contents:

■ **Candy & Fudge**
■ **Dried Fruits, Nuts, & Seeds**
■ **Pretzels**
■ **Popcorn**

Other popular snacks found elsewhere in this book:

■ **Bagels** - see the *Breads & Spreads* chapter
■ **Cookies, Doughnuts, Ice Cream/Frozen Yogurt, and Muffins** - see the
  Desserts chapter
■ **French Fries, Hot Dogs & Corn Dogs** - see the *Burgers & Fast Food* chapter
■ **Nachos, Tortilla Chips** - see the *Mexican Restaurants* chapter
■ **Pizza** - see the *Pizza* chapter
■ **Potato Chips** - see the *Deli & Sandwich Shops* chapter
■ **Sodas, Milkshakes, and Coffee Drinks** - see the *Beverages* chapter

Candy & Fudge

Stores selling candy in bulk are very popular in shopping malls, amusement parks, theatres, and airports. Since there is no nutritional information on the label, we are likely to consume more calories than we realize. On the next page is a calorimeter for the most popular candies listing the calories and fat grams per 1, 2, and 3 oz portions. Following this chart is more detailed nutritional information per ounce and per individual piece. Since your candy purchase is often shown in pounds rather than ounces, following is a conversion chart.

Conversion Chart:

Ounces		Pounds
1	=	0.06
2	=	0.13
3	=	0.19
4	=	0.25
5	=	0.31

Ounces		Pounds
6	=	0.38
7	=	0.44
8	=	0.5
9	=	0.56
10	=	0.63
11	=	0.69

Ounces		Pounds
12	=	0.75
13	=	0.81
14	=	0.88
15	=	0.94
16	=	1.0

Candy & Fudge Calorimeter: Calories & fat per serving

Calories per oz	Candy & Fudge	Calories & Fat (g)		
		1 oz (0.06#)	2 oz (0.13#)	3 oz (0.19#)
160	Chocolate Covered Almonds	160 12g	320 24g	480 36g
160	Hershey® Kisses w/almonds, Semi-Sweet Chocolate, Chocolate w/nuts	160 10g	320 20g	480 30g
150	M&M® Peanut, Nonpareil Chocolate Wafers, Hershey® Kisses, Hershey® Minatures, Reese's Peanut Butter Cups, Milk Chocolate	150 9g	300 18g	450 27g
140	M&M®, Malted Milk Balls, Reese's® Pieces	140 6g	280 12g	420 18g
130	Boston Baked Beans, Chocolate Covered Raisins, Candy Coated Almonds, Fudge w/nuts, Yogurt Cov'd Pretzels	130 5g	260 10g	390 15g
120	Choc Coated Peppermint Patties, Fudge (choc or vanilla), Peanut Brittle	120 4g	240 8g	360 12g
120	Caramels	120 2g	240 5g	360 8g
110	Tootsie Rolls, Caramels w/cream centers	110 2g	220 4g	330 7g
110	Cinnamon Flavored Candies, Drops (lemon & watermelon w/sugar coating), Smarties, Starlight Mints (sugar free & regular), Sweet Tarts	110 0g	220 0g	330 0g
100	Bubble Gum, Candy Corn, Dinner Mints, Gum Drops, Gummy Bears or Worms, Hard Candies, Jaw Breakers, Jelly Beans, Licorice, Orange Slices	100 0g	200 0g	300 0g
70	Gumballs, Sugar Free Gummy Bears & Hard Candies	70 0g	140 0g	210 0g

In the following table, notice that fat, sodium, and exchanges are listed *per ounce*. The calorie column lists the number of calories in each *individual* piece.

Candy Calorimeter: Calories per ounce & per piece

Candy	PER PIECE		PER OUNCE		
	Calories EACH	Fat (g) EACH	Fat (g) PER OZ	Sodium (mg) PER OZ	Exchanges PER OZ
70 calories/oz:					
Gumballs, regular ½ inch	5	0	0	0	1CHO
Gumballs, larger 1¼ inch	30	0	0	0	1CHO
Gummy bears, sugar-free	6	0	0	0	1CHO
Hard candies, sugar-free	9	0	0	0	1CHO
100 calories/oz:					
Bubble gum	25	0	0	0	1½CHO
Candy corn	6	0	$0.^5$	3	1½CHO
Dinner mints	3	0	0	0	1½CHO
Gum drops, spice drops	11	0	$0.^2$	1	1½CHO
Gummy bears, American or European style	7	0	0	17	1½CHO
Gummy worms	25	0	0	17	1½CHO
Gummy worms, sugar-coated	35	0	0	20	1½CHO
Hard candies	23	0	0	92	1½CHO
Jaw breakers, ½ inch	6	0	0	na	1½CHO
Jaw breakers, 1 inch	40	0	0	na	1½CHO
Jaw breakers, 1¾ inch	200	0	0	na	1½CHO
Jelly beans, regular sized	9	0	$0.^1$	3	1½CHO
Jelly beans, sm gourmet sized	4	0	$0.^1$	3	1½CHO
Licorice sticks, 6"	33	$0.^3$	1	71	1½CHO
Licorice pieces	8	0	1	85	1½CHO
Mints, mini soft non-pareils	2	0	$0.^6$	na	1½CHO
Orange slices	50	0	0	10	1½CHO
110 calories/oz:					
Caramels with cream centers	47	1	$2.^3$	na	1½CHO+½FAT
Cinnamon flav'd candies, sm	2	0	0	0	1½CHO
Drops, lemon or watermelon	15	0	0	3	1½CHO
Smarties	25	0	0	0	1½CHO
Starlight mints	20	0	0	19	1½CHO
Starlight mints, sugar-free	20	0	0	na	1½CHO
Sweet tarts	4	0	0	0	2CHO
Sweet tarts, jumbo	37	0	0	na	2CHO
Tootsie® roll midget	27	$0.^5$	$2.^1$	28	1½CHO+½FAT

*Carbs=Carbohydrate, na=not available   **Exchanges: ST=Starch, Mlk=Milk (skim) FR=Fruit, CHO=Other Carbohydrates, V=Vegetable, MT=Meat (medium fat), FAT=Fat

Candy Calorimeter: Calories per ounce & per piece (cont.)

Candy	PER PIECE		PER OUNCE		
	Calories EACH	Fat (g) EACH	Fat (g) PER OZ	Sodium (mg) PER OZ	Exchanges PER OZ
120 calories/oz:					
Caramels	36	1	2	65	1½CHO+½FAT
Chocolate covered thin mints, small	28	0.8	4	na	1¼CHO+1FAT
Fudge, vanilla or chocolate	na	na	4	50	1CHO+1FAT
Peanut Brittle	na	na	3	10	1CHO+½FAT
130 calories/oz:					
Boston baked beans	6	0.2	5	0	1½CHO+1FAT
Chocolate covered raisins	6	0.2	5	14	1½CHO+1FAT
Candy coated almonds	16	0.7	5	na	1½CHO+1FAT
Fudge with nuts	na	na	5	na	1CHO+1FAT
Yogurt-covered pretzels	na	na	5	200	1CHO+1FAT
140 calories/oz:					
M&M®	4	0.2	6	17	1¼CHO+1FAT
Malted milk balls, large	40	1.9	6	na	1¼CHO+1FAT
Malted milk balls, small	11	0.4	5	na	1¼CHO+1FAT
Reese's® pieces	4	0.2	6	47	1¼CHO+1FAT
150 calories/oz:					
M&M® peanut	13	0.7	9	15	1CHO+1½FAT
Nonpareils, chocolate wafers	21	1	8	na	1CHO+1½FAT
Hershey®'s kisses	26	1.5	9	25	1CHO+2FAT
Hershey®'s minatures	46	2.8	9	20	1CHO+2FAT
Milk Chocolate	na	na	9	10	1CHO+2FAT
Reese's® peanut butter cups, miniatures	42	2.4	9	84	1CHO+2FAT
160 calories/oz:					
Chocolate covered almonds	20	2	12	na	¾CHO+2½FAT
Chocolate w/nuts	na	na	10	20	1CHO+2FAT
Hershey®'s kisses w/almonds	26	1.6	10	19	1CHO+2FAT
Semi-sweet Chocolate	na	na	10	5	1CHO+2FAT

Dried Fruit, Nuts & Seeds

Dried fruit, although containing virtually no fat, is high in calories. Fruit has the same amount of calories whether it is dried or fresh. But, It is easier to eat more calories in the form of dried fruit because the volume is smaller.

Nuts and seeds are also concentrated sources of calories because of their high fat content. If you have purchased the dried fruit, nuts, or seeds from a vendor that weighed your purchase in pounds, refer to the chart in the candy section on how to convert pounds into ounces.

Dried Fruits & Nuts

	Calories	Fat (g)	Sodium (mg)	Carbs* (g)	Exchanges**
Dried Fruits (1oz):					
Apple Rings, 4	69	0	25	17	1FR
Apricots, 8	67	0	2	16	1FR
Dates, 3½	78	0.^{1}	1	19	1FR
Figs, 1½	72	0.^{3}	3	18	1FR
Mixed Fruit	74	0.^{1}	26	18	1FR
Peaches, 2	68	0.^{2}	2	17	1FR
Pears, 1½	74	0.^{2}	2	18	1FR
Pineapple Ring, 1	30	0	na	7	½FR
Prunes, 3	67	0.^{1}	1	16	1FR
Raisins, 3T	86	0.^{1}	4	22	1½FR
Nuts & Seeds (1 oz – roughly ¼ c or a small handful):					
Almonds, unsalted, 24	167	15	3	5	¾MT+2½FAT
Almonds, hickory smoked, 24	166	15	120	5	¾MT+2½FAT
Almonds, oil roasted, 22	176	16	3	5	¾MT+2½FAT
Cashews, dry roasted, 18	163	13	4	9	¼ST+½MT+2FAT
Cashews, oil roasted, 18	163	14	5	9	¼ST+½MT+2FAT
Chestnuts, roasted	70	0.^{6}	1	14	1ST
Coconut, dried sweetened (1/3 c)	125	9	6	11	¾CHO+2FAT
Hazelnuts (filberts), dry roasted	188	19	1	5	4FAT
Hazelnuts, roasted & salted	180	18	40	5	3½FAT
Macadamia Nuts, dry roasted	193	21	117	3	4FAT
Macadamia Nuts, oil roasted	204	22	2	3	4FAT
Mixed Nuts, oil roasted	175	16	3	6	½ST+3FAT
Peanuts, dry roasted, 3T	164	14	228	6	1MT+2FAT
Peanuts, honey roasted	170	13	180	8	¼ST+1MT+1½FAT
Peanuts, Spanish oil roasted	162	14	121	5	1MT+1½FAT
Pistachio Nuts, dry roasted, 47	172	15	2	7	¼ST+½MT+2½FAT
Pecans, oil roasted, 15 halves	195	20	0	5	4FAT
Sunflower Seeds, dry roasted	165	14	1	6	1MT+2FAT
Walnuts	176	17	3	5	1MT+2½FAT

Carbs=Carbohydrate, na=not available   **Exchanges:** ST=Starch, Mlk=Milk (skim)
FR=Fruit, CHO=Other Carbohydrates, V=Vegetable, MT=Meat (medium fat), FAT=Fat

Pretzels

A large chewy pretzel (about the width of this book) has been marketed in kiosks at airports, amusement parks, and movie theatres for years. New to the scene is a softer pretzel prepared plain, with butter & salt, and in a variety of other flavors. Freestanding pretzel shops selling the newer varieties are opening all over the country. These latest pretzels are about the same size as the chewy pretzel but weighs less because it is not as dense.

Pretzels	Calories	Fat (g)	Sodium (mg)	Carbs* (g)	Exchanges**
Chewy Soft Pretzel	300	1	650	60	4ST
Tender Soft Pretzel, w/out butter *or* salt	310	2	na	68	4ST
w/butter & salt	375	8	na	68	4ST+1FAT
w/butter, sugar & cinnamon	440	12	na	80	5ST+½CHO+1½FAT
Iced & prepared w/raisins	490	6	na	100	6ST+½CHO
w/butter & poppyseeds	390	14	na	64	4ST+2FAT
w/butter & sesame seeds	400	14	na	64	4ST+2FAT
almond pretzel	390	8	na	70	4½ST+1FAT

Popcorn

Popcorn is often considered a healthy food due to its high fiber content (about 1 g/cup). When air-popped, popcorn has just 30 calories a cup. Unfortunately, movie theatres, malls, and convenience stores are not using air-popped or "light" popcorn. The end result is a snack that is high in fat and calories (55 calories/cup).

✔ **Select the popcorn prepared with a healthier vegetable oil** (such as cannola or safflower) rather than coconut oil, if you have a choice. Coconut oil is one of the most saturated, "unhealthy" oils available.

✔ **Order it without butter**. The "butter" that is added is usually a butter-flavored oil and contains 125 calories per tablespoon. A medium sized popcorn may contain more than four tablespoons!

Cut the Butter:	Calories	Fat (g)
10 cups Popcorn w/3T butter	925	80
10 cups Popcorn Plain	550	38
Total:	**375**	**42**

---

*Carbs=Carbohydrate, na=not available   **Exchanges:** ST=Starch, Mlk=Milk (skim) FR=Fruit, CHO=Other Carbohydrates, V=Vegetable, MT=Meat (medium fat), FAT=Fat

Popcorn

	Calories	Fat (g)	Sodium (mg)	Carbs* (g)	Exchanges**
Popcorn (without butter):					
1 cup	55	4	40	5	¼ST+¾FAT
3 cups	154	11	120	15	¾ST+2FAT
8 cups	440	30	320	38	2ST+6FAT
12 cups	660	46	480	57	3ST+9FAT
20 cups	1100	76	800	95	5ST+15FAT
24 cups	1320	91	960	114	6ST+18FAT
Butter-Flavored Oil:					
1 Tablespoon (approx. 1 squirt)	125	14	0	0	3FAT
4 Tablespoon	600	56	0	0	11FAT

Popcorn is sold in cups, bags, and boxes. Here are some tips to determine how many cups of popcorn is in your serving.

CUPS:

If your popcorn was served in a cup, estimate how many fluid ounces it holds. Compare it to the cup sizes shown under the *Beverages* chapter or look for a size printed on the cup. The ounces may be labeled on the outside of the cup or on the bottom band (a code of "NO. 22P" is 22 oz). Then divide the number of ounces by 8 to see how many cups it will hold. For example, a 22 oz cup holds nearly three cups (22 ÷ 8 = 2.75 cups).

Ounces		Cups		Ounces		Cups
8	=	1		22	=	2¾
12	=	1½		44	=	5½
16	=	2		64	=	8

BOXES:

The small, standard size found in many stores and in most airports measures 5½" wide X 8½"high X 2" deep (the size of the front cover of this book and two inches deep). This contains approximately 8 cups of popcorn when the cover is closed. If it is open and overflowing, count on at least 9 cups.

BAGS:

Watch out, it's easy to overstuff bags. The measurements below are when the bag is filled, not overfilled.

Cups	Height		Width		Depth
12	9"	X	5"	X	3½"
20	9¾"	X	7½"	X	3½"
24	12"	X	7¼"	X	3½"

For visual assistance, the 12 cups bag is about the size of the front cover of this book, but three and a half inches thick.

*Carbs=Carbohydrate, na=not available   **Exchanges:** ST=Starch, Mlk=Milk (skim) FR=Fruit, CHO=Other Carbohydrates, V=Vegetable, MT=Meat (medium fat), FAT=Fat

PART 3

American Style Dinners

Appetizers

Appetizers are small samples of foods designed to pacify your appetite until your meal arrives. But, how many of us can afford the calories of both an appetizer *and* an entrée? Consider the following:

✓ **Avoid fried appetizers or make the fried appetizer your entrée.** If you enjoy fried foods, ask if there is an appetizer portion (or half portion) available. Appetizers are smaller than the entrée portion and, therefore, have fewer calories.

✓ **Have the leaner appetizers as your entrée.** Think about ordering a lean appetizer such as shrimp cocktail, crabmeat cocktail, or oysters on the half shell with a salad instead of an entrée. Cocktail sauce is also low in fat.

Appetizers can make Lower Calorie Meals:	Calories	Fat (g)
6 Shrimp Cocktail w/2T Cocktail Sauce	220	3
Garden Salad w/fat-free dressing	80	1
2 oz Italian Bread w/2t Whipped Margarine	210	8
Total:	**510**	**12**
Marguerita Pizza, ½ of 12" ("no oil & light on the cheese")	450	9
Minestrone Soup, 8 oz	95	3
Total:	**545**	**12**

✓ **Limit the sauces** that come with appetizers. Most sauces are high in fat and calories. Order them on the side; dip your fork into the sauce and then into the food for a taste with every bite. For nutritional information on sauces not found in this chapter, refer to the *Entrees and Sauces* chapter.

Appetizers

	Calories	Fat (g)	Sodium (mg)	Carbs* (g)	Exchanges**
Artichoke, 1 med cooked	55	0	80	10	1½V
Bruschetta -1oz bread grilled w/ oil	270	10	154	15	1ST+2FAT
Buffalo Wings, 6	450	30	3000	10	½CHO+5MT+1FAT
Blue cheese dressing, 2T	160	16	310	0	3FAT
Calamari, fried, 3 oz	200	8	250	7	½ST+2MT
Caviar, 2T	80	4	480	0	1MT
Melba toast, 4	40	0	90	7	½ST
Ceviche, 4 oz	150	5	na	0	4MT(lean)
Chicken Quesadillas, 6½"	465	26	1010	30	2ST+3MT+2FAT
Clams, raw, 3	50	1	110	0	2MT(very lean)
Crostini (thin French bread toast rounds with pate), 2	170	10	190	8	½ST+1MT+1FAT
Egg Rolls, 1 med	250	15	490	18	¾ST+1V+2½FAT
Sweet and Sour Sauce, 2T	55	0	70	14	1CHO
Fried Mozzarella Sticks, 4 (3 oz)	300	21	950	6	½ST+3MT+1FAT
Marinara sauce, ¼ c	50	1	300	7	1V
Fried Whole Onion	895	68	900	70	1V+3ST+13½FAT
Fried Zucchini, Mushrooms, ½ c	190	10	200	25	1V+1ST+2FAT
Herbed Pork Pâté, 2T	70	3	110	0	1MT
Butter Crackers, 3	80	4	110	12	¾ST+½FAT
Liver Pate, 2T	80	7	190	0	½MT+½FAT
Nachos w/ beans & cheese, 6 lg	480	30	630	20	1ST+2MT+3FAT
Nachos w/ beans, cheese, & meat, 6 lg	690	48	1200	20	1ST+3MT+5FAT
Nuts, 1 oz (about ¼ c)	180	14	180	5	1MT+2FAT
Olives, 10 lg pickled green	45	5	926	0	1FAT
10 med pickled, ripe, greek style	65	7	na	0	1½FAT
1 super colossal ripe	13	1.[1]	145	0	¼FAT
Oysters Rockefeller, 3	85	6	150	4	1V+1FAT
Oysters, raw, 6	120	2	150	0	4MT(very lean)
Marguerita Pizza, 12" (thin crust w/vegetables, sauce & cheese)	1100	46	3000	110	7ST+1V+4MT+4FAT
Popcorn, 1c	55	4	40	5	¼ST+¾FAT
Quesadillas, 6½"diameter	430	24	760	30	2ST+2MT+2½FAT
Roasted Peppers marinated in olive oil	45	3	na	4	½V+½FAT
Shrimp Cocktail, 4 large	120	2	172	0	3MT(very lean)
Cocktail sauce, 2T	40	0	320	10	½CHO
Stuffed Jalapenos	70	4	200	8	½ST+1FAT
Stuffed Mushrooms, 1 regular	40	3	175	3	½ V+½FAT
Porcini, 1 lg	150	15	200	6	1V+2FAT
Stuffed Potato Skins, 4 skins (6 oz)	560	40	600	35	2ST+1MT+6½FAT
Sour cream, ¼ c	104	10	24	0	2FAT

*Carbs=Carbohydrate, na=not available   **Exchanges: ST=Starch, Mlk=Milk (skim)
FR=Fruit, CHO=Other Carbohydrates, V=Vegetable, MT=Meat (medium fat), FAT=Fat

Appetizers (continued)

	Calories	Fat (g)	Sodium (mg)	Carbs* (g)	Exchanges**
Tortilla Chip, 1 regular-sized	18	1	8	3	na
Tortilla Chip, 7 regular	126	7	56	18	1ST+1FAT
Nacho Cheese Sauce, 2T	100	8	580	1	½MT+1FAT
Guacamole, ¼ c	110	10	420	3	2FAT
Salsa, ¼ c	20	0	440	4	1V

*Carbs=Carbohydrate, na=not available   **Exchanges: ST=Starch, Mlk=Milk (skim)
FR=Fruit, CHO=Other Carbohydrates, V=Vegetable, MT=Meat (medium fat), FAT=Fat

Beverages

Chapter Content:
■ Cold Beverages: Sodas, Juices, Milk, Iced Tea, Lemonade, Eggnog, & Shakes
■ Coffee, Coffee Beverages, & other Hot Beverages
■ Alcoholic Beverages

Beverages contain anywhere from 0 - 125 calories *per ounce*. Notice that alcoholic beverages top the list. That's because alcohol has 7 calories per gram, rather than the 4 calories per gram for all other carbohydrates.

Beverage Calorimeter: Calories per fluid ounce

125	Creme de Menthe
100	Coffee Liqueurs
85	100 Proof Liqueurs
60	Manhattan, Martini
40	Nonalcoholic Eggnog, Table Wines
30	Ice Cream Shake, Sherry
25	Champagne, Dry White Wine, Frozen Yogurt Shakes
20	Whole Milk, Fruit Juices (Cranberry, Grape, Prune), Fruit Smoothies
17	Fruit Punches
15	2% Low Fat Milk, Fruit Juices (Apple, Grapefruit, Orange), Orange Sodas, Lemonade, Orange Breakfast Drinks
12	Regular Colas, 1% Low Fat Milk, Beer
10	Skim Milk & Buttermilk (made with skim milk) Flavored Coffees, Sweetened Tea, Coffee with cream & sugar
0	Water, Sparkling Waters without added sugar, Club Soda, Perrier, Diet Sodas, Unsweetened Tea & Coffee

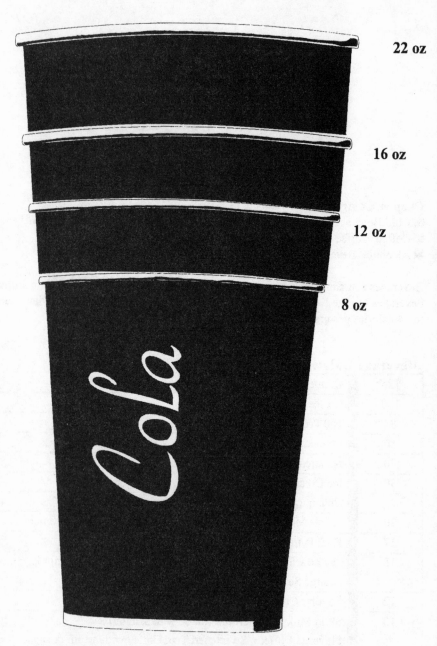

Don't know the serving size of your favorite beverage? Use these actual beverage cup sizes for comparison.

Cold Beverages

Fountain Beverages

✓**All sodas are fat-free but only the diet sodas are calorie-free.** A can of soda has about 150 calories - all derived from sugar! While 150 calories may not sound like much, the calories can have a cumulative effect. All other things being equal, if you are currently drinking six cans of regular soda a day and switch to diet soda, you will be consuming 900 calories a day less. That amounts to a weight loss of almost two pounds each week!

The Diet Soda Difference:		Calories	Fat (g)
12 oz Soda X 6 per day		900	0
12 oz Diet Soda X 6 per day		0	0
	Savings:	**900**	**0**

900 calories X 365 days in a year = 328,500 calories
328,500 ÷ 3500 = weight loss of 94 pounds of fat in a year

How many calories do you consume from soda? It depends on the beverage chosen, size of cup, and the amount of ice put into the glass. To quickly assess the calories in your favorite fountain beverage, refer to the following calorimeter.

Fountain Beverage Calorimeter: Calories per serving

Calories/ 12 oz Can	Fountain Beverages	Calories Per Cup with 20% Ice				
		8 oz	12 oz	16 oz	22 oz	32 oz
210	Orange Sunkist® Soda	110	170	225	310	450
195	Mandarin Orange Slice®	105	155	210	285	415
180	Hawaiian Punch®	95	145	190	265	385
170	A&W® Root Beer, Mountain Dew®, Surge®	90	135	180	250	365
160	Barq's® Root Beer, RC® Cola	85	130	170	235	340
150	Big Red®, Dr. Pepper®, Pepsi®, Lemon Lime Slice®	80	120	160	220	320
140	Coca Cola®, Mr. Pibb®, 7Up®, Sprite®	75	110	150	205	300
0	Diet Sodas	0	0	0	0	0

*** For fat, sodium, and exchanges per 12 oz can, refer to the nutritional information on the next page.**

Milk

✓ **Many restaurants provide skim or low fat milk,** even if it is not listed on the menu. Making this healthy change is recommended for everyone over the age of two.

Skim Milk vs Whole Milk:	Calories	Fat (g)
8 oz Whole Milk	150	8
8 oz Skim Milk	90	0
Savings:	**60**	**8**

Fruit Juice

✓ **Fruit juice contains just as many calories as soda.** It may be healthier to switch from drinking soda to fruit juice because, unlike soda, fruit juices contain vitamins and minerals. But fruit juice doesn't contain fewer calories than non-diet soda. So don't expect the change to cause a weight loss. If you want to lose weight, eat *fresh* fruit for vitamins, minerals, and fiber. Then drink a non-caloric beverage such as water or a diet beverage.

Compare these Two Beverages:	Calories	Fat (g)
12 oz Cola Beverage	140	0
12 oz Orange Juice	170	0

Shakes

✓ **Shake made with skim milk are a better choice.** Even the fat-free shakes are high in calories because of their high sugar content! A 12 oz shake contains almost 10 teaspoons worth! Can you afford the extra calories?

Fat-Free not Calorie-Free:	Calories	Fat (g)
12 oz Ice Cream Shake	385	8
12 oz Fat-Free Shake	275	0
Savings:	**110**	**8**

COLD BEVERAGES

	Calories	Fat (g)	Sodium (mg)	Carbs* (g)	Exchanges**
Fruit/Vegetable Juices (6 oz):					
Tomato Juice	40	0	0	10	2V
Apple Juice	85	0	13	21	1½FR
Cranberry Juice	110	0	8	28	2FR
Grape Juice	120	0	5	30	2FR
Grapefruit Juice	70	0	2	18	1FR
Orange Juice	85	0	1	21	1½FR
Prune Juice	130	0	8	33	2FR

COLD BEVERAGES (continued)

	Calories	Fat (g)	Sodium (mg)	Carbs* (g)	Exchanges**
12 oz can (w/out ice):					
A&W Root Beer	170	0	45	43	2¾CHO
Barq's® Root Beer	160	0	70	40	2½CHO
Big Red®	150	0	30	38	2½CHO
Coca Cola®	140	0	50	35	2½CHO
Diet Coke®	0	0	40	0	FREE
Diet Dr. Pepper®	0	0	55	0	FREE
Diet Pepsi®	0	0	35	0	FREE
Diet Rite Cola	0	0	0	0	FREE
Diet 7Up®	0	0	35	0	FREE
Diet Sprite®	0	0	40	0	FREE
Dr. Pepper®	150	0	55	38	2½CHO
Hawaiian Punch®	180	0	170	45	3CHO
Mr. Pibb®	140	0	45	35	2¼CHO
Mountain Dew®	170	0	70	43	2¾CHO
Pepsi®	150	0	35	38	2½CHO
RC Cola	160	0	50	40	2½CHO
7Up®	140	0	75	35	2¼CHO
Slice®, Mandarin Orange	195	0	55	49	3¼CHO
Slice ®, Lemon Lime	150	0	55	38	2½CHO
Sprite®	140	0	70	35	2¼CHO
Sunkist Orange Soda	210	0	60	53	3½CHO
Surge	170	0	40	43	2¾CHO
Milk (8 oz):					
Skim Milk	90	0	120	12	1Mlk
2% Low Fat Milk	120	5	120	12	1Mlk+1FAT
Whole Milk	150	8	120	12	1Mlk+1½FAT
Other Cold Beverages (12 oz):					
Iced Tea, sweetened	120	0	80	30	2CHO
Lemonade	130	0	130	33	2CHO
Shakes & Egg Nog:					
Fruit Smoothie, 16 oz	320	<1	10	75	5FR
Fruit & fat-free milk Smoothie, 16 oz	250	<1	125	50	1Mlk+2½FR
Fruit & frozen yogurt Smoothie, 16 oz	400	5	120	80	2½FR+3CHO
Ice Cream Shakes, 22 oz	625	29	320	72	4CHO+1Mlk+6FAT
12 oz Ice Cream Shake	385	8	270	51	3CHO+½Mlk+1FAT
Fat-Free Yogurt Shakes, 12 oz	275	0	160	51	3CHO+½Mlk
Egg Nog, non-alcoholic, 4 oz	190	13	75	9	½CHO+¼Mlk+½MT +2½FAT

Coffee and other Hot Beverages

✓ **Coffee, espresso, and tea have negligible calories.** It is what you add to these drinks, however, that will impact your weight and waist!

✓ **Know what's in your beverage** so you'll know what substitutions to ask for.

- ■ Espresso - Strong coffee brewed under pressure
- ■ Cappuccino - Espresso and steamed milk
- ■ Latte - Espresso and steamed milk (but more milk than w/cappuccino)
- ■ Mocha - Espresso, steamed milk, and chocolate syrup

✓ **Ask for your beverage to be prepared with skim or low fat milk.** Nearly every restaurant and coffee shop offers these lower fat alternatives for your coffee and espresso drinks. Remember, drinking just 10 calories more than your body needs will put on an extra pound of fat each year!

Whiten your Coffee with Milk:	Calories	Fat (g)
Instead of: 1 oz Coffee Cream	60	6
1 oz Non-Dairy Creamer	45	3
1 oz Whole Milk	20	1
Choose: 1 oz Skim Milk	10	0
Savings:	**10-50**	**1-6**

Have your Latte Prepared with Skim Milk:	Calories	Fat (g)
12 oz Latte made with whole milk	195	10
12 oz Latte made with skim milk	115	$0.^5$
Savings:	**80**	**$9.^5$**

✓ **Enjoy your beverage without whipping cream.** Depending on whether skim, 2% or whole milk is used in the preparation of the drink, the addition of whipping cream can nearly double the calories!

Skip the Whipped Cream:	Calories	Fat (g)
12 oz Mocha (2% milk) w/ ¼ c whipping cream	280	18
12 oz Mocha (2% milk) w/out whipping cream	180	6
Savings:	**100**	**12**

✓ **There are sixteen calories in a teaspoon of sugar.** That may not sound like a whole lot of calories, but consider this. If you add just a teaspoon of sugar in every cup you drink, and you drink 3 cups a day, that adds up to an extra 48 calories each day. Multiply that by 365 days in the year and you end up with an extra five pounds of fat each year.   Can you afford the calories?

Get used to the Taste of Sweetners:	Calories	Fat (g)
3 t of sugar a day	48	0
3 t sugar/day X 365 days in a year	17,520	0

17,520 calories ÷ 3500 calories in a pound = 5 pounds of fat!

✓ **For those of you concerned about the dangers of non-caloric sweeteners, consider this.** There *may* be risks associated with the excess consumption of non-caloric sweeteners - we just don't know enough yet. But researchers do know of *definite risks* associated with carrying around too much weight such as increased risk of heart disease, high blood pressure, diabetes, and certain types of cancer. If you are still concerned about the safety of non-caloric sweeteners, cut out the sugar and sweeteners completely. The coffee or tea may taste different initially, but by the end of two weeks your taste buds will have adjusted to the difference.

Hot Beverages Calorimeter: Calories per ounce & serving size

Calories per oz	Hot Beverages	Calories & Fat grams (g)			
		8 oz	12 oz	16 oz	20 oz
18	Latte (whole milk)	145 / 6g	215 / 10g	290 / 12g	360 / 16g
17	Mocha (whole milk)	135 / 5g	205 / 8g	270 / 10g	340 / 14g
15	Latte or Mocha (low fat milk) / Hot Chocolate	120 / 4g	180 / 6g	240 / 7g	300 / 9g
12	Mocha (skim milk)	100 / 1g	145 / 2g	190 / 3g	240 / 4g
10	Flavored Coffees (sugar sweetened)	80 / 1g	120 / $1.^5$g	160 / 2g	200 / $2.^5$g
9	Latte (skim milk)	72 / 0g	110 / $0.^5$g	145 / $0.^6$g	180 / $0.^8$g
7	Cappuccino (whole milk)	55 / 3g	85 / 5g	110 / 6g	140 / 8g
6	Cappuccino (low fat milk)	50 / 2g	70 / 3g	100 / 4g	120 / 5g
5	Cappuccino (skim milk)	40 / 0g	60 / 0g	80 / 0g	100 / 0g
0	Coffee, Espresso, Tea (plain)	0 / 0g	0 / 0g	0 / 0g	0 / 0g

Hot Beverages

	Calories	Fat (g)	Sodium (mg)	Carbs* (g)	Exchanges**
Coffee & Espresso:					
Coffee, black, 8 oz	5	0	0	0	FREE
Coffee, decaf, black, 8 oz	5	0	0	0	FREE
Coffee, flavored w/ sugar, 8 oz	72	1	4	16	1CHO
Espresso, 1 shot	5	0	0	1	FREE
Latte:					
Latte w/skim milk, 8 oz	65	0	95	9	¾Mlk
12 oz	115	0.5	160	15	1¼Mlk
16 oz	140	0.6	190	18	1½Mlk
20 oz	190	0.8	250	24	2Mlk
Latte w/2% milk, 8 oz	95	4	90	9	¾Mlk+1FAT
12 oz	155	6	155	15	1¼Mlk+1FAT
16 oz	190	7	185	18	1½Mlk+1½FAT
20 oz	250	9	245	24	2Mlk+2FAT
Latte, w/whole milk, 8 oz	120	6	90	9	¾Mlk+1FAT
12 oz	195	10	155	15	1¼Mlk+2FAT
16 oz	235	12	185	18	1½Mlk+2½FAT
20 oz	310	16	245	24	2Mlk+3FAT
Cappuccino:					
Cappuccino w/skim milk, 8 oz	40	0	50	5	½Mlk
12 oz	60	0	80	6	½Mlk
16 oz	80	0	95	9	¾Mlk
20 oz	100	0	125	12	1Mlk
Cappuccino w/2% milk, 8 oz	50	2	50	5	½Mlk+½FAT
12 oz	75	3	80	6	½Mlk+½FAT
16 oz	100	4	95	9	¾Mlk+1FAT
20 oz	125	5	125	12	1Mlk+1FAT
Cappuccino, w/whole milk, 8 oz	55	3	50	5	½Mlk+½FAT
12 oz	85	5	80	6	½Mlk+1FAT
16 oz	110	6	95	9	¾Mlk+1FAT
20 oz	140	8	125	12	1Mlk+1½FAT
Mocha (w/out whipping cream):					
Mocha, w/skim milk, 8 oz	100	1	75	17	½Mlk+¾CHO
12 oz	150	2	125	24	¾Mlk+1CHO+½FAT
16 oz	200	3	175	35	1Mlk+1½CHO+½FAT
20 oz	230	4	200	42	1Mlk+2CHO+1FAT
Mocha, w/2% milk, 8 oz	120	4	75	17	½Mlk+¾CHO+1FAT
12 oz	180	6	125	24	¾Mlk+1CHO+1FAT
16 oz	240	7	175	35	1Mlk+1½CHO+1½FAT
20 oz	280	10	200	42	1Mlk+2CHO+2FAT
Mocha, w/whole milk, 8 oz	130	5	75	17	½Mlk+¾CHO+1FAT
12 oz	210	8	125	24	¾Mlk+1CHO+1½FAT
16 oz	280	10	175	35	1Mlk+1½CHO+2FAT
20 oz	320	14	200	42	1Mlk+2CHO+3FAT

*Carbs=Carbohydrate, na=not available   **Exchanges: ST=Starch, Mlk=Milk (skim)
FR=Fruit, CHO=Other Carbohydrates, V=Vegetable, MT=Meat (medium fat), FAT=Fat

Hot Beverages (continued)

	Calories	Fat (g)	Sodium (mg)	Carbs* (g)	Exchanges**
Other Hot Beverages:					
Tea, 1 bag	2	0	5	0	FREE
Hot Chocolate, 8 oz	110	2	130	21	½Mlk+1CHO+½FAT
Hot Chocolate, made w/2% milk	120	4	120	21	½Mlk+1CHO+1FAT
Condiments:					
Half & half, 1T	20	$1.^7$	6	0	½FAT
Honey, 1 tsp	21	0	0	6	¼CHO
Honey, 1T	64	0	0	16	1CHO
18% Butterfat Cream, 1 T	30	$2.^5$	5	<1	½FAT
Light Table Cream, 1T	30	3	6	<1	½FAT
Milk, skim, 1T	5	0	8	<1	FREE
Milk, 2%, 1T	$7.^5$	$0.^3$	8	<1	FREE
Milk, whole, 1T	10	$0.^5$	8	<1	FREE
Nondairy lightener, liquid, 1T	22	$1.^5$	7	2	½FAT
Nondairy lightener, powdered, 1tsp	10	1	3	1	FREE
Sugar, 1t	16	0	0	4	¼CHO
Heavy Cream, 1T	50	6	6	<1	1FAT
Whipping Cream, whipped, 2T	50	6	6	<1	1FAT
Whipped Topping, pressurized, 2T	23	$1.^8$	4	<1	½FAT
Whipped Topping, pressurized, ¼ c	46	$3.^6$	8	$2.^5$	1FAT
Accompaniments:					
Biscotti, 7" long, ⁷/₈" wide, $1.^3$ oz	112	5	41	16	1ST+1FAT

How Much Caffeine am I Consuming?

Coffee provides 75% of all the caffeine consumed in America. Caffeine is also found in tea, caffeinated fountain beverages, chocolate, and some drugs. Although there is no hard evidence to support these concerns, some people are concerned about its possible connections to cancer, high blood pressure, and coronary heart disease. Caffeine is a stimulant; if you are sensitive to its effects you may want to limit your intake to two cups a day.

	Caffeine (mg)		Caffeine (mg)
Coffee Beverages:		**Other Beverages:**	
Espresso, 1 oz	35	Chocolate milk, 1 oz	5
Double	70	Cocoa or hot chocolate, 8 oz	5
Espresso, decaf, 1 oz	5	Cola, 12 oz	50
Double	10	Tea, decaf, 8 oz	5
Coffee, 8 oz	100	Tea, 8 oz	50
Coffee, Gourmet, 8 oz	150	Tea, green or instant, 8 oz	30
Caffè Latte, Cappuccino, *or* Mocha, 8 oz	35	Tea, bottled, 12 oz or from instant mix, 8 oz	15
Caffè Latte, Cappuccino, *or* Mocha, 16 or 20 oz	70	Chocolate, dark, bittersweet, or semi-sweet, 1 oz	20

*Carbs=Carbohydrate, na=not available   **Exchanges: ST=Starch, Mlk=Milk (skim)
FR=Fruit, CHO=Other Carbohydrates, V=Vegetable, MT=Meat (medium fat), FAT=Fat

Alcoholic Beverages

In the second chapter we mentioned that carbohydrates and proteins have 4 calories per gram, while fats have 9. Where does alcohol fit it? Alcohol, a fermented carbohydrate, is a concentrated source of calories at 7 calories per gram. Although most alcoholic beverages are fat-free, the calories from alcohol can still be damaging to your weight! Here are some general guidelines for Dining Lean with alcoholic beverages.

✓ **Save the alcoholic drinks for special occasions** if you can't afford the extra calories.

Drink Calorie-free Beverages instead of Mixed Drinks:		
	Calories	Fat (g)
8 oz Screwdriver, Gin & Tonic, Bloody Mary, *or* Bourbon & Soda	200	0
8 oz Diet Soda, Coffee, Tea, Water, Club Soda, *or* Mineral Water	0	0
Savings:	**200**	**0**

Skip the Liqueurs in Coffee:		
	Calories	Fat (g)
Coffee + 1½ oz Creme de Menthe	180	0
Black Coffee	0	0
Savings:	**180**	**0**

✓ **Choose the lighter versions of your favorite beverages.**

Order Light Beer:		
	Calories	Fat (g)
12 oz Beer	150	0
12 oz Light Beer	100	0
Savings:	**50**	**0**

Instead of a Wine Cooler, Order Club Soda/Wine:		
	Calories	Fat (g)
8 oz Wine Cooler	160	0
4 oz Wine + 4 oz Club Soda	80	0
Savings:	**80**	**0**

✓ **Find another favorite beverage – one with fewer calories.**

Order Simple rather than Fancy:		
	Calories	Fat (g)
8 oz Margarita *or* Piña Colada	320-480	0 - 6
1 oz Rum + 7 oz Cola	190	0
Savings:	**130-290**	**0 - 6**

Estimate your portion size and then use the Calorimeter below to learn more about the calories in your favorite alcoholic beverages. There is no fat in most alcoholic beverages. If there is fat, it is noted on the Calorimeter and in the nutritional information that follows.

Alcoholic Beverage Calorimeter: Calories & fat per serving

Calories per oz	Alcoholic Beverages	Calories & fat (g)			
		1½ oz	4 oz	8 oz	12 oz
125	Creme de Menthe	188	500	1000	1500
120	Southern Comfort	180	480	960	1440
110	Drambuie	165	440	880	1320
105	Coffee w/Cream*	155	420	840	1260
		7g	19g	38g	57g
100	Liqueurs: Anisette Liqueurs, Crème d'Amande, Crème de Banana, Crème de Cacao	150	400	800	1200
95	Liqueurs: Benedictine, B&B, Rock & Rye, Tía Maria	145	380	760	1140
85	100 Proof Liquor Liqueurs: Kirsch, Sloe Gin, Peppermint Snapps	125	340	680	1020
80	Tequila Liqueurs: Amaretto, Pernod, Triple Sec, Apricot Brandy, Cherry Heering, Creme de Cassis, Grand Marnier	120	320	640	960
75	90 Proof Liquor Liqueurs: Curaçao	115	300	600	900
70	Brandy	105	280	560	840
65	80 Proof Liquor	100	260	520	780
60	Manhattan, Martini	90	240	480	720
58	Piña Coladas*, Grasshopper*, Golden Cadillac*, Velvet Hammer*, Brandy Alexandra*	85	230	465	700
		3g	7g	14g	21g
55	SloeGin Fizz, Old Fashioned	85	220	440	660
50	Glögg*	75	200	400	600
		1g	2g	4g	6g

* These alcoholic beverages contain fat. The others do not.

Alcoholic Beverage Calorimeter (continued)

Calories per oz	Alcoholic Beverages	Calories & fat (g)			
		1½ oz	4 oz	8 oz	12 oz
45	Hot Buttered Rum*, Irish Coffee*	70 3g	180 7g	360 14g	540 21g
45	Wines: Muscatel, Port, Vermouth (sweet), Dessert Wines (sweet)	70	180	360	540
40	Margarita, Whiskey Sour, Mexican Sunset Wines: Dessert Wines (dry), Madeira Tokay, Dubonnet, Sweet Wines	60	160	320	480
38	Brandy Cream*	60 3g	150 7g	300 14g	450 21g
35	Tequila Sunrise, Daquiri, Dry Vermouth	55	140	280	420
30	Sherry Wines: Cold Duck, Sparkling Burgundy, Sauterne	45	120	240	360
25	Bourbon/Soda, Bloody Mary, Campari/Soda, Gin/Tonic, Screwdriver Wines: Beaujolais, Champagne, Chablis, Chianti, Rhine, Rhone, Bordeaux, Burgundy, Rosé, White Burgundy, Cabernet Sauvignon, Chardonnay, French Colombard, Riesling, Sylvaner, Red Zinfandel	40	100	200	300
20	Tom Collins, Highball, Mint Julep, Sparkling Wine Coolers Wines: Sauvignon Blanc, White Zinfandel, Chablis, Chenin Blanc, Table Wines, Liebfraumilch	30	80	160	240
15	Wine Spritzer	25	60	120	180
13	Dark Beer & Ale, Malt Liquors	20	50	104	156
12	Beer	20	50	96	144
9	Light Beer	15	35	72	108

* These alcoholic beverages contain fat. The others do not.

Alcoholic Beverages containing fat

	Calories	Fat (g)	Sodium (mg)	Carbs* (g)	Exchanges**
Brandy Alexander, 5 fl oz	275	10	15	na	na
Brandy Cream, 4 fl oz	150	7	na	na	na
Coffee w/cream, 1½ fl oz	155	7	na	na	na
Glögg, 4 fl oz	190	2	na	na	na
Golden Cadillac, 4 fl oz	230	7	na	na	na
Grasshopper, 4 fl oz	230	7	na	na	na
Hot Buttered Rum, 6 fl oz	255	9	na	na	na
Irish Coffee, 6 fl oz	280	11	na	na	na
Piña Colada, 4½ fl oz	260	3	na	na	na
Velvet Hammer, 4 fl oz	230	7	9	na	na

Soups

You've just arrived at the restaurant and you're feeling famished. What can you order that will be served fast? Soups, if chosen wisely, can stave off your appetite until your main course arrives. The following guidelines are for your consideration when ordering soups.

✓ **Choose broth-based soups.** Broth-based soups have fewer calories than cream-based soups and can help satiate you so that you don't overeat during the rest of the meal. Unfortunately, all restaurant soups are high in sodium.

✓ **Milk-based soups are significantly lower in calories than cream-based soups.** Be sure to ask about the ingredients of the soup. You are more likely to find the higher fat cream based soups at the more upscale restaurants than at a salad bar. Some restaurants are serving healthy "cream" soups made with skim milk and pureed vegetables. These would be acceptable low fat options. Just ask.

✓ **Thicker soups (such as gumbo) may have be prepared with roux** (a thickener made from fat and flour). The fat increases the caloric content more than it would appear by sight.

✓ **Skip the garnish.** Some soups, in upscale restaurants, are "garnished" with a dollop of sour cream (50 calories and 5 grams fat) or a swirl of light cream (30 calories and 3 grams of fat per tablespoon). Your Tortilla soup may have fried tortilla strips and avocado cubes added prior to being served. Baked potato soup might be topped with crumbled bacon. You may want to consider asking for your soup to be served plain unless you can afford the extra calories!

✓ **Don't eat the bowl.** In some restaurants, soup is served in a bread bowl, a round loaf of bread with the top removed and the inside partially scooped out. This bowl, though low in fat, contains over 600 calories!

✓ **Select a cup, not a bowl.** Save the calories for other courses you want to enjoy.

✓ **Select a larger bowl of one of the lower calorie soups and make it a meal!**

Make Soup into a Light Meal:	Calories	Fat (g)
12 oz Vegetable Soup	120	5
2 oz Focaccio bread w/1t olive oil	220	11
TOTAL:	340	16

Soup Calorimeter: Calories & fat per serving

Calories per oz	Soup	Calories & Fat (g)		
		8 oz cup	12 oz sm bowl	16 oz lg bowl
45	French Onion Soup (topped with melted cheese), Cheese Soup (thick), Baked Potato Soup	360 22g	540 33g	720 44g
39	Chile con Carne (w/beans & meat)	310 13g	465 20g	620 26g
33	French Onion Soup (simple), New England Clam Chowder, Fish Chowder, Seafood Gumbo, Vichyssoise	260 15g	390 23g	520 30g
29	Cheese Soup (w/milk), Oyster Stew, Cream of Chicken, Lobster Bisque, Tomato Bisque, Tortilla Soup	225 14g	340 21g	450 28g
25	Manhattan Clam Chowder, Split Pea w/ham, Cream of Potato	200 8g	300 12g	400 16g
23	Black Bean, Chili w/beans (no meat), Bouillabaisse, Lentil / Cream of: Asparagus, Broccoli, Celery, *or* Mushroom	180 7g	270 11g	360 15g
15	Chicken Noodle, Chicken Rice, Tomato	120 3g	180 5g	240 6g
13	Minestrone	100 3g	150 5g	200 6g
10	Vegetable, Gazpacho	80 3g	120 5g	160 6g

Soups* (1 c)

	Calories	Fat (g)	Sodium (mg)	Carbs* (g)	Exchanges**
Baked Potato Soup	350	22	na	21	½Mlk+1ST+1MT +3FAT
Bean Soup *or* Black Bean Soup	180	6	na	22	1½ST+1MT
Bouillabaisse, w/out rice	155	5	na	10	1V+2MT(lean)
Cheese Soup, made w/milk	230	15	na	14	½ST+½Mlk+½MT +2½FAT
Cheese Soup (thick)	360	27	na	11	½Mlk+1V+1½MT +4FAT
Chicken Noodle *or* Chicken Rice	120	3	na	15	1ST+½MT
Chili Con Carne w/Beans	310	13	na	30	2ST+2MT+½FAT
Chile w/Beans, no meat	180	6	na	22	1½ST+1MT
Clam Chowder, Manhattan	210	9	na	16	2V+½ST+1MT+1½FAT
Clam Chowder, New England *or* Fish Chowder	260	13	na	18	½Mlk+½ST+1MT +1½FAT
Cream of Asparagus, Broccoli, Celery, *or* Mushroom	180	9	na	18	¾ST+½Mlk+2FAT
Cream of Chicken	185	12	na	9	¼ST+½Mlk+½MT +2FAT
Cream of Potato Soup	190	10	na	15	1ST+2FAT
French Onion Soup	260	15	na	20	1ST+1V+1MT+1½FAT
French Onion Soup w/melted cheese	380	22	na	30	2ST+1MT+3FAT
Gazpacho	90	2	na	10	2V+½FAT
Gumbo, Seafood	250	16	na	6	½Mlk+1MT+2FAT
Lentil	190	5	na	22	1½ST+1MT
Lobster Bisque	220	15	na	5	1V+1MT+2FAT
Minestrone	95	3	na	15	3V+½FAT
Oyster Stew	220	15	na	6	½Mlk+1MT+2FAT
Pasta e Fagioli	280	8	na	35	2ST+1V+1MT
Split Pea w/Ham	190	6	na	35	2ST+1FAT
Tomato	135	3	na	20	1ST+1V+½FAT
Tomato Bisque	225	12	na	11	½ST+1V+½Mlk +2FAT
Tortilla Soup	240	14	na	17	1V+¾ST+½MT+2FAT
Vegetable Soup	70	2	na	10	2V+½FAT
Vichyssoise (chilled potato soup)	270	18	na	21	1ST+½Mlk+3½FAT
Bread Bowl (size to fit 12 oz of soup)	625	3	na	120	8ST

* Sodium content varies greatly depending on the recipe. Most average 1000 mg/8 oz.

---

*Carbs=Carbohydrate, na=not available   **Exchanges: ST=Starch, Mlk=Milk (skim)
FR=Fruit, CHO=Other Carbohydrates, V=Vegetable, MT=Meat (medium fat), FAT=Fat

Salads

People watching their weight often have the misconception that all salads are low calorie, low fat meals. Salad *can* be low fat, but often the dieter chooses the wrong items and ends up with far more calories than a hamburger and fries. Take a look at how a healthy salad can become a disaster.

A Healthy Meal:

	Calories	Fat (g)
Raw Vegetables, 2 c	100	0
Cottage Cheese, ¼ c	60	5
Chickpeas, 2T	20	0
Shredded Cheese, 2T	60	5
Fat Free Salad Dressing, 2T	40	0
Croutons, 1 Spoon	45	3
Fresh Fruit, ½ c	50	0
TOTAL:	**375**	**13**

Can Double in Calories *Fast*:

	Calories	Fat (g)
All of the above, without the fat-free dressing	335	13
plus Regular Salad Dressing (2 ladles or 4T)	320	32
TOTAL:	**655**	**45**

And Get Even Higher in Calories:

	Calories	Fat (g)
All of the above, plus…	655	45
Potato Salad, ¼ c	100	7
Broccoli/Cauliflower in Ranch dressing, ¼ c	80	8
Blueberry Muffin, 2 oz (small)	200	8
Margarine, 1½ t	53	6
TOTAL:	**1088**	**74**

Indeed, a salad with all those little extras has almost as much fat as a stick of butter, and chances are, those people thought they were eating healthy. Next time you're at the salad bar, use these suggestions to make informed decisions:

Salad Bars

✓ **At the salad bar, pile on the raw vegetables, beans (non-marinated), and fresh fruit**. These are all low in fat and calories. These selections lead people to mistakenly believe that all salads are low calorie. It's the mayonnaise, oil , and salad dressings that converts a healthy meal into a harmful meal.

✓ **Keep the prepared salads to a minimum.** While plain pasta, cabbage, potatoes, chicken, and tuna fish are low in calories, the addition of mayonnaise (at 100 calories a tablespoon) will more than double the calories. This also applies for oil-prepared salads.

Look how Mayonnaise affects the Total Calories:	Calories	Fat (g)
Cole Slaw prepared w/mayonnaise, ½ c	85	6
Cabbage, ½ c	8	0
Savings:	77	6

✓ **Choose lean protein.** There are many high-fat protein selections on the salad bar: cheese, eggs, and tuna fish salad. If you want to add healthy protein to your meal, think about adding cottage cheese or non-marinated beans. You may also want to order grilled chicken to top your salad.

Eat Your Protein Plain:	Calories	Fat (g)
Chicken Salad, ¼ c	125	9
Grilled Chicken Breast, ¼ c	50	1
Savings:	75	8

✓ **Select only small amounts of nuts and seeds.** Did you know that just a small handful of nuts or seeds (¼ c) contains 200 calories? As a healthy alternative, add water chestnuts or raw jicama for crunch. Jicama is a low calorie white vegetable that looks much like raw potato.

Choose Jicama Instead of Nuts:	Calories	Fat (g)
Nuts, ¼ c	200	18
Jicama, ¼ c	12	0
Savings:	188	18

✓ **Request fat-free salad dressings**. Salad bars and restaurants typically stock them. Other low calorie, no-fat options for a salad include picante sauce, salsa, lemon, and flavored vinegars (such as red wine, balsamic, or tarragon vinegar).

✓ **How big is that ladle?** Most salad dressing ladles contain two tablespoons of dressing. Some hold four! How many ladles of salad dressing are you using?

✓ **Keep in mind that all portions listed are for level measures** – not heaping! Generally, a heaping tablespoon contains two level tablespoons.

Salads

	Calories	Fat (g)	Sodium (mg)	Carbs* (g)	Exchanges**
Vegetables:					
Raw Vegetables & Sprouts, 1c	25	0	5	5	1V
Avocado, ¼	85	7	5	0	2FAT
Green Peas, 2T	15	0	50	4	¼ST
Jicama, ¼ c	12	0	1	3	½V
Olives, Black, 2	10	1	80	0	FREE, 10=1FAT
Green, 2	9	1	180	0	FREE, 10=1FAT
Pickles, 2 slices	1	0	60	0	FREE
Pickle, 1 medium	7	0	928	0	FREE
Pimento Stuffed Green Olives, 5	25	3	470	0	½FAT
Meats & Protein (2T unless noted):					
Chopped Egg	30	2	30	0	½MT
Whole Boiled Egg, 1	80	6	70	0	1MT
Cottage Cheese	25	1	100	0	½MT
Ham	25	1	250	0	½MT
Parmesan Cheese	50	3	290	0	¾MT
Pepperoni, sliced, 6 pc	30	3	70	0	½FAT, 9 pc=1FAT
Shredded Cheese	50	4	250	0	¾MT
Garnishes (2T):					
Bacon Bits	45	3	570	4	¼ST+½FAT
Chickpeas (Garbanzo beans)	20	0	75	4	¼ST
Chow Mein Fried Noodles	20	1	15	4	¼ST
Croutons	30	1	75	8	½ST
Granola	65	2	35	8	½ST+½FAT
Kidney Beans	27	1	73	8	½ST
Nuts, unsalted	200	18	0	1	3½FAT
Raisins	56	0	2	30	1FR
Sunflower Seeds	80	7	1	1	1½FAT
Salad Dressings (1T):					
Blue Cheese	80	8	155	<1	1½FAT
French	80	9	200	4	¼CHO+1½FAT
Honey Mustard	85	9	150	1	2FAT
Italian	80	9	145	1	2FAT
Oil and Vinegar	70	8	0	0	1½FAT

*Carbs=Carbohydrate, na=not available **Exchanges:** ST=Starch, Mlk=Milk (skim) FR=Fruit, CHO=Other Carbohydrates, V=Vegetable, MT=Meat (medium fat), FAT=Fat

Salads (continued)

Salad Dressings (1T) continued:

	Calories	Fat (g)	Sodium (mg)	Carbs* (g)	Exchanges**
Olive Oil	120	14	0	0	3FAT
Ranch	60	5	130	3	1FAT
Blue Cheese	80	8	160	<1	1½FAT
French	70	6	180	4	¼CHO+1FAT
Thousand Island	60	5	110	6	¼CHO+1FAT
Vinaigrette	90	9	8	0	2FAT
Low Calorie Dressings	30-50	3-5	120	1 - 4	½-1FAT
Fat-Free Salad Dressing	6-30	0	135	1 - 7	FREE
Picante Sauce or Salsa	5	0	110	1	FREE
Vinegar	2	0	0	0	FREE
Lemon, ¼	4	0	0	0	FREE

Prepared Salads

✓ **Ask about the salad's ingredients**. You may want to request that some of the higher calorie ones such as avocado, anchovies, bacon, croutons, boiled egg, or cheese not be added.

Be Picky about What is in your Salad:		
	Calories	Fat (g)
Cobb Salad w/dressing	465	31
Cobb Salad w/dressing, no bacon	330	27
Savings:	**35**	**4**

✓ **Ask for your salad to be served in a plate or bowl rather than in a taco shell.** Taco salads are frequently served in a fried tortilla shell. The regular sized fried tortilla, without the filling, can contain about 400 calories. A lower calorie/fat alternative is to have the salad served on a plate.

On a Plate, Please:		
	Calories	Fat (g)
Taco Salad in Taco Shell	930	69
Taco Salad served on a Plate	510	39
Savings:	**420**	**30**

✓ **Request salad dressings *on the side*** so that you can control the amount of dressing that is added. Restaurants typically add an average of three tablespoons (240 calories) of dressing on a small salad and as much as a half cup (640 calories and 64 grams of fat) on a large salad meal!

✓ **Request low calorie dressing** rather than the dressing the salad is typically prepared with. Salad dressings, to prevent wilting, are not added until just prior to serving. Consider ordering the spinach salad with a lowfat honey mustard dressing instead of the usual hot bacon dressing.

*Carbs=Carbohydrate, na=not available   **Exchanges:** ST=Starch, Mlk=Milk (skim) FR=Fruit, CHO=Other Carbohydrates, V=Vegetable, MT=Meat (medium fat), FAT=Fat

Prepared Salads

	Calories	Fat (g)	Sodium (mg)	Carbs* (g)	Exchanges**
Prepared Salads (¼ c):					
Ambrosia Salad	75	3	170	12	¾FR+½FAT
Broccoli/Cauliflower/Ranch	80	8	175	5	1V+1½FAT
Carrot Raisin Salad	80	5	95	15	1FR+1FAT
Chicken Salad	125	9	350	0	1½MT
Cole Slaw w/mayonnaise	85	6	100	5	1V+1FAT
Cole Slaw w/vinaigrette	55	4	5	5	1V+1FAT
Egg Salad	123	11	170	0	1MT+1FAT
Fruit Delight	55	2	2	8	½FR+½FAT
Kidney Bean Salad	55	2	155	8	½ST+½FAT
Macaroni Salad	100	7	180	8	½ST+1½FAT
Marinated Mixed Vegetable Salad	60	4	150	5	1V+1FAT
Oriental Fruit Salad	80	3	30	15	1FR+½FAT
Pea Salad	70	6	90	5	1V+1FAT
Potato Salad w/ mayo	100	7	330	8	½ST+1½FAT
Potato Salad w/vinaigrette	75	4	130	8	½ST+1FAT
Rotelli Pasta Salad	120	6	150	15	1ST+1FAT
Snow Salad	70	4	20	8	½FR+1FAT
Spaghetti Salad	125	7	2	12	¾ST+1½FAT
Three Bean Salad	90	4	180	8	½ST+1FAT
Tuna Salad	190	10	410	8	½CHO+2 MT
Waldorf Salad	70	5	70	8	½FR+1FAT
Fresh Tossed Salads (per 1 c):					
Caesar Salad w/ dressing	170	13	550	8	¼ST+1V+½MT+2FAT
Caesar Salad w/out dressing	90	4	475	8	¼ST+1V+½MT
Chicken Caesar w/ dressing	260	20	750	8	¼ST+1V+2MT+2FAT
Chicken Caesar w/out dressing	140	7	450	8	¼ST+1V+1MT+½FAT
Cobb Salad w/ dressing	365	31	675	5	1V+1½MT+4½FAT
Crab Louis w/ dressing	290	21	410	5	1V+2MT+2FAT
Crab Louis w/out dressing	150	5	455	5	1V+2MT(lean)
Garden Salad w/out dressing	50	2	45	5	1V+½FAT
Green Side Salad w/out dressing	50	3	75	5	1V+½FAT
Greek Salad w/ dressing	120	9	320	5	1V+2FAT
Oriental Chicken w/out dressing	160	5	150	13	½ST+1V+2MT(lean)
Oriental Chicken w/ dressing	275	17	725	13	½ST+1V+2MT+1½FAT
Roma Tomato, Mozzarella, & Basil	120	9	180	5	1V+½MT+1FAT
Spinach Salad w/dressing	120	10	210	5	1V+2FAT

*Carbs=Carbohydrate, na=not available   **Exchanges: ST=Starch, Mlk=Milk (skim)
FR=Fruit, CHO=Other Carbohydrates, V=Vegetable, MT=Meat (medium fat), FAT=Fat

Breads & Spreads

Chapter Contents:

■ General Recommendations
■ Estimating the Calories & Fat Grams in Bread
■ Bread Portion Sizes: Bagels, Biscuits, Bread, Breadsticks, Cornbread, Gingerbread, Croissants, English Muffins, Foccacio, French & Italian Bread, French Roll, and Rolls
■ Nutritional Information: Breads & Spreads

Breads and muffins contain anywhere from 70-125 calories per ounce. That doesn't sound like much until you realize how fast an ounce goes down! Most of us eat far more than a single ounce serving. Here are some suggestions to help you keep your weight down.

✓ **Unbuttered breads such as sliced bread or toast, English muffins, bagels, and French bread have 70-80 calories per ounce and little or no fat.** Biscuits and croissants are higher in fat and calories.

Order the English Muffin rather than a Biscuit:		Calories	Fat (g)
Biscuit, 1½ oz (small)		190	11
English Muffin, 1½ oz (standard sized)		130	1
	Savings:	60	10

Have a Bagel instead of a Croissant:		Calories	Fat (g)
Croissant, 3 oz		360	20
Bagel, 3 oz		240	2
	Savings:	120	18

✓ **Limit the amount of bread you eat.** A 1 oz unbuttered breadstick has just 80 calories and 1 gram of fat. However, most restaurants are serving larger breadsticks in the range of 1½ to 2 oz each. And do you stop at just one breadstick? Can your body afford all those calories?

✓ **Just take the portion you can healthily afford to eat and then ask that the rest of the bread be taken away** or simply move it from your end of the table. Don't torture yourself by staring at the bread basket all evening!

✓ **Always order your bread** *dry* **so you can decide how much of the toppings to add.** Ask for that roll or breadstick *plain* (without the butter glaze on the top). In time, your taste buds will adjust to the unbuttered taste.

✓ **Add only small amounts of fat to your bread.** Use thin slivers of fat rather than hunks. A thin layer of jelly or jam has less calories and fat than a comparable portion of butter or margarine.

Put Jelly on your Toast instead of Margarine:	Calories	Fat (g)
2 Pieces Toast with 1 T margarine	240	12
2 Pieces Toast with 1 T jelly	195	1
Savings:	**45**	**11**

✓ **Vegetable margarine or oil has as many calories as butter, but is a healthier fat** because it is mostly unsaturated (lower in saturated fats). Like all other non-animal foods, vegetable margarine and oil also contains no cholesterol.

✓ **Watch the cream cheese.** Are you spreading your bagel with cream cheese because of the promotion that "cream cheese has half the calories of butter or margarine"? While it is true that cream cheese has half the calories of butter or margarine, we tend to use more than twice as much!

Cream Cheese vs Margarine is Often No Difference:	Calories	Fat (g)
Bagel with 2T cream cheese	340	13
Bagel with 1T margarine	340	13
Savings:	**0**	**0**

Estimating the Calories & Fat grams in Bread

How many calories are in the breads that you enjoy? To find out you'll need two nuggets of information found in this chapter:

❶ Calories per ounce found on the Bread Calorimeter below and

❷ Portion size of the bread you ate. The most accurate way to find this out is to take the food back to the home or the office and weigh your portion on a postage scale. Since that is not always practical, many portion sizes of your favorite breads are described or depicted on the next few pages.

Bread Calorimeter: Calories & fat per serving

Calories per oz	Breads	Calories & Fat (g)				
		1 oz	2 oz	3 oz	4 oz	5 oz
125	Biscuits	125	250	375	500	625
		8g	15g	23g	30g	38g
120	Croissants, plain	120	240	360	480	600
		7g	13g	20g	26g	33g
110	Gingerbread Muffins (lemon poppy seed, chocolate chip)	110	220	330	440	550
		6g	11g	17g	22g	28g
100	Muffins (fruit or grain)	100	200	300	400	500
		4g	8g	13g	17g	21g
90	Buttered Breadsticks Cornbread, Focaccio Yeast Rolls, glazed w/butter	90	180	270	360	450
		3g	6g	9g	12g	15g
90	Bagel (chocolate chip)	90	180	270	360	450
		2g	4g	7g	9g	11g
80	Bagel (except chocolate chip) Breadstick, English Muffin Hamburger & Hot Dog Bun Italian Bread, Low Fat Muffins Pita Bread, Submarine Roll Yeast Rolls, unbuttered	80	160	240	320	400
		1g	1g	2g	2g	3g
70	French Roll & Baguette Sandwich Bread Slices	70	140	210	280	350
		1g	2g	3g	4g	5g

Bread Portion Sizes

How many ounces are you eating? The descriptions and depictions below should help you to determine your portion size:

Bagels

While bagels in your grocery store usually weigh 2 - 3 ounces, gourmet bagels are 4 - 5 ounces! Mini bagels are 1 ounce in size. The outline of the 5 ounce bagel, at almost five inches in diameter, wouldn't even fit in the borders of this printed page. Compare your bagel to the diameter of the bagels shown here.

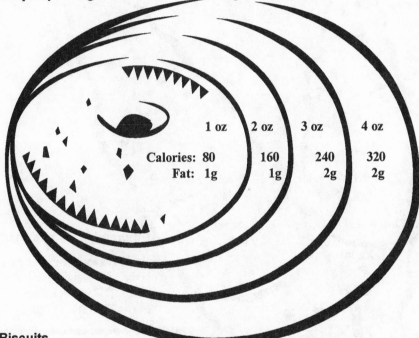

	1 oz	2 oz	3 oz	4 oz
Calories:	80	160	240	320
Fat:	1g	1g	2g	2g

Biscuits

Biscuits are very heavy; therefore, portion sizes are deceptively smaller than you may think. A 1 oz biscuit is about the size of a small biscuit packed in the smallest tubes in the refrigerated section in the grocery store. Most restaurant biscuits weigh at least 2 oz.

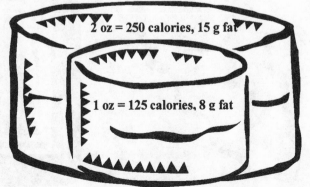

2 oz = 250 calories, 15 g fat

1 oz = 125 calories, 8 g fat

Bread

Most of us are familiar with the standard 1 oz slice of bread (½" thick) at the grocery store. Compare the bread slices at the restaurant to this size. Restaurants also serve a thicker, 1½ oz slice of bread (¾" thick) that is often referred to as "Texas Toast." Figure on the mini loaf of bread to contain 3 - 4 ounces.

Breadsticks

Depicted here are the two most common sizes of breadsticks served in restaurants. The 1 oz breadstick is about 5½" long while the 1½ oz breadstick is 7½" long and thicker.

1 oz

1½ oz

Buttered: 115 calories
5 g fat

175 calories
8 g fat

Plain: 80 calories
1 g fat

120 calories
2 g fat

Cornbread & Gingerbread

Portion sizes for cornbread & gingerbread are about the same:
1 oz = 2" X 1¾" (1" high)
2 oz = 2" X 3½" (1" high)

Cornbread
1 oz = 90 calories
3 g fat

Gingerbread
1 oz = 110 calories
6 g fat

1" thick

Croissants

The 1 oz dinner croissant is very small – just 3½" long. The 3 oz croissant is more sandwich sized at 5½" long. This is how they may look from a side view.

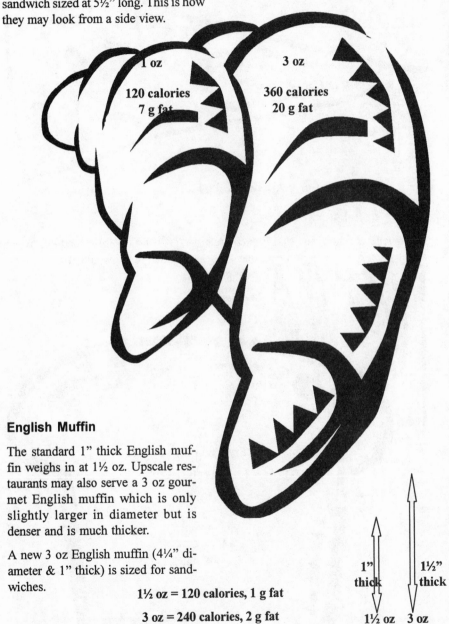

1 oz

**120 calories
7 g fat**

3 oz

**360 calories
20 g fat**

English Muffin

The standard 1" thick English muffin weighs in at 1½ oz. Upscale restaurants may also serve a 3 oz gourmet English muffin which is only slightly larger in diameter but is denser and is much thicker.

A new 3 oz English muffin (4¼" diameter & 1" thick) is sized for sandwiches.

1½ oz = 120 calories, 1 g fat

3 oz = 240 calories, 2 g fat

**1"
thick**

**1½"
thick**

1½ oz   3 oz

Focaccio

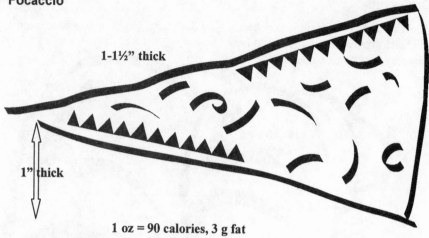

1-1½" thick

1" thick

1 oz = 90 calories, 3 g fat

French *or* Italian Bread

A baguette is a long and thin French bread. A 1½" slice of this bread will weigh about 1 oz. A ¾" slice of the regular French or Italian bread would also be 1 oz.

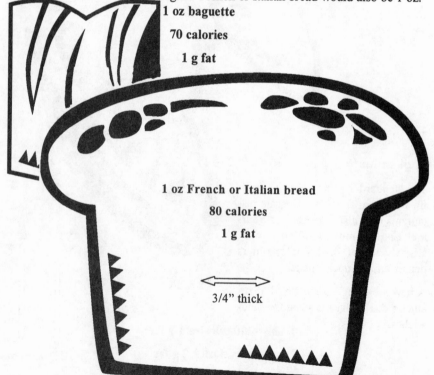

1 oz baguette

70 calories

1 g fat

1 oz French or Italian bread

80 calories

1 g fat

3/4" thick

French Roll

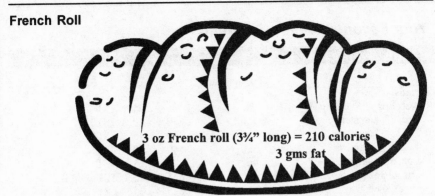

3 oz French roll (3¾" long) = 210 calories
3 gms fat

3 oz submarine roll (6" long) = 210 calories, 3 gms fat

Pita Bread & Submarine Rolls – see the *Deli & Sandwich Shops* chapter.

Hamburger Bun – see the *Burgers & Fast Foods* chapter.

Muffins – see the *Desserts* chapter.

Rolls

Yeast rolls are light and fluffy dinner rolls. A 1 oz roll is quite small – about the size of the "brown and serve" rolls found in the bread section of your local grocery store. Most restaurants serve larger rolls - about 1½ to 2 oz in size. Compare your favorite yeast rolls to the ones pictured here. The glazed (buttered) rolls have more fat and calories.

2 oz Glazed: 210 calories
10 g fat

Plain: 160 calories
2 g fat

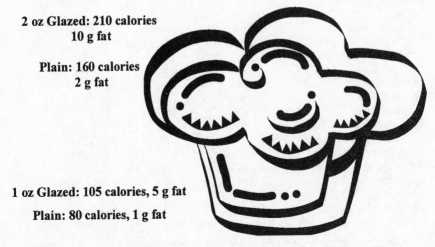

1 oz Glazed: 105 calories, 5 g fat
Plain: 80 calories, 1 g fat

Your Favorite Breads & Spreads

Breads & Spreads

	Calories	Fat (g)	Sodium (mg)	Carbs* (g)	Exchanges**
Breads:					
Bagel, 1 oz, 2½" diameter	80	0	135	15	1ST
2 oz, 3" diameter	160	0.⁵	270	30	2ST
3 oz, 3½" diameter	240	1	400	45	3ST
4 oz, 4¼" diameter	320	2	540	60	4ST
5 oz, 5" diameter	400	3	675	75	5ST
Chocolate chip, 5 oz	450	11	675	75	5ST+1FAT
Poppy seed, 5 oz	415	4	675	75	5ST
Sesame seed, 5 oz	427	5	675	75	5ST
Biscuits, 1 oz, 2" around	125	8	275	12	¾ST+1½FAT
1½ oz, 2" X 2¾" square	190	11	400	19	1¼ST+2FAT
2 oz, 3" around	250	17	533	22	1½ST+3FAT
3 oz	375	22	750	30	2ST+4FAT
Bread, regular slice ½" thick, 1 oz	70	1	150	15	1ST
Thicker slice ¾" thick	110	1	225	22	1½ST
Small loaf, 4 oz	280	5	640	52	3½ST+1FAT
Breadstick, 1 oz plain	80	1	120	15	1ST
1 oz buttered	116	5	160	15	1ST+1FAT
1½ oz plain	120	2	180	22	1½ST
1½ oz buttered	175	8	240	22	1½ST+1½FAT
Cornbread, 1¾" X 2"X 1", 1 oz	90	3	480	15	1ST+½FAT
1½ oz piece, 2½" X 2"X1"	135	5	720	19	1¼ST+1FAT
2 oz piece, 3½" X 2"X1"	180	6	960	26	1¾ST+1FAT
Cracker, Butter Crackers, 3	80	4	110	12	¾ST+½FAT
Melba Toast, 2	20	0	45	4	¼ST
Saltine Cracker, 2	24	1	70	4	¼ST
Sesame Breadstick, 1	15	0	20	4	¼ST
Croissant, 1 oz dinner	120	7	130	12	¾ST+1½FAT
2 oz	240	13	260	22	1½ST+2FAT
3 oz sandwich-sized	360	20	400	34	2¼ST+4FAT
English Muffin, regular, 1½ oz	130	1	140	22	1½ST
Gourmet *or* Sandwich size, 3 oz	220	2	420	38	2½ST
Focaccio Bread, 1 oz	90	2	200	15	1ST+¼FAT
French Baguette, 1 oz	70	1	110	15	1ST
French Roll, 2 oz, 4" long	140	2	220	30	2ST
3 oz, 6" long	210	3	470	38	2½ST
Gingerbread, 1¾" X 2"X 1", 1 oz	90	3	480	15	1ST+½FAT
1½ oz piece, 2½" X 2"X1"	135	5	720	19	1¼ST+1FAT
2 oz piece, 3½" X 2"X1"	180	6	960	26	1¾ST+1FAT
Italian Bread, 1 oz	75	1	150	15	1ST
Spoon Bread, ½ c	150	6	260	21	1ST+½Mlk+1FAT

Carbs=Carbohydrate, na=not available **Exchanges:** ST=Starch, Mlk=Milk (skim)
FR=Fruit, CHO=Other Carbohydrates, V=Vegetable, MT=Meat (medium fat), FAT=Fat

Breads & Spreads (continued)

Breads (continued):

	Calories	Fat (g)	Sodium (mg)	Carbs* (g)	Exchanges**
Yeast Roll, small unbuttered, 1oz	80	2	140	15	1ST+½FAT
Yeast Roll, sm 1oz, glazed w/butter	105	5	140	15	1ST+1FAT
Yeast Roll, large unbuttered, 2 oz	160	4	280	30	2ST+½FAT
Yeast Roll, lg 2oz, glazed w/butter	210	10	280	30	1ST+2FAT
Spreads:					
Apple Butter, 1T	20	0	0	4	¼FR
Butter, 1t	36	4	41	0	1FAT
Butter, 1T	108	12	123	0	2½FAT
Country Gravy, ¼ c	85	7	250	4	¼ST+1½FAT
Cream Cheese, 2T	100	10	85	0	2FAT
Cream Cheese, 2T low fat	70	5	150	0	½MT+½FAT
Honey Butter, 1t	28	2	20	2	½FAT
Honey Butter, 1T	84	6	60	8	½CHO+1FAT
Honey, 1t	21	0	0	4	¼CHO
Honey, 1T	64	0	1	15	1CHO
Jelly, Jams, *or* Preserves, 1t	18	0	1	4	¼CHO
Jelly, Jams, *or* Preserves, 1T	54	0	2	15	1CHO
Margarine, 1t	35	3	45	0	¾FAT
Margarine, 1T	100	11	100	0	2½FAT
Oil, 1t	40	5	1	0	1FAT
Oil, 1T	120	14	6	0	3FAT
Whipped Butter, 1T	81	9	93	0	2FAT
Whipped Margarine, 1T	70	7	70	0	1½FAT

Entrees & Sauces

Chapter Contents:

- General Guidelines
- Estimating the Calories & Fat Grams in Your Entree
- Beef, Pork, & Lamb Calorimeter
- Chicken & Other Poultry Calorimeter
- Seafood Calorimeter
- Other Meats Calorimeter
- Fats, Gravies, and Sauces

Most of the calories and fat grams in a single meal are found in the entree. Here are some general guidelines for dining lean during this course.

✓ **Select fish, chicken, and turkey** that have been grilled, baked, or roasted.

Pick the Leaner Choices More Often:		
	Calories	Fat (g)
Per 6 oz portion:		
Grilled Fish (average varieties)	240	6
Roasted White Turkey, w/out skin	270	6
Roasted White Chicken, w/out skin	300	8
Sirloin Steak, trimmed	360	16
Roasted Dark Chicken, w/out skin	360	16
Roasted White Chicken *or* Turkey, w/skin	360	16
Roasted Dark Chicken *or* Turkey, w/skin	420	20
Fried Chicken Breast	420	20
Sirloin Steak, untrimmed	480	28
Fried Chicken Thigh	480	30
Fried Fish	540	30
Sausage	600	48

Healthy ↑

Not So Healthy ↓

✓ **Eat half the meat**. Health authorities recommend we eat no more than 6 ounces of meat, poultry, and seafood a day. That's two portions of 3 oz (the size of a deck of cards) each. This recommendation is based upon the need to replace our daily protein losses as well as our need to cut back on our fat and cholesterol intake. Restaurants often serve protein portions much larger than 6 ounces so be prepared to split the entree with another person or request a "doggie bag" to take half of the meat home.

✓ **Order broiled or grilled chicken or seafood instead of fried.** Some fat is usually added when seafood is broiled or grilled, but not as much as when the food is fried.

Fried Seafood is Often Twice as High in Calories:		Calories	Fat (g)
6 oz Fried Scallops		510	26
6 oz Broiled Scallops w/2t butter		252	10
	Savings:	**258**	**16**

✓ **Remove the skin off poultry to save a substantial amount of calories.**

Take it Off:		Calories	Fat (g)
Roasted Chicken leg & thigh		300	16
Roasted Chicken leg & thigh, without the skin		170	8
	Savings:	**1130**	**8**

✓ **Trim all visible fat off meats and poultry.** Yes, much of the fat is marbled into the meat. But trimming your meat will make a huge difference in your waistline. Leaner cuts of beef that have been trimmed of all visible fat can be as low in fat and calories as chicken.

Cut the Fat:		Calories	Fat (g)
8 oz Brisket, lean & fat		800	72
8 oz Brisket, lean only		550	30
	Savings:	**250**	**42**

✓ **Eat more fish and shellfish.** As a group, they comprise the leanest "meat" category, however, the calories and fat grams ranges widely within this group. Even the fattiest fish are fairly low in calories and are considered healthy. The fish oil is very unsaturated and is one of the "healthy" fats. One class of fats present in fish, omega-3 fatty acids, appears to be able to lower serum cholesterol and triglycerides.

What about cholesterol? Isn't shellfish high in cholesterol? The recent refinement of measuring procedures has demonstrated that shellfish does not have as much cholesterol as was once thought. The cholesterol content of clams, mussels, oysters, scallops, Alaska King crab, and lobster are in the same range as chicken and beef. Shrimp and squid *are* higher in cholesterol (see the cholesterol chart on the next page), but they are so low in fat that they can still be included in a low fat/low cholesterol diet once or twice a week.

✓ **Request your fish to be prepared with little or no butter or oil.** It's not uncommon for restaurants to use a tablespoon or two of butter or oil to grill, blacken, or pan-fry fish. Consider asking for your fish to be seasoned with lemon, wine, and spices instead.

Added Fats can Double the Calories:	Calories	Fat (g)
6 oz Cod, Pollock, or Scrod	180	2
Plus 1T butter	108	12
Total:	**288**	**14**

✓ **Send the melted butter back.** Enjoy the sweet taste of lobster – without the butter dip. Clarified butter contains 120 calories per tablespoon!

✓ **Avoid *Prime* cuts of beef.** There are three grades of beef based on the fat content of the meat. Select is the leanest, choice is in the middle, and prime is the fattiest cut. If you are buying lean meat in the grocery store, you are probably getting the select grade. You'll be hard pressed to find the select grade in many restaurants; choice is far more common. Upscale steakhouses often buys prime cuts of beef because they feel that the extra marbling of fat adds more flavor. The extra fat contributes an additional 5-10 % more calories and 10-25% more fat than the choice grade.

✓ **Order a lean cut of beef.** At the grocery store you can recognize the leanest cuts of beef and pork by the use of "round" or "loin" in the name. In restaurants different names are used:

Club	Kabob	Medallions	Sirloin Steak
Delmonico	Kansas City	New York	Strip Steak
Filet Steak	London Broil	Roast Beef	Tenderloin, pork
Filet Mignon (without the bacon)			

✓ **Order a boneless cut of beef, pork, or lamb.** Typically, bone-in cuts are higher in fat than boneless cuts.

✓ **Order a smaller cut.** A smaller beef cut of 3-4 oz may be available as an appetizer or on a sandwich plate. A petite steak of 4 oz would fit nutritional guidelines better than a typical 8-10 oz entrée portion. Since many upscale restaurants cut their own beef they may be able to cut a steak any size that you request.

✓ **Request little or no oil when preparing the meat.** Steaks, fajitas, chicken, and fish are often brushed with oil during cooking. While some *may* be necessary to prevent sticking on the grill, most is added for appearances only. Watch out - the Chicken Fajitas often have butter poured over them before serving. Now you know why the fajitas sizzle on your way to the table! Tell them you'd rather have "pretty thighs" than a "pretty piece of meat."

No Oils, Please:	Calories	Fat (g)
Grilled Chicken Breast, 6 oz brushed with 2t oil	360	20
Grilled Chicken Breast, 6 oz with "no oil"	300	8
Savings:	**60**	**12**

✓ **Watch the cholesterol.** Variety cuts of beef, pork, and lamb are considered delicacies and are comparable in calories and fat grams to other meat cuts. But some organ meats have very high amounts of cholesterol. Since the American Heart Association recommends no more than 300 mg of cholesterol each day, it is recommended that these organ meats be consumed only once a month.

Cholesterol/3 oz	Animal Protein (3 oz)	Cholesterol (mg)
<100	Fish, Clams, Crab, Mussels, Sardines, Salmon, Scallops	20-70
	Lobster	60-90
	Chicken	70
	Beef: steak, roast, ear, feet, jowl, tail, tongue, tripe	80
100-199	Caviar, 1T or Roe, 1 oz	100
	Crayfish	120
	Pork Chitterlings, Pork Tongue	125
	Shrimp	130
	Beef & Pork Hearts, Pork Stomach	170
200-299	Squid	200
	Beef Lungs, Beef Thymus	240
	Pork Pancreas	270
300-399	Pork Liver, Beef Spleen	300
	Beef Kidney & Liver, Pork Lungs	330
400-499	Pork Kidney	410
	Pork Spleen	430
>500	Beef Brains	1700
	Pork Brains	2200

Estimating the Calories & Fat Grams in your Entrée

To calculate the calories and fat grams of your meat entrée, follow these 3 steps:

❶ **Find your entrée in the next four calorimeters**. Note that menu items may be detailed as fried, untrimmed, trimmed, with skin, and w/out skin. *Italicized print* denotes fried items. The calories and fat of the all other entrée are considered to be baked, roasted, or grilled without any additional fat. Unless you requested otherwise, the restaurant probably added some fat as described in step 3. The four calorimeters include:

■ Beef, Pork, & Lamb

■ Poultry – Chicken, Turkey, Duck, Goose, Pheasant, & Quail

■ Seafood – Shellfish & Fish

■ Other Meats – Organ meats, Variety cuts, Wild game, & Exotic meats

❷ **Read across the calorimeter to find the number of calories and fat gram for *your* cooked portion size.** The *cooked* portion size will be significantly smaller than the uncooked portions quoted on the menu or by the server. The following are some expected weights for the most commonly served portions after cooking losses. Trimming the fat and bone as well as removing the skin will reduce the portion size further.

Boneless Meats	
Raw Wt (oz)	Cooked Wt (oz)
4 =	3
6 =	4½
8 =	6
10 =	7½
12 =	9
14 =	10½
16 =	12
20 =	15

Meat with Bones	
Raw Wt (oz)	Cooked Wt (oz)
8 =	4
12 =	6
16 =	8
20 =	10

Meat with Bones	
Raw Wt (oz)	Cooked Wt (oz)
8 =	4
12 =	6
16 =	8
20 =	10

❸ **Account for the fat or sauces that were added to your entrée**. Unless you have requested otherwise, most restaurants are adding butter, margarine, or oil to your entrée. Expect a teaspoon of these fats to be added for every 3 oz cooked portion. See the Gravies, Sauces, & Spread Calorimeter, that follows the four entrée calorimeters, for more details on these and other sauces.

Beef, Pork, & Lamb Calorimeter: Calories & fat per *cooked* portion

Calories per oz	Beef, Pork, & Lamb	Calories & Fat (g)			
		3 oz	4½ oz	6 oz	7½ oz
130	**Beef** (untrimmed): Short Ribs	390	585	780	975
		36g	54g	72g	90g
110	**Beef** (untrimmed): Brisket	330	495	660	825
		28g	42g	56g	70g
100	**Beef & Pork**: Sausage **Beef** (untrimmed): Beef Ribs, Meatloaf **Lamb** (untrimmed): Lamb Chops **Pork** (untrimmed): Pork Chops, Pork Ribs, Spareribs	300 24g	450 36g	600 48g	750 60g
90	**Beef**: *Chicken Fried Steak* **Beef** (untrimmed): Porterhouse Steak, T-bone, Prime Rib, Filet Mignon **Pork** (untrimmed): Pork Loin, Tenderloin	270 19g	405 28g	540 37g	675 47g
80	**Beef** (untrimmed): Sirloin Steak **Beef** (trimmed): Beef Short Ribs **Pork** (trimmed): Ribs	240 14g	360 21g	480 28g	600 34g
70	**Lamb** (untrimmed): Leg of Lamb **Veal** (untrimmed): Roast **Beef** (untrimmed): London Broil, Roast Beef, Kabobs **Beef** (trimmed): Prime Rib, Rib Steak, Rib Eye Steak, Brisket, Corned Beef, Fajitas, Ribs, Porterhouse, T-bone **Pork** (trimmed): Pork Loin, Pork Chop	210 13g	315 20g	420 26g	525 33g
60	**Beef** (trimmed): Sirloin Steak, New York, Club, Demonico, Strip Steak, Kansas City, Filet Mignon, Filet Steak, Medallions, London Broil, Kabob, Roast Beef, Pot Roast, Stew & Soup Meat, Stir Fry Meat **Pork** (trimmed): Ham, Pork Tenderloin	180 8g	270 12g	360 16g	450 20g
50	**Lamb** (trimmed): Chops, Leg of Lamb	150 6g	225 10g	300 13g	375 16g

* Add 10% to calories and fat grams if meat is labeled as a *prime* cut.

If no cooking method is specified and your meat was:
  Pan grilled - add 1t butter (40 calories, 4 gms fat) for each 3 oz portion
  Fried - add 1T butter (120 calories, 12 gms fat) for each 3 oz portion

Seafood Calorimeter: Calories & fat per *cooked* portion

Calories per oz	Seafood	Calories & Fat (g)			
		3 oz	4½ oz	6 oz	7½ oz
100	Bass (stuffed & baked)	**300**	**450**	**600**	**750**
	Fried Eel, Fried Mackerel, Fried Smelt	16g	24g	32g	40g
90	*Fried: Catfish, Ocean Perch, Red Snapper, Shrimp*	**270**	**405**	**540**	**675**
		15g	23g	30g	38g
85	*Fried: Croaker, Pomfret, Scallops*	**255**	**385**	**510**	**640**
		13g	20g	26g	33g
75	Greenland Halibut, Shad, Pacific Herring, Atlantic Mackerel, Sablefish	**225**	**340**	**450**	**565**
		16g	23g	31g	39g
75	*Fried: Clams, Oysters*	**225**	**340**	**450**	**565**
		13g	20g	26g	33g
75	*Fried: Bass*	**225**	**340**	**450**	**565**
		10	15g	20g	25g
70	*Fried Abalone*	**210**	**315**	**420**	**525**
		8g	12g	16g	20g
65	Pompano, Chinook & Sockeye Salmon	**195**	**295**	**390**	**490**
	Fried: Fish Cakes, Squid	10g	15g	20g	25g
60	Atlantic Herring, Other Mackerel, Whale	**180**	**270**	**360**	**450**
	Fried: Haddock, White Perch	8g	12g	16g	20g
55	Milkfish, Coho & Atlantic Salmon, Trout (other varieties), Bluefish Tuna, Yellowtail	**165**	**250**	**330**	**415**
	Fried: Cuddlefish	7g	11g	14g	18g
50	Halibut, Carp, Orange Roughy, Spot, Whitefish, Shark	**150**	**225**	**300**	**375**
		6g	10g	13g	16g
45	Freshwater Bass, Bluefish, Catfish, Mullet, Chum & Pink Salmon, Sturgeon, Swordfish, Rainbow Trout	**135**	**205**	**270**	**340**
		4g	6g	8g	10g
40	Abalone, Cisco, Halibut, Spiny Lobster, King Mackerel, Sea Trout, Sheepshead, Shrimp, Smelt, Yellowfin & Skipjack Tuna	**120**	**180**	**240**	**300**
		2g	3g	4g	6g
35	Striped Bass, Mussels, Northern Lobster, Oysters, Pacific Rockfish, Perch, Red Snapper, Sea Bass, Squid, Tilefish, Turbot, White Sucker, Whiting, Wolfish	**105**	**160**	**210**	**265**
		2g	3g	4g	5g
30	Clams, Cod, Crab, Crayfish, Cuttlefish, Ling, Lingcod, Monkfish, Ocean Pout, Octopus, Pike, Pollock, Scallops, Scrod, Skate, Sunfish	**90**	**135**	**180**	**225**
		1g	2g	2g	3g

If no cooking method is specified above and your meat was:
Pan grilled - add 1t butter (40 calories, 4 gms fat) for each 3 oz portion
Fried - add 1T butter (120 calories, 12 gms fat) for each 3 oz portion

Chicken & Poultry Calorimeter: Calories & fat per *cooked* portion

Calories per oz	Chicken & Poultry	Calories & Fat (g)			
		3 oz	4½ oz	6 oz	7½ oz
100	**Chicken:** *Fried Chicken Wing* **Duck** w/skin	300 24g	450 36g	600 48g	750 60g
90	**Goose** w/skin	270 19g	405 28g	540 37g	675 47g
80	**Chicken:** *Fried Dark Chicken*	240 15g	360 23g	480 30g	600 38g
70	**Chicken:** Dark Chicken w/skin, *Fried Chicken Fingers, Fried White Chicken* **Goose** w/out skin **Turkey:** Dark Turkey w/skin	210 10g	315 15g	420 20g	525 35g
60	**Pheasant:** w/skin **Turkey:** White Turkey w/skin **Chicken:** White Chicken w/skin, Dark Chicken w/out skin **Duck:** w/out skin **Squab** (pigeon) w/out skin	180 8g	270 12g	360 16g	450 20g
55	**Turkey:** Dark Turkey w/out skin **Quail** w/out skin	165 6g	250 9g	330 11g	415 15g
50	**Chicken:** Breast w/out skin **Pheasant** w/out skin	150 4g	225 6g	300 8g	375 10g
45	**Turkey:** White Turkey w/out skin	135 3g	205 5g	270 6g	340 8g
40	**Guinea Hen** w/out skin	120 3g	180 5g	240 6g	300 8g

Other Meats Calorimeter: Calories & fat per *cooked* portion

Calories per oz	Other Meats	Calories & Fat (g)			
		3 oz	4½ oz	6 oz	7½ oz
110	**Pork:** Tail	330 31g	495 46g	660 61g	825 77g
90	**Beef:** Sweetbreads, Thymus **Pork:** Chitterlings **Sheep:** Tongue	270 22g	405 33g	540 44g	675 55g
80	**Beef:** Pancreas, Tongue **Pork:** Tongue	240 16g	360 24g	480 32g	600 40g
80	**Chicken:** *Fried Giblets*	240 12g	360 18g	480 23g	600 30g

If no cooking method is specified above and your meat was:
Pan grilled - add 1t butter (40 calories, 4 gms fat) for each 3 oz portion
Fried - add 1T butter (120 calories, 12 gms fat) for each 3 oz portion

Other Meats Calorimeter (continued)

Calories per oz	Other Meats	Calories & Fat (g)			
		3 oz	4½ oz	6 oz	7½ oz
70	**Lamb:** Liver, Tongue	**210**	**315**	**420**	**525**
		14g	21g	28g	35g
70	**Lamb:** Heart	**210**	**315**	**420**	**525**
	Other Meats: Beaver, Eel, Raccoon	12g	54g	72g	90g
60	**Beef:** Brains	**180**	**270**	**360**	**450**
	Pork: Pickled Pig's Feet	13g	20g	26g	33g
60	**Beef:** *Panfried Liver* **Pork:** Pancreas **Squab (pigeon):** Giblets **Other Meats:** Opossum, Rabbit	**180**	**270**	**360**	**450**
		8g	12g	16g	20g
55	**Pork:** Pig's Feet	**165**	**250**	**330**	**415**
		11g	17g	22g	28g
55	**Chicken:** Heart **Duck:** Liver **Goose:** Gizzard **Turkey:** Heart **Pheasant:** Giblets	**165**	**250**	**330**	**415**
		6g	9g	12g	15g
50	**Beef:** Brains	**150**	**225**	**300**	**375**
	Pork: Stomach, Ears	10g	15g	20g	25g
50	**Beef:** Heart, Liver **Calf:** Sweetbreads, Tongue **Goose & Pork:** Liver **Lamb:** Sweetbreads **Turkey:** Giblets, Gizzard, Liver	**150**	**225**	**300**	**375**
		4g	6g	9g	11g
45	**Chicken:** Giblets, Gizzard, Liver **Other Meats**: Muskrat, Reindeer, Turtle, Venison	**135**	**205**	**270**	**340**
		4g	6g	8g	10g
40	**Pork:** Brains	**120**	**180**	**240**	**300**
		8g	12g	16g	20g
40	**Beef:** Kidneys, Spleen, Tripe **Lamb** Spleen **Pork:** Heart, Kidneys, Spleen	**120**	**180**	**240**	**300**
		4g	5g	7g	9g
35	**Beef:** Lungs	**105**	**160**	**210**	**265**
		3g	5g	6g	8g
30	**Pork:** Lungs **Lamb:** Lungs **Other Meats**: Frog Legs, Snail	**90**	**135**	**180**	**225**
		2g	3g	5g	6g

If no cooking method is specified above and your meat was:
    Pan grilled - add 1t butter (40 calories, 4 gms fat) for each 3 oz portion
    Fried - add 1T butter (120 calories, 12 gms fat) for each 3 oz portion

Entrees

	Calories	Fat (g)	Sodium (mg)	Carbs* (g)	Exchanges**
Beef, trimmed (3 oz):					
Corned Beef, trimmed	210	13	945	0	3MT
Fajitas	210	13	750	0	3MT
London Broil, Kabob, Roast Beef, Pot Roast, Stew, Soup, & Stir Fry Meat	180	8	20	0	3MT(lean)
Short Ribs	240	14	15	0	3MT
Prime Rib, Rib & Rib Eye Steak, Brisket, Ribs, Porterhouse, T-bone	210	13	20	0	3MT+1FAT
Steaks: Sirloin, New York, Club, Delmonico, Strip, Kansas City, Filet Mignon, Filet	180	8	20	0	3MT(lean)
Beef & Veal, untrimmed (3 oz):					
Beef Stroganoff, 3 oz beef	410	27	620	7	1V+ 3MT+2½FAT
Brisket	330	27	20	0	3MT+2½FAT
Chicken Fried Steak	270	19	500	16	1ST+2½MT+1FAT
London Broil, Roast Beef, Kabobs	210	13	20	0	3MT
Meatballs, 6 - 1½" balls	400	25	632	13	1ST+3MT+2FAT
Pepper Steak, 3 oz steak + veggies	275	13	485	12	2V+3MT
Porterhouse, T-bone, Prime Rib, Filet Mignon	270	19	20	0	3MT+1FAT
Ribs	300	24	15	0	3MT+1½FAT
Sauerbraten	240	14	160	0	3MT
Sausage	300	24	960	1	3MT+1½FAT
Short Ribs	390	36	15	0	3MT+4FAT
Sirloin Steak	240	14	20	0	3MT
Steak au Poivre, 3 oz	220	12	120	0	3MT
Swiss Steak, 3 oz steak w/veggies	240	10	400	29	1½ST+1V+3MT(lean)
Veal, untrimmed: Roast	210	13	20	0	3MT
Weiner Schnitzel, 3 oz breaded veal w/sauce	335	17	550	17	1ST+3MT
Pork (3 oz):					
Pork, untrimmed: Chops, Spareribs	300	24	25	0	3MT+1½FAT
Pork, untrimmed: Loin, Tenderloin	270	19	20	0	3MT+1FAT
Pork, trimmed: Ribs	240	14	20	0	3MT
Loin Chop	210	13	20	0	3MT
Pork Ham, trimmed	180	8	1190	0	3MT(lean)
Pork Tenderloin, trimmed	180	8	20	0	3MT(lean)
Lamb (3 oz):					
Lamb Chops, untrimmed	300	24	15	0	3MT+1½FAT
Lamb, untrimmed: Leg of Lamb	210	13	20	0	3MT
Lamb, trimmed: Chops, Leg of Lamb	150	6	20	0	3MT(lean)

*Carbs=Carbohydrate, na=not available   **Exchanges: ST=Starch, Mlk=Milk (skim)
FR=Fruit, CHO=Other Carbohydrates, V=Vegetable, MT=Meat (medium fat), FAT=Fat

Chicken & Other Poultry

	Calories	Fat (g)	Sodium (mg)	Carbs* (g)	Exchanges**
Fried Chicken (per average piece):					
Wing	190	12	385	6	¼ST+1½MT+1FAT
Thigh	310	21	575	7	½ST+4MT
Breast	360	18	760	17	1ST+3½MT
Drumstick	150	10	265	5	¼ST+1¾MT
Chicken Fingers, 5 (9oz)	620	34	1450	23	1½ST+6MT+1FAT
Buffalo Wings, 1	70	5	300	3	½MT+½FAT
Ranch Dressing, 1T	75	8	80	3	1½FAT
Fried Chicken (3 oz):					
Dark w/skin	244	15	440	6	½ST+3MT
Dark w/out skin	205	10	160	0	2½MT
White w/skin	211	10	440	7	½ST+2¾MT
White w/out skin	165	5	140	0	3MT(lean)
Roasted Chicken (per average piece):					
Dark w/skin	330	22	765	0	4½MT
Dark w/out skin	210	10	725	0	4MT(lean)
Breast and wing w/skin	370	19	1160	0	6½MT(lean)
Breast w/out skin	160	4	800	0	5MT(very lean)
Roasted Chicken (3 oz):					
Dark w/skin	217	14	75	0	3MT
Dark w/out skin	174	8	81	0	3MT(lean)
White w/skin	190	9	64	0	3MT(lean)
White w/out skin	148	4	66	0	3MT(lean)
Other Poultry (3 oz cooked, without added salt):					
Duck, w/skin	288	24	60	0	3MT+1½FAT
Duck, w/out skin	171	10	56	0	3MT
Dark Turkey w/skin	189	10	65	0	3MT
Dark Turkey w/out skin	160	6	66	0	3MT(lean)
White Turkey w/skin	169	7	54	0	3MT(lean)
White Turkey w/out skin	135	3	55	0	3MT(very lean)
Goose w/skin	270	19	23	0	3MT+1FAT
Goose w/out skin	204	11	65	0	3MT
Guinea Hen w/out skin	126	3	na	0	3MT(very lean)
Pheasant w/out skin	152	4	42	0	3MT(lean)
Quail w/out skin	153	5	58	0	3MT(lean)
Squab (pigeon) w/out skin	162	9	na	0	3MT(lean)
Other Chicken Dishes:					
Chicken and Dumplings, 2 c	410	20	470	28	1½ST+1V+3MT+1FAT
Chicken Divan, 1¼ c	350	22	390	13	½ST+1V+3MT+1½FAT
Chicken Tetrazzini, ½ c spaghetti + ½ c chicken with sauce	490	23	505	27	1½ST+1V+3MT+1½FAT

*Carbs=Carbohydrate, na=not available   ****Exchanges:** ST=Starch, Mlk=Milk (skim) FR=Fruit, CHO=Other Carbohydrates, V=Vegetable, MT=Meat (medium fat), FAT=Fat

Fish & Shellfish

	Calories	Fat (g)	Sodium (mg)	Carbs* (g)	Exchanges**
4 oz Raw Fish/3 oz cooked (no fat added):					
Abalone	120	0.8	340	0	3MT(very lean)
Bass, Freshwater	128	4	80	0	3MT(very lean)
Bass, Striped	108	3	80	0	3MT(very lean)
Bluefish	140	5	68	0	3MT(lean)
Carp	144	6	56	0	3MT(lean)
Catfish, Channel	132	5	72	0	3MT(very lean)
Clams	84	1	64	0	3MT(very lean)
Cisco	112	2	64	0	3MT(very lean)
Cod	92	0.8	68	0	3MT(very lean)
Crab, Alaska King	96	0.8	948	0	3MT(very lean)
Crab, Blue & Dungeness	96	1	336	0	3MT(very lean)
Crab, Queeen	100	1	612	0	3MT(very lean)
Crayfish	100	1	60	0	3MT(very lean)
Cuttlefish	88	0.8	420	0	3MT(very lean)
Halibut	124	3	60	0	3MT(very lean)
Halibut, Greenland	212	16	92	0	3MT
Herring, Atlantic	180	10	100	0	3MT(lean)
Herring, Pacific	220	16	84	0	3MT
Ling	100	0.8	152	0	3MT(very lean)
Lingcod	96	1	68	0	3MT(very lean)
Lobster, Northern	104	1	336	0	3MT(very lean)
Lobster, Spiny	128	2	200	0	3MT(very lean)
Mackerel, Atlantic	232	16	104	0	3MT
Mackerel, King	120	2	180	0	3MT(very lean)
Mackerel, other varieties	176	9	100	0	3MT(lean)
Milkfish	168	8	92	0	3MT(lean)
Monkfish	84	2	20	0	3MT(very lean)
Mullet, Striped	132	4	72	0	3MT(very lean)
Mussels, Blue	96	2	324	0	3MT(very lean)
Ocean Pout	88	1	68	0	3MT(very lean)
Octopus	92	1	260	0	3MT(very lean)
Orange Roughy	144	8	72	0	3MT(lean)
Oysters	88	3	124	0	3MT(very lean)
Perch	104	2	72	0	3MT(very lean)
Pike	100	0.8	48	0	3MT(very lean)
Pollock	92	1	80	0	3MT(very lean)
Pompano	188	11	72	0	3MT(lean)
Red Snapper	112	2	72	0	3MT(very lean)
Rockfish, Pacific	108	2	68	0	3MT(very lean)
Salmon, Atlantic & Coho	164	7	48	0	3MT(lean)
Salmon, Chinook & Sockeye	196	11	52	0	3MT(lean)
Salmon, Chum & Pink	136	4	60	0	3MT(lean)
Sablefish	220	16	64	0	3MT
Scallops	100	0.8	184	0	3MT(very lean)
Scrod, Atlantic	92	0.8	60	0	3MT(very lean)
Sea Bass	108	2	76	0	3MT(very lean)

*Carbs=Carbohydrate, na=not available   **Exchanges:** ST=Starch, Mlk=Milk (skim)
FR=Fruit, CHO=Other Carbohydrates, V=Vegetable, MT=Meat (medium fat), FAT=Fat

Fish & Shellfish (continued)

	Calories	Fat (g)	Sodium (mg)	Carbs* (g)	Exchanges**
SeaTrout	116	4	64	0	3MT(lean)
Shad	220	16	60	0	3MT
Shark	148	5	88	0	3MT(lean)
Sheepshead	124	3	80	0	3MT(very lean)
Shrimp (½ c cooked)	120	2	172	0	3MT(very lean)
Smelt, Rainbow	112	3	68	0	3MT(very lean)
Spot	140	6	32	0	3MT(lean)
Squid	104	2	52	0	3MT(very lean)
Sturgeon	120	4	92	0	3MT(very lean)
Sucker, White	104	3	44	0	3MT(very lean)
Sunfish	100	0.8	92	0	3MT(very lean)
Swordfish	136	4	100	0	3MT(lean)
Tilefish	108	3	60	0	3MT(very lean)
Trout, Rainbow	132	4	32	0	3MT(very lean)
Trout, other varieties	168	8	60	0	3MT(lean)
Tuna, Bluefish	164	6	44	0	3MT(lean)
Tuna, Yellowfin & Skipjack	120	1	40	0	3MT(very lean)
Turbot, European	108	3	168	0	3MT(very lean)
Whitefish	152	7	56	0	3MT(lean)
Whiting	104	2	80	0	3MT(very lean)
Wolfish	108	3	96	0	3MT(very lean)
Yellowtail	164	6	44	0	3MT(lean)

Fried Fish, 3 oz:

	Calories	Fat (g)	Sodium (mg)	Carbs* (g)	Exchanges**
Abalone, Fried	216	8	668	0	3MT(lean)
Bass, Striped, Fried	224	10	280	7	½ST+3MT(lean)
Bass, Stuffed & Baked	296	18	na	7	½ST+3MT+½FAT
Catfish, Breaded & Fried	260	15	316	7	½ST+3MT
Clams, Breaded & Fried	228	12	412	7	½ST+3MT
Croaker, Breaded & Fried	252	14	396	7	½ST+3MT
Cuddlefish, Fried	168	9	180	0	3MT(lean)
Eel, Breaded & Fried	288	16	104	7	½ST+3MT
Fish Cakes, Fried	196	9	200	7	½ST+3MT(lean)
Haddock, Breaded & Fried	188	7	200	0	3MT(lean)
Mackerel, Fried	312	16	192	7	½ST+3MT
Ocean Perch, Breaded & Fried	260	15	172	7	½ST+3MT
Oysters, Breaded & Fried	224	14	472	7	½ST+3MT
Pomfret, Fried	256	12	160	0	3MT
Red Snapper, Fried	260	14	104	0	3MT
Scallops, Breaded & Fried	244	12	528	7	½ST+3MT
Shrimp, Breaded & Fried	276	14	388	7	½ST+3MT
Smelt, Breaded & Fried	284	14	608	7	½ST+3MT
Squid, Breaded & Fried	200	8	248	7	½ST+3MT(lean)
White Perch, Fried	188	9	200	0	3MT(lean)

Other Fish Dishes:

	Calories	Fat (g)	Sodium (mg)	Carbs* (g)	Exchanges**
Shrimp Paella, 2 c	430	10	685	47	3ST+4MT(lean)

*Carbs=Carbohydrate, na=not available   **Exchanges: ST=Starch, Mlk=Milk (skim)
FR=Fruit, CHO=Other Carbohydrates, V=Vegetable, MT=Meat (medium fat), FAT=Fat

Variety Cuts & Other Meats

	Calories	Fat (g)	Sodium (mg)	Carbs* (g)	Exchanges**
Poultry Variety Cuts (3 oz cooked):					
Giblets: Chicken, fried	237	12	97	0	4MT(lean)
Chicken, simmered	135	4	50	0	3MT(lean)
Pheasant	159	6	na	0	3MT(lean)
Squab (pigeon)	176	8	na	0	3MT(lean)
Turkey, simmered	143	4	51	0	3MT(lean)
Gizzard: Chicken, simmered	131	3	57	0	3MT (very lean)
Goose	159	6	na	0	3MT(lean)
Turkey, simmered	140	3	46	0	3MT (very lean)
Heart: Chicken, simmered	159	7	41	0	3MT(lean)
Turkey, simmered	152	5	47	0	3MT(lean)
Liver: Chicken, simmered	135	5	44	0	3MT(lean)
Duck	155	5	na	0	3MT(lean)
Goose	143	5	151	0	3MT(lean)
Turkey, simmered	145	5	55	0	3MT(lean)
Beef Variety Cuts (3 oz cooked):					
Brains, simmered	138	11	103	0	2MT
Brains, pan fried	168	14	135	0	2MT+½FAT
Heart	150	5	54	0	3MT (very lean)
Kidney, simmered	123	3	41	0	3MT (very lean)
Liver, braised	132	4	60	0	3MT (very lean)
Liver, pan fried	186	7	100	8	½ST+3MT(lean)
Lungs, braised	103	3	87	0	3MT (very lean)
Pancreas, braised	231	15	51	0	3MT
Spleen, braised	123	4	49	0	3MT (very lean)
Sweetbreads, cooked	272	20	99	0	3MT+1FAT
Calf Sweetbreads, cooked	143	3	na	0	3MT (very lean)
Thymus, braised	273	21	99	0	3MT+1FAT
Tongue, simmered	243	18	51	0	3MT+½FAT
Calf Tongue, braised	135	5	na	0	3MT(lean)
Tripe	112	5	53	0	3MT(lean)
Pork Variety Cuts (3 oz cooked):					
Chitterlings, simmered	261	25	33	0	3MT+2FAT
Ears, simmered	141	9	141	0	3MT(lean)
Feet, cured, pickled	174	14	na	0	2MT+1FAT
Feet, simmered	165	11	na	0	2MT
Brains, braised	117	8	78	0	1MT+½FAT
Heart, braised	126	4	31	0	3½MT(very lean)
Jowl	748	80	30	0	1MT+14FAT
Kidney, braised	129	4	69	0	3MT(very lean)
Liver, braised	141	4	42	0	3MT(very lean)
Lungs, braised	84	3	69	0	2MT(very lean)
Pancreas, braised	189	9	36	0	3MT(very lean)
Spleen, braised	129	3	na	0	3MT(very lean)
Stomach	135	11	59	0	3MT

*Carbs=Carbohydrate, na=not available   ****Exchanges:** ST=Starch, Mlk=Milk (skim) FR=Fruit, CHO=Other Carbohydrates, V=Vegetable, MT=Meat (medium fat), FAT=Fat

Other Meats (continued)

	Calories	Fat (g)	Sodium (mg)	Carbs* (g)	Exchanges**
Pork Variety Cuts (3 oz cooked):					
Tail, simmered	339	31	na	0	2MT+4FAT
Tongue, braised	231	16	93	0	3MT
Sheep & Lamb Variety Cuts (3 oz cooked):					
Lamb Heart, braised	222	12	na	0	3MT
Lamb Liver, broiled	222	11	71	0	3MT
Lamb Lungs	87	2	na	0	2MT(very lean)
Lamb Spleen	132	5	na	0	3MT(lean)
Lamb Sweetbreads, cooked	149	5	na	0	3MT(lean)
Lamb Tongue, braised	216	15	na	0	3MT
Sheep Tongue, braised	276	22	na	0	3MT+1FAT
Other Meats (3 oz cooked):					
Beaver	211	12	na	0	3MT
Eel	200	13	55	0	3MT
Frog Legs	83	0.3	na	0	3MT(very lean)
Muskrat	131	4	na	0	3MT(lean)
Opossum	189	9	na	0	3MT(lean)
Rabbit	185	9	35	0	3MT(lean)
Raccoon	219	12	na	0	3MT
Reindeer	145	4	na	0	3MT(lean)
Snail	75	1	na	0	3MT(very lean)
Turtle	120	4	na	0	3MT(lean)
Venison	143	5	na	0	3MT(lean)

Fats, Gravies, & Sauces

✔ **Always ask for your entrée to be prepared with as little fat as necessary.** Most of the cooked meats, poultry, and seafood listed in the previous calorimeters were calculated without the typical addition of fats. Unless you requested otherwise, estimate that an additional teaspoon (t) of butter, margarine, or oil has been used for the preparation of each cooked 3 oz portion of non-fried entrée. For reference there are three teaspoons in a tablespoon.

✔ **Request the use of a non-stick spray whenever possible.** Ounce for ounce, non-stick sprays have just as many calories as the oil it is derived from. But is sprayed in such a thin layer that the non-stick spray adds on fewer calories. Each typical five-second spray contains about 12 calories.

---

*Carbs=Carbohydrate, na=not available   **Exchanges:** ST=Starch, Mlk=Milk (skim)
FR=Fruit, CHO=Other Carbohydrates, V=Vegetable, MT=Meat (medium fat), FAT=Fat

✓ **Ask for sauces on the side**, including barbecue sauce. Most sauces are either very high in fat or high in sugar. Leaner sauces include salsas, black bean sauce, and those made from chicken stock and pureed vegetables. Or ask the chef to substitute a different sauce.

Substitute Lower Calorie Sauces:	Calories	Fat (g)
Po Boy: Roll, *Fried* Shrimp+¼c ***Tartar Sauce***	890	54
Po Boy: Roll, *Grilled* Shrimp+¼c ***Cocktail Sauce***	<u>535</u>	<u>11</u>
Savings:	**355**	**43**

✓ **Request low fat sauces**. There are six types of sauces from highest fat and calorie to the lowest:

■ Butter – melted butter or margarine to which seasonings are added (includes herb butter, lemon butter, pesto sauces).

■ Vinaigrette – blend of oil, vinegar, and seasonings (includes Beurre Blanc, Beurre Noir, Vinaigrettes, and Italian dressing).

■ Mayonnaise-Type – created from an mixture of margarine, butter, or oil and eggs (includes Bearnaise, Dill sauce, Hollandaise, Lemon Caper sauce, Tartar sauce, Roumoulade, and Tarragon sauce.

Calories per Tablespoon:

100	Butter					
90		Vinaigrette				
80			Mayonnaise			
70						
60						
50				White Sauce		
40					Brown Sauce	Tomato Sauce
30						
20						
10						
0						

■ White Sauce – roux-based sauce made from margarine or butter, flour, and milk, cream, or light stock (includes Bechamel sauce, Cheese sauce, Mornay sauce, and Veloute).

■ Brown Sauce – roux-based sauce made with margarine or butter, flour, and brown stock (includes Bordelaise, Brown gravy, and Mushroom sauce).

■ Tomato – tomato sauce seasoned with spices and herbs (includes Cocktail Sauce, Barbecue sauce, Marinara, Salsas, and Veracruz sauce).

Sauces, Spreads, & Gravies Calorimeter

Calories per t	Fats, Gravies, Sauces & Spreads	Calories & Fat (g)			
		1T	2T	3T	4T
40	Oil (all types), Clarified Butter	**120** 14g	**240** 28g	**360** 42g	**480** 56g
37	Butter	**110** 12g	**220** 24g	**330** 37g	**440** 48g
33	Aioli, Herb Butter sauce, Mayonnaise, Margarine, Rémoulade sauce	**100** 11g	**200** 22g	**300** 33g	**400** 44g
27	Lemon Butter sauce, Whipped Butter, Salad Dressings	**80** 9g	**160** 18g	**240** 28g	**320** 37g
25	Beurre Blanc, Buerre Noir, Butter Wine sauce, Hollandaise, Meuniere, Pesto, Tartar sauce, Whipped Margarine	**75** 8g	**150** 15g	**225** 23g	**300** 30g
20	Béarnaise, Creamy Dill sauce, Creamy Horseradish sauce	**60** 6g	**120** 12g	**180** 18g	**240** 24g
15	Creamy Dijon sauce, Tarragon sauce, Honey Mustard Cream sauce	**45** 4g	**90** 8g	**130** 12g	**185** 16g
12	Alfredo sauce, Lemony Dill sauce, Chili Cream sauce	**35** 4g	**70** 7g	**110** 11g	**145** 14g
10	Au Jus (drippings), Béchamel, Caper sauce, Cheese sauce, Cream sauce, Guacamole, Mornay sauce, Newburg sauce, Oyster sauce, Sour Cream	**30** 3g	**60** 5g	**90** 8g	**120** 10g
8	Chutneys, Cranberry sauce, Orange sauce, Sweet & Sour sauce	**25** 0g	**50** 0g	**75** 0g	**100** 0g
7	Bolognese (cream based), Mustard sauce, Gravy, Mushroom sauce, Veracruz	**20** 2g	**42** 3g	**65** 5g	**85** 6g
6	Chili sauce, Cocktail sauce, Ketchup, Sweet Pickle Relish, White Sauce-thin	**20** 0g	**40** 0g	**60** 0g	**75** 0g
5	Bolognese (tomato based), Mustard, Veloute, Tomato Coulis	**15** 1g	**30** 2g	**45** 3g	**60** 4g
5	Barbecue, Steak sauce, Teriyaki sauce	**15** 0g	**30** 0g	**45** 0g	**60** 0g
4	Bordelaise, Marinara	**12** $0.^7$g	**24** 1g	**36** 2g	**48** 3g
3½	Soy sauce, Worcestershire	**10** 0g	**20** 0g	**30** 0g	**40** 0g
2½	Madeira, Brown sauce, Tomato sauce	**8** $0.^2$g	**15** $0.^3$g	**23** $0.^5$g	**30** $0.^6$g
2	Canned Au Jus, Burgundy Wine sauce, Horseradish, Hot sauce, Picante sauce, Salsa	**5** 0g	**10** 0g	**15** 0g	**20** 0g

Gravies, Sauces, & Spreads

Per 2T:	Calories	Fat (g)	Sodium (mg)	Carbs* (g)	Exchanges**
Aioli Sauce (garlic oil)	195	21	5	0	4FAT
Alfredo Sauce	75	7	180	<1	1½FAT
Au Jus, canned	5	0	150	0	FREE
Au Jus, drippings	60	6	100	0	1FAT
Barbecue	30	0	500	2	½CHO
Béarnaise	120	12	220	3	2½FAT
Béchamel	51	5	70	1	1FAT
Buerre Blanc	154	16	2	0	3½FAT
Buerre Noir	136	15	148	0	3FAT
Bolognese, cream-based	50	$3.^5$	45	2	1FAT
Bolognese, tomato-based	32	$1.^6$	146	3	¼ST+¼FAT
Bordelaise	22	$1.^5$	150	2	¼FAT
Brown Sauce	15	$0.^1$	30	2	FREE
Burgundy Wine Sauce	10	$0.^3$	5	1	FREE
Butter, unsalted	216	24	4	0	5FAT
Butter, salted	216	24	246	0	5FAT
Butter Wine Sauce	140	14	140	2	3FAT
Caper Sauce	60	5	265	3	1FAT
Cheese Sauce	60	4	180	3	1FAT
Chili Cream Sauce	72	8	33	0	1½FAT
Chili Sauce	35	0	380	9	½ST
Chutney	55	0	0	14	½FR+½CHO
Cocktail Sauce	40	0	320	10	½CHO
Cranberry Sauce	52	0	10	13	1FR
Cream Sauce, thick	108	12	40	0	2½FAT
Cream Sauce, thin	50	4	180	1	1FAT
Creamy Dijon Sauce	96	8	90	3	1½FAT
Creamy Dill Sauce	126	13	90	1	2½FAT
Gravy	40	3	150	2	½FAT
Hollandaise	135	14	105	3	3FAT
Honey Mustard Cream Sauce	91	9	30	2	1½FAT
Horseradish, 1T	6	0	14	1	FREE
Creamy Horseradish Sauce	110	10	220	4	2FAT
Hot Sauce, 1t	0	0	20	0	FREE
Guacamole	55	5	210	2	1FAT
Ketchup	36	0	360	4	½CHO
Lemony Dill Sauce	72	7	283	0	1½FAT
Lemon Butter Sauce	176	19	250	0	4FAT
Madeira	15	$0.^5$	30	0	FREE
Margarine	200	23	200	0	4½FAT
Marinara	25	1	150	4	½V+¼FAT
Mayonnaise	200	22	160	0	4½FAT
Meuniére	130	14	510	0	3FAT
Mornay	64	5	160	4	1FAT

*Carbs=Carbohydrate, na=not available   **Exchanges:** ST=Starch, Mlk=Milk (skim)
FR=Fruit, CHO=Other Carbohydrates, V=Vegetable, MT=Meat (medium fat), FAT=Fat

Gravies, Sauces, & Spreads (continued)

Per 2T continued:

	Calories	Fat (g)	Sodium (mg)	Carbs* (g)	Exchanges**
Mushroom Sauce	40	3	87	3	½FAT
Mustard, 1T	15	1	190	1	FREE
Mustard Sauce	43	3	200	3	½FAT
Newburg	55	5	200	2	1FAT
Oil, Clarified Butter	240	28	6	0	5FAT
Orange Sauce	53	0	10	13	1CHO
Oyster Sauce	55	4	150	5	1FAT
Pesto	155	15	244	3	3FAT
Picante Sauce	10	0	220	2	FREE
Rémoulade Sauce	200	22	210	0	4½FAT
Salad Dressings, average	160	16	300	4	3FAT
Salsa	10	0	150	2	½V
Sour Cream	52	5	12	<1	1FAT
Soy Sauce, 1t	3	0	340	0	FREE
Soy Sauce, reduced sodium, 1t	3	0	170	0	FREE
Steak Sauce	30	0	200	4	¼CHO
Sweet and Sour Sauce	55	0	70	11	½CHO
Sweet Pickle Relish	40	0	210	9	½CHO
Tarragon Sauce	90	8	153	1	1½FAT
Tartar Sauce	140	16	440	0	3FAT
Teriyaki Sauce, 1T	15	0	610	3	FREE
Teriyaki Sauce, reduced sodium, 1T	15	0	320	3	FREE
Tomato Coulis	30	2	70	4	½V+½FAT
Tomato Sauce	14	0.[4]	20	3	FREE
Velouté	30	2	25	3	½FAT
Veracruz	42	4	177	2	½V+½FAT
Whipped Butter	162	18	186	0	3½FAT
Whipped Margarine	140	14	140	0	3FAT
White Sauce, thin	36	3	96	3	½FAT
Worcestershire	22	0	465	4	¼CHO

---

*Carbs=Carbohydrate, na=not available   **Exchanges:** ST=Starch, Mlk=Milk (skim)
FR=Fruit, CHO=Other Carbohydrates, V=Vegetable, MT=Meat (medium fat), FAT=Fat

Accompaniments

The previous chapter's recommendation to eat only half of your entrée may bring about a concern of "that's not much of a meal." In the majority of restaurants, the entrée covers the plate while the vegetables and starch (if even offered) appear to be simply plate garnishments.

For better health each of us should strive for eating smaller servings of animal protein along with larger portions of accompaniments (including starchy foods and vegetables). Starchy foods (such as rice, potatoes, bread, and pasta) are low in fat when prepared simply. Vegetables are high in fiber, vitamins, and minerals; the American Cancer Society suggests we eat at least five servings of fruits and vegetables each day. When prepared without a lot of butter or oil, vegetables, are also low in calories and fat. Here are some other guidelines for dining lean.

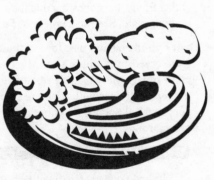

✔ **Split your entrée with a friend and order extra vegetables, starches,** and or a salad. Most restaurants will comply. Ordered this way, the foods fill the plate just as they would have before but the meal is lower in fats and calories and just as filling.

✔ **Ask for steamed vegetables and request no butter or other fats to be added**. Don't be fooled by assuming that the term "steamed" vegetables refers to fat-free vegetables. Most restaurants use the low fat steaming method for cooking vegetables and then add on butter, margarine, oil, or cheese sauce prior to serving. Some vegetables, however, are prepared ahead of time in bulk and may not be available without butter. In that case, ask the server to drain the vegetables well when serving.

Take a look at what a difference adding fat to vegetables makes.

No fat, please:

	Calories	Fat (g)
Steamed asparagus (½ c) with 1t melted butter	60	4
Steamed asparagus (½ c)	25	0
Savings:	**35**	**4**

Skip the Cheese Sauce:

	Calories	Fat (g)
Broccoli (½ c) with Cheese Sauce (3T)	115	6
Steamed broccoli (½ c)	25	0
Savings:	**90**	**6**

✓ **Canned vegetables will be higher in sodium than fresh or frozen vegetables.** Canned vegetables contain approximately 300-400 mg sodium per ½ cup cooked portion.

✓ **The addition of french fries or onion rings can easily double the calories** of your meal. Consider asking for a lower calorie substitute, splitting an order with a friend, or requesting that they only put a half order of the fried vegetable on your plate. See the *Burgers & Fast Food* chapter for more details.

✓ **Order your mashed potatoes without gravy or with gravy on the side.** Gravies served by a quick service restaurant are usually prepared from low fat gravy mixes. More upscale restaurants use meat drippings, butter, and/or cream to prepare gravies with far more calories and fat. To be on the safe side, enjoy your mashed potatoes without gravy or have it served on the side so you can use sparingly.

Get It on the Side:

	Calories	Fat (g)
Mashed Potatoes (½ c) with Gravy (2T)	160	8
Mashed Potatoes (½ c)	120	5
Savings:	**40**	**3**

✓ **Order the baked potato "dry."** Ask for butter, sour cream, and other condiments on the side (to be used wisely or not at all). Other low fat/low calorie toppings include salsa alone or combined with sour cream, mustard, or low fat ranch dressing.

The Baked Potato Difference:

	Calories	Fat (g)
Loaded Baked Potato, 9 oz plus toppings	572	39
Dry Baked Potato, 9 oz	185	0
Savings:	**387**	**39**

Baked Potato Calorimeter: Calories & Fat per serving

	Calories & Fat (g) per serving				
	3 oz	6 oz	9 oz	12 oz	16 oz
Plain	80	160	270	360	470
	0g	0g	0g	0g	0g
w/ butter only	116	232	378	522	686
	4g	8g	12g	18g	24g
	(1t)	*(2t)*	*(1T)*	*(1½T)*	*(2T)*
w/sour cream only	88	177	296	399	522
	1g	2g	3g	4g	5g
	(1t)	*(2t)*	*(1T)*	*(1½T)*	*(2T)*
w/cheese only	99	198	327	446	584
	2g	4g	5g	8g	10g
	(2t)	*(4t)*	*(2T)*	*(3T)*	*(¼ c)*
w/butter & sour cream	124	249	404	561	738
	5g	10g	15g	22g	29g
	(1t each)	*(2t each)*	*(1T each)*	*(1½T ea)*	*(2T each)*
w/butter, sour cream & cheese	143	287	461	647	852
	7g	14g	20g	30g	39g

All of the potato condiments are in level amounts (shown in italics), not heaping spoonfuls. Your potato may have more or less.

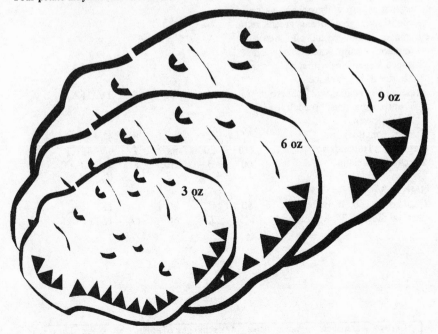

For green salads, coleslaw, and potato salad, please review the *Salads* chapter.

Accompaniments

	Calories	Fat (g)	Sodium (mg)	Carbs* (g)	Exchanges**
Sauces:					
Butter, 1t	36	4	40	0	1FAT
Cheese Sauce, 2T	60	4	180	2	1FAT
Vegetables (½ c unless noted):					
Avocado, ¼	85	7	5	5	1½FAT
Artichoke, 1	50	0.[2]	80	12	2V
Broiled Tomato, ½ w/butter & cheese	80	6	na	6	1V+1FAT
Creamed Spinach	185	15	550	11	2V+3FAT
Greens, spinach, *or* cabbage seasoned with bacon or meat	60	4	300	7	1V+1FAT
Greens, spinach, *or* cabbage sauteed in oil	120	12	150	7	1V+2½FAT
Grilled Vegetables: eggplant, onions, peppers, squash, tomatoes	135	12	210	8	1V+2½FAT
Mushrooms, ¼ c sautéed in butter	110	11	125	2	2FAT
Okra & Tomatoes	40	2	300	8	1V+½FAT
Onion Rings, 1 ring	82	6	91	6	½ST+1FAT
Fried Whole Onion	2000	180	na	45	4ST+4V+36FAT
Ratatouille, ¾ c	75	4	80	11	1½V+1FAT
Spinach Soufflé	140	9	na	10	2V+2FAT
Steamed Vegetables w/out added fat: asparagus, broccoli, cabbage, carrots, cauliflower, green beans, greens, okra, spinach, yellow & zucchini squash, tomatoes, turnip, wax beans	25	0.[1]	5	7	1V
Steamed Vegetables w/melted butter *or* butter sauce	60	4	45	7	1V+1FAT
Steamed Vegetables w/2T cheese sauce: asparagus, broccoli, cauliflower	85	4	185	8	1V+1FAT
Stewed Tomatoes	55	2	na	9	1V+½FAT
Vegetables Hollandaise	210	20	na	7	1V+4FAT
Zucchini Marinara	60	3	310	8	1V+½FAT
Starchy Vegetables (½ c):					
Corn on the cob, 3", no butter	80	1.[5]	20	17	1ST
Corn on the cob, 3", w/butter	115	5.[5]	60	17	1ST+1FAT

---

*Carbs=Carbohydrate, na=not available   **Exchanges:** ST=Starch, Mlk=Milk (skim)
FR=Fruit, CHO=Other Carbohydrates, V=Vegetable, MT=Meat (medium fat), FAT=Fat

Accompaniments (continued)

	Calories	Fat (g)	Sodium (mg)	Carbs* (g)	Exchanges**
Potato, Baked, medium 9 oz	270	0	17	52	3¼ST
1T butter	110	12	123	0	2½FAT
1T sour cream	26	3	6	0	½FAT
1T shredded cheese	30	3	45	0	½MT
1T crumbled bacon	30	2	80	0	½FAT
Potato, 9 oz loaded w/ all above	466	20	271	52	3¼ST+½MT+3½FAT
Potato, Baked, large 16 oz	470	0	30	93	5½ST
2T butter	215	24	245	0	5FAT
2T sour cream	52	5	12	0	1FAT
2T shredded cheese	60	5	90	0	1MT
2T crumbled bacon	60	5	160	0	1FAT
Potato, 16 oz loaded w/all above	857	39	537	93	5½ST+1MT+7FAT
2T Bacon bits	60	2	260	0	1MT
Twice Baked, 8 oz	380	14	140	40	2½ST+1MT+1½FAT
Potatoes, mashed w/butter	120	5	300	17	1ST+1FAT
Hashbrowns, homefries, puffs	165	10	50	15	1ST+2FAT
New Potatoes, buttered	120	5	60	19	1ST+1FAT
Au Gratin	160	9	530	19	1ST+2FAT
Scalloped Potatoes	140	5	420	18	1ST+1FAT
French Fries	150	8	80	20	1ST+1½FAT
Fries covered w/ ¼ c cheese sce	270	16	440	20	1ST+3FAT
Potato Pancakes, one 4"	170	10	400	20	1ST+2FAT
Starchy vegetables (corn, green peas) seasoned w/out butter	70	0.¹	5	18	1ST
Starchy vegetables (corn, green peas) seasoned w/butter	105	4	45	18	1ST+1FAT
Sweet Potatoes w/butter, marshmallows	200	2	na	36	2¼ST+½FAT
Starches (½ c):					
Beans, Baked or Black beans	120	1	500	27	1½ST
Boston Baked Beans	170	3	600	34	1ST+1CHO+½FAT
Refried Beans	250	13	325	18	1ST+2½FAT
Blackeyed Peas w/bacon or meat	135	4	450	17	1ST+1FAT
Couscous, no butter	170	0	4	36	2ST
Couscous, w/ butter	205	4	45	36	2ST+1FAT
Noodles/pasta w/out butter or sauce	80	0	3	20	1ST
Noodles or pasta, buttered	115	4	40	20	1ST+1FAT
Spaetzle, German noodle dish	190	5	160	26	1½ST+1FAT
Polenta, no butter	120	0	180	32	2ST
Fried Polenta, 2" X 2½" X ½"	90	4	130	17	1ST+1FAT
Popovers, Herbed, 1	160	7	130	19	1¼ST+1½FAT
Parmesan, 1	170	8	90	20	1¼ST+1½FAT
Red Beans w/rice, no meat	160	1	na	20	2ST
Red Beans w/rice, w/meat	280	10	na	18	2ST+2FAT

*Carbs=Carbohydrate, na=not available   **Exchanges: ST=Starch, Mlk=Milk (skim)
FR=Fruit, CHO=Other Carbohydrates, V=Vegetable, MT=Meat (medium fat), FAT=Fat

Accompaniments (continued)

	Calories	Fat (g)	Sodium (mg)	Carbos* (g)	Exchanges**
Starches (½ c) continued:					
Rice, steamed white	120	0	200	25	1½ST
Fried Rice	185	6	450	24	1½ST+1FAT
Rice Pilaf	160	3	520	22	1½ST+½FAT
Dirty Rice (w/sausage), ½ c	195	9	500	22	1¼ST+1MT+½FAT
Risotto w/butter	170	5	280	23	1½ST+1FAT
Risotto w/cheese	180	6	na	21	1½ST+½MT+1FAT
Stuffing	205	9	650	17	1ST+2FAT
Condiments (2T):					
Corn Relish	26	0	120	6	1V
Gravy	40	3	150	1	½FAT

Desserts

Chapter Contents:

■ Fruit, Frozen Yogurt, Soft Serve, & Ice Cream
■ Calculating the Calories & Fat for Frozen Desserts
■ Other Desserts

If you can still afford some calories after you have eaten your meal, enjoy some dessert. Below are some general guidelines for selecting desserts within your calorie and dietary fat budget.

✓ **Choose fresh fruit** "without cream or other topping." Often this is enough to satisfy a sweet tooth. Ask for it, even it's it not on the menu. And be sure to ask about whipping cream, powdered sugar, or that unplanned cookie that might be arriving with that healthy fruit. Can you afford those calories?

Fruit & Toppings

	Calories	Fat (g)	Sodium (mg)	Exchanges
Fresh Fruit*, ½ c	20-70	0	<10	½-1FR
Fruit packed in sugar or prepared with sugar*, ½ c	75-120	0	<10	1-2FR
Whipping Cream, pressurized, 2T	23	2	4	½FAT
Whipping Cream, pressurized, ¼ c	46	4	8	1FAT
Whipping Cream, whipped, 2T	50	6	6	1FAT
Heavy Cream or Crème Fraiche, 2T	104	11	12	2FAT

*Nutritional information for a wide variety of fruit is listed in the *Breakfast* chapter.

✓ **Enjoy a cup of flavored tea or coffee** for a satisfying finish to a meal with the benefit of fewer calories than a rich dessert.

✓ **Enjoy a small cup of low fat or fat-free frozen yogurt**. It's sweet, satisfying and, other than fruit, one of the lowest calorie desserts. Frozen yogurt is considerably lower in calories and fat grams than ice cream. Here's a comparison of small portion, just a half cup, without toppings! How much ice cream can you eat?

Yogurt's the Better Choice:	Calories	Fat (g)
Ice Cream, ½ c	200-300	8-24
Non Fat Frozen Yogurt, ½ c	100	0
Savings:	**100-200**	**8-24**

✓ **Order frozen yogurt instead of soft serve**. Surprise! Surprise! If restaurants have a self-serve machine and it is not labeled as frozen yogurt, assume that it is soft serve - which is higher in calories.

Ask for Frozen Yogurt:		Calories	Fat (g)
Soft Serve, ½ c		140	5
Soft Frozen Yogurt, ½ c		100	0
	Savings:	**40**	**5**
DQ® CC Cookie Dough Blizzard®, medium		950	36
DQ® Heath® Breeze®		710	18
	Savings:	**240**	**18**

✓ **Select lower fat ice cream, sherbet, or sorbet**. Many ice cream shops are offering lower fat ice creams that still taste rich and creamy.

Choose Low Fat Ice Cream:		Calories	Fat (g)
Ice Cream, ½ c		200-300	8-24
Low Fat Ice Cream, ½ c		130	2
	Savings:	**70-170**	**6-22**

Choose Sorbet over Sherbet:		Calories	Fat (g)
Sherbet, ½ c		135	2
Sorbet, ½ c		110	1
	Savings:	**25**	**1**

✓ **Ask your taste buds**. Let's be honest. When we know the frozen yogurt has fewer calories, do you ever overindulge? That maybe OK if you really feel satisfied. Ask yourself:

Which Would You Rather Have?	Calories	Fat (g)
Frozen *Non Fat* Yogurt, 1½ c	300	0
Ice Cream, ½ c	300	18

✓ **Order it served in a cup or small cone.** The small-sized cake or sugar cones have negligible fat and few calories. The large waffle cones are considerably higher in fats and calories. Chocolate, nut dips, and candy sprinkles add even more.

Have a Small Cone:		
	Calories	Fat (g)
Waffle Cone, chocolate covered	300	10
Cake Cone	25	0
Savings:	275	10

✓ **Watch the sauces and toppings.** Unless you've selected fresh fruit, the toppings will add significantly to the total calories. Most companies use a 2T ladle to spoon on the sauces and toppings. One ladle may be used on the smaller cups, while the larger cups often have 2 or more ladles.

Have It Plain:		
	Calories	Fat (g)
Large Frozen Yogurt Sundae (4T hot fudge sauce, 2T nuts, & ½ c whipped cream)	710	31
Large Cup Frozen Yogurt	270	5
Savings:	440	26

✓ **Sugar free doesn't mean calorie free.** Regular frozen yogurt is typically sweetened with sugar. Sugar-free frozen yogurts and ice creams often use aspartame (Nutrasweet), sorbitol, or fructose. Each sugar-free product has a few less calories, but perhaps not as much as you might think.

Sugar Free Saves a Few Calories:		
	Calories	Fat (g)
Baskin 31 Robbins® Nonfat Ice Cream, ½ c	100-120	0
Baskin 31 Robbins® No Sugar Added, ½ c	80-100	1-3
Savings:	20-40	1-3g more

Calculating the Calories & Fat Grams in Frozen Yogurt

When restaurants provide nutritional information it is often in terms of a 1/2 cup portion. Be honest about the portion size you were served. Often your cup is considerably larger.

> **Quiz:** You are buying soft-serve frozen yogurt. The brochure states that each 4 fluid ounces contains 100 calories. You notice the cup sizes are labeled: Small (5 oz), Medium (8 oz), and Large (12 oz). You select the 8 oz cup. How many calories are in your yogurt?

200 calories, you say? Wrong. It has 300! How?

The brochure stated that the product contains 100 calories per *fluid* ounce. The labeled cup sizes describe the *weight* ounces of the yogurt when the cup is filled. *Fluid* ounces and *weight* ounces are not always the same. They *are* the same for water, juice, and milk. In other words, one measuring cup of water, juice, or milk has both 8 *fluid* (volume) ounces and 8 *weight* ounces. That's probably why we assume that fluid ounces and weight ounces are the same for *everything*. They are not the same with everything and they are not the same for frozen yogurt.

When your cup of frozen yogurt is **weighed** (for quality control or for pricing) keep in mind that you can not calculate the calories directly from this number. In the process of making frozen yogurt (and other soft serve products), air is incorporated into the product. Companies refer to this in terms of "percent overrun."

Since most companies have a 50% overrun, simply multiply the weight ounces by 1½. Therefore, a cup of frozen yogurt weighing 4 oz (4 *weight* ounces) will equate to 6 *fluid* ounces. Here's a chart to make calculations easier.

Calories in Frozen Yogurt & Soft Serve* per serving size

Size of Cup or Cone	Calories & fat (g) per 4 fluid oz serving as labeled:							
	40	60	80	100	110	120	140	150
4 oz (6 fl oz)	60 0g	90 0g	120 0g	150 1g	165 2g	180 3g	210 5g	225 8g
5 oz (7½ fl oz)	75 0g	115 0g	150 0g	190 1g	205 2g	225 4g	265 6g	280 10g
6 oz (9 fl oz)	90 0g	135 0g	180 0g	225 2g	250 3g	270 5g	315 7g	340 12g
7 oz (10½ fl oz)	105 0g	160 0g	210 0g	265 2g	290 3g	315 6g	370 8g	395 14g
8 oz (12 fl oz)	120 0g	180 0g	240 0g	300 2g	330 4g	360 6g	420 9g	450 16g
9 oz (13½ fl oz)	135 0g	205 0g	270 0g	340 3g	370 5g	405 7g	475 11g	510 18g
10 oz (15 fl oz)	150 0g	225 0g	300 0g	375 3g	415 5g	450 8g	525 12g	565 20g

*Assuming 50% overrun. If the liquid ingredients are inadequately frozen, the final product will be very runny. Because there is less air in a runny product, you can fit more yogurt into the cup. More yogurt means even more calories than the chart above demonstrates.

Cone with 4 wt oz (6 fl oz)

Cones & Toppings

	Calories	Fat (g)	Sodium (mg)	Carbs* (g)	Exchanges**
Cones (1):					
Cake	25	0	35	6	¼CHO
Sugar	60	0	50	15	½CHO
Lg. Waffle	120	2	55	23	1½CHO+½FAT
Waffle Cone/Fresh Baked	150	2	5	33	2CHO+½FAT
Waffle Cone, chocolate covered	300	10	50	52	3½CHO+2FAT
Waffle Cone, chocolate covered w/nuts	400	19	50	52	3½CHO+4FAT
Fruit Toppings (2T):					
Fresh strawberries	6	<1	0	2	FREE
Fresh blueberries	10	<1	1	3	¼FR
Fruit Cocktail, canned in own juice	14	0	1	4	¼FR
Raisins	56	<1	5	14	1FR
Shredded coconut, dried & sweetened	45	3.5	24	3	¼CHO+½FAT
Syrups & Toppings (2T):					
Chocolate syrup	90	1	30	20	1½CHO
Hot Fudge topping	120	5	35	19	1½CHO+1FAT
No Sugar Added/ Fat-Free Hot Fudge	90	0	96	23	1½CHO
Butterscotch topping	130	1	110	29	2CHO
Caramel topping	120	3	90	23	1½CHO
Strawberry topping	60	0	5	15	1CHO
Blueberry or Pineapple topping	70	0	15	17	1CHO
Walnuts in syrup	130	1	na	26	1½CHO
Marshmallow creme	90	0	20	23	1½CHO
Whipped topping	23	1.8	2	2	½FAT
Grenadine, 1T	60	0	0	15	1CHO
Candy & Nut Toppings (slightly rounded 2T):					
Chocolate or Yogurt-covered raisins	120	5	30	20	½FR+1CHO+1FAT
Sprinkles ("Jimmies")	140	5	0	24	1½CHO+1FAT
Cookies, crumbled	135	5	95	23	1½CHO+1FAT
Butterfinger, crumbled	130	5	57	23	1½CHO+1FAT
Heath bar, crumbled	140	9	106	15	1CHO+2FAT
Reese's pieces	140	6	47	19	1¼CHO+1FAT
Plain M&M's®	140	6	15	19	1¼CHO+1FAT
Peanut M&M's®	150	7	15	18	1¼CHO+1½FAT
Granola	60	3	30	8	½CHO+½FAT
Nuts, unsalted	100	9	0	3	2FAT

*Carbs=Carbohydrate, na=not available ****Exchanges:** ST=Starch, Mlk=Milk (skim) FR=Fruit, CHO=Other Carbohydrates, V=Vegetable, MT=Meat (medium fat), FAT=Fat

✓ **Order one dessert and several forks** so everyone at the table can share. Our taste buds are the most sensitive in the first few bites; that's when a sweet and rich dessert offers the most satisfaction. Having just a few bites is also sensible because most desserts have anywhere from 300 to over 1000 calories per restaurant serving.

✓ **Ask the server for a smaller portion of dessert**. They will still charge you for the whole piece, but you've saved the calories. Remember you can't eat what isn't there.

✓ **Choose one of the lower calorie desserts** such as Angel food and sponge cake which have the least amount of calories per ounce. Reduced fat brownies, cakes, and muffins may also be offered. While these low fat and fat-free baked goods have significantly less fat than their regular counterparts, the calories are still fairly high due to the fact that low fat desserts are often higher in sugar. In addition, even low fat desserts are served in very large portions.

✓ **Skip the piecrust**. Most of the fat and calories in pies, cobblers, and turnovers come from the piecrust. The fruit filling is rather low in calories. So if you like the pie filling more than the crust, don't feel guilty about leaving the crust behind. You'll save more than half the calories.

✓ **Choose the sugar-free pie**. It can save you some calories, but perhaps not as many as you think. It still has a piecrust and 40% of the pie's calories come from the fat in the piecrust. But, of course, every little bit counts!

Choose Pies Made with Equal®:	Calories	Fat (g)
Denny's Apple Pie	430	20
Denny's Apple Pie sweetened with Equal®	370	20
Savings:	60	0

✓ **Muffins are very misleading.** Which has less calories and fat: muffins or doughnuts? The muffin, you say? Probably not. It's true that muffins are not fried and may even have fewer calories per ounce than doughnuts. But the muffin may end up having more fat and calories simply because an average doughnut is about 2-3 ounces while muffins often weigh more (4-6 oz).

Which Would You Rather Have?	Calories	Fat (g)
Muffin, 4 oz (baseball size)	400	17
Yeast Doughnut, 2 ½ oz (regular sized)	250	11
Savings:	150	6

Enjoy the Low Fat Muffins:	Calories	Fat (g)
Regular Blueberry Muffin, 4 oz	400	17
Low Fat Blueberry Muffin, 4 oz	320	1
Savings:	80	16

Calculating the Calories and Fat in Baked Goods

Shops selling frozen yogurt and low fat ice creams often have nutritional information. Most other desserts do not. So how do you find out the number of calories and grams of fat in the other desserts? It's easy.

You can calculate the calories of *any* desserts as long as you know

❶ the weight of the item and

❷ the calories per ounce as shown on the Desserts Calorimeter on these two pages.

If bringing a scale with you is not an option, estimate the weight by comparing your dessert to the portion sizes depicted throughout this chapter.

Desserts Calorimeter: Calories & fat per serving

Calories Per oz		Calories & Fat (g)				
		1 oz	2 oz	3 oz	4 oz	5 oz
160	Shortbread	**160**	**320**	**480**	**640**	**800**
		9g	19g	28g	37g	47g
135	Almond & Choc Almond Biscotti Brownie, Cake Doughnuts Chocolate Croissant Chocolate Chip Cookie Pound Cake, Macaroons Peanut Butter Brownie *or* Cookie	**135** 8g	**270** 15g	**405** 23g	**540** 30g	**675** 38g
125	Cookies: butter, oatmeal, sugar	**125**	**250**	**375**	**500**	**625**
		5g	10g	16g	21g	26g
120	Plain & Almond Croissant	**120**	**240**	**360**	**480**	**600**
	Choc Cream Filled Doughnuts	7g	13g	20g	26g	33g
110	Cheesecake Coffeecake, Cinn Rolls & Danish Muffins: chocolate chip, lemon poppy seed Gingerbread, Madeleines Pecan Pie, Scones Sweet Cheese Croissant	**110** 6g	**220** 11g	**330** 17g	**440** 22g	**550** 28g

Desserts Calorimeter: Calories & fat per serving (continued)

Calories Per oz		Calories & Fat grams (g)				
		1 oz	2 oz	3 oz	4 oz	5 oz
100	Biscotti, plain Fritters, Glazed Fritters Cakes/Cupcakes (plain or frosted) Muffins: fruit or grain Yeast Doughnuts (includ glazed, frosted, crème & jelly filled) Fruit Tarts & Turnovers Pies: Boston Cream, Buttermilk, German Choc, Choc Cream	**100** 4g	**200** 8g	**300** 13g	**400** 17g	**500** 21g
80	Tiraminsu	**80** 5g	**160** 10g	**240** 14g	**360** 19g	**400** 24g
80	Pies: Fruits including Lemon & Lime, Coconut Custard, Mincemeat	**80** 3g	**160** 6g	**240** 10g	**360** 13g	**400** 17g
80	Angel Food Cake Lowfat Muffins Sponge Cake	**80** $0.^3$g	**160** $0.^6$g	**240** $0.^9$g	**320** $1.^2$g	**400** $1.^5$g
60	Pies: Banana Custard, Banana Cream, Custard, Pumpkin	**60** 3g	**120** 6g	**180** 9g	**240** 12g	**300** 15g

Brownie

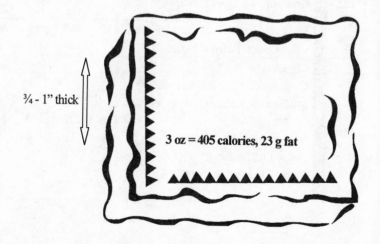

¾ - 1" thick

3 oz = 405 calories, 23 g fat

Cakes

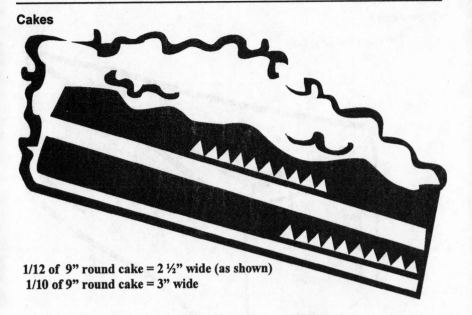

1/12 of 9" round cake = 2 ½" wide (as shown)
1/10 of 9" round cake = 3" wide

Cakes, frosted or unfrosted, contain approximately 100 calories per ounce. The amount of ounces per slice vary greatly. Refer to the Cake Calorimeter below or the nutritional information at the end of this chapter for more details.

Cake Calorimeter: Calories & Fat grams per portion

9" Round Cake	Calories & Fat (g)	
	1/12 cake	1/10 cake
Angel Food Cake	160	190
	0g	0g
Carrot Cake	521	625
	23g	28g
Chocolate Cake	575	690
	25g	30g
Italian Rum Custard	360	430
	20g	24g
Pound Cake	280	340
	13g	16g
Sponge Cake	190	230
	3g	4g
Yellow Cake	540	650
	23g	28g

Cheesecake

3 oz = 330 calories, 23 g fat

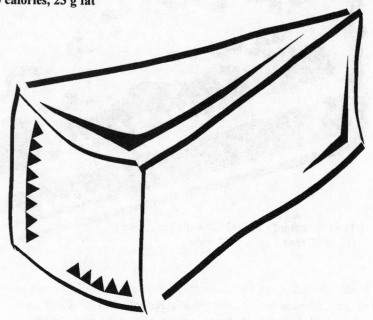

Coffee Cake, Cinnamon Rolls

3 oz =
330 calories
17 g fat

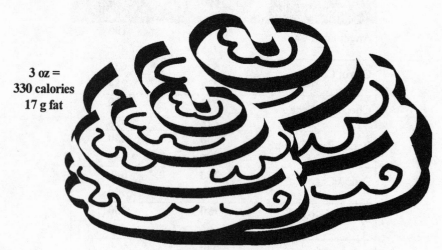

7½ oz = 825 calories, 42 g fat

Cookies

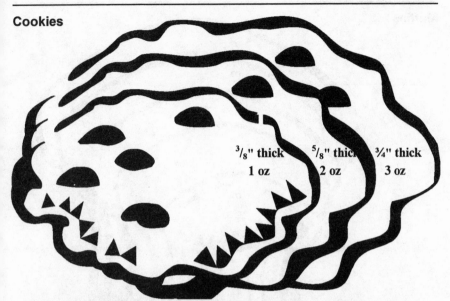

$^3/_8$" thick
1 oz

$^5/_8$" thick
2 oz

$^3/_4$" thick
3 oz

Cookie Calorimeter: Calories & Fat grams per cookie

Cookie	Calories & Fat (g)		
	1 oz	2 oz	3 oz
Peanut Butter, Chocolate Chip, Macadamia Nut, *or* Chocolate Chunk	135	270	405
	8g	15g	23g
Butter, Oatmeal, Oatmeal Raisin, *or* Sugar	125	250	375
	5g	10g	16g

Doughnuts

2 oz Yeast Raised Doughnut
200 calories, 8 g fat

2 oz Cake Doughnut
270 calories, 15 g fat

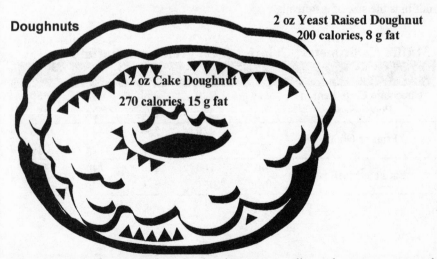

Note that ounce for ounce, the cake doughnuts are smaller and more compact and yet have more calories and fat than yeast raised doughnuts.

Muffins

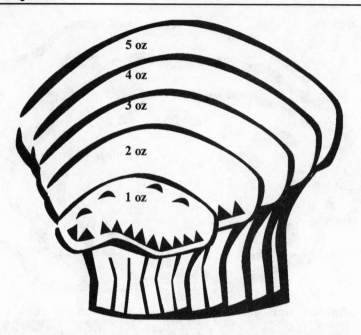

The calories in your muffin vary greatly depending on its size. A 1 oz muffin is very small – almost bite size. The 4 oz muffin is about the size of a baseball; the 5 oz muffin is the size of a softball.

Muffin Calorimeter: Calories & fat grams per muffin

Muffin	Calories & Fat (g)				
	1 oz	2 oz	3 oz	4 oz	5 oz
Chocolate Chip, Lemon Poppy Seed	**110**	**220**	**330**	**440**	**550**
	6g	11g	17g	22g	28g
Fruit or Grain	**110**	**220**	**330**	**440**	**550**
	4g	8g	13g	17g	21g
Fat Free Muffins	**80**	**160**	**180**	**240**	**300**
	$0.^3$g	$0.^6$g	$0.^9$g	$1.^2$g	$1.^5$g

Pies

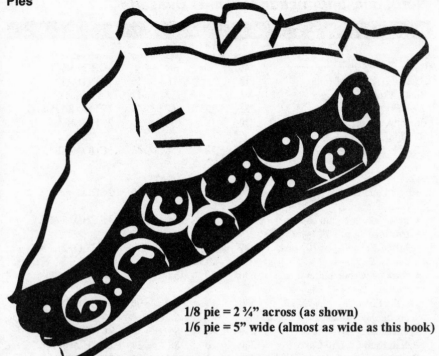

1/8 pie = 2 ¾" across (as shown)
1/6 pie = 5" wide (almost as wide as this book)

Pie Calorimeter: Calories & Fat grams per portion

9" Pie	Calories & Fat (g)	
	¹/₈ pie	¹/₆ pie
Apple	**270**	**360**
	13g	17g
Banana Cream	**270**	**360**
	12g	16g
Blueberry	**290**	**390**
	13g	17g
Cherry	**350**	**465**
	17g	23g
Chocolate Cream	**290**	**380**
	18g	24g
Coconut Cream	**275**	**365**
	14g	19g
Key Lime	**345**	**460**
	15g	20g
Lemon Meringue	**350**	**465**
	15g	20g
Pecan	**430**	**570**
	24g	32g

Nutritional Information for Other Desserts

Desserts

	Calories	Fat (g)	Sodium (mg)	Carbs* (g)	Exchanges**
Baklava, 2" X 2"	440	30	na	30	2CHO+6FAT
Biscotti, 1.³ oz, 6½" long	112	5	41	15	1ST+1FAT
Blintz, Cheese, 3" long	80	2	135	12	¾ST+½MT
Cherry, 3	385	17	na	45	2ST+1FR+3½FAT
Brownie, 2½ oz, 2"X2¼"X1" high	330	19	100	30	2CHO+4FAT
3½ oz, 2"X3"X1" high	475	28	150	45	3CHO+5½FAT
Cakes:					
Angel Food Cake, ¹/₁₂ of tube (2½" slice)	160	0	0	30	2CHO
Carrot Cake w/cream cheese frosting, ¹/₁₀ of 9" 2 layer	625	28	na	68	4½CHO+5½FAT
Chiffon Cake, ¹/₁₂ of 10" tube pan	290	12	160	200	2½CHO+2½FAT
Chocolate w/choc butter cream frosting, ¹/₁₀ of 9" 2 layer	690	30	na	75	5CHO+6FAT
Devil's Food Cake, ¹/₁₂ of 9" double layer cake	530	19	240	90	6CHO+4FAT
Fruitcake, ½" X 4" slice	210	7	85	30	2CHO+1½FAT
Italian Rum Custard Cake, ¹/₁₂	360	20	80	34	2¼CHO+4FAT
Pound Cake, 1" sl (rectangular pan) or 2½" wide (9" tube)	280	13	130	30	2CHO+2½FAT
Strawberry Shortcake, 2 ½" biscuit	430	24	240	45	1ST+1FR+1CHO+5FAT
Sponge Cake, 2½" slice	190	3	160	30	2CHO+½FAT
Pineapple Upside Down Cake, 3" X 3" X 2" high	360	14	na	38	1½CHO+1FR+3FAT
Yellow Cake, ¹/₁₂ of 9" cake	540	23	na	60	4CHO+4½FAT
Unfrosted Cake, 3" square X 2" high	210	10	200	30	2CHO+2FAT
Frosted Cake, 3" square X2" high	375	18	270	53	3½CHO+3½FAT
Cake Icing, chocolate, 2T	140	5	50	23	1½CHO+1FAT
Vanilla, 2T	150	3	20	30	2CHO+½FAT
Cheesecake, 3 oz slice, 1½" wide slice from 9" tube, 1½" high	330	23	318	23	1½CHO+½MT+4FAT
6 oz slice, 3" wide slice from 9" tube, 1½" high	660	46	636	45	3CHO+1MT+7½FAT
9 oz slice, 3" wide slice, 2½" high	990	69	955	68	4½CHO+1MT+12FAT
Chocolate Mousse, 1c	380	32	na	15	1CHO+6½FAT
Chocolate Pots de Crème, ²/₃ c	270	21	30	23	1½CHO+4FAT

*Carbs=Carbohydrate, na=not available   **Exchanges: ST=Starch, Mlk=Milk (skim)
FR=Fruit, CHO=Other Carbohydrates, V=Vegetable, MT=Meat (medium fat), FAT=Fat

Desserts (continued)

	Calories	Fat (g)	Sodium (mg)	Carbs* (g)	Exchanges**
Cobblers & Crisps:					
Fruit Cobbler, 1c	330	9	210	53	1FR+2½CHO+2FAT
Fruit Crisp, 1 c	260	8	100	45	1FR+2CHO+1½FAT
Cookies (Peanut Butter, Chocolate Chip, Macadamia Nut, Chocolate Chunk):					
1 oz	135	8	100	16	¾CHO+1½FAT
2 oz	270	15	200	34	1½CHO+3FAT
3 oz	405	23	300	50	2¼CHO+4½FAT
Cookies (Butter, Oatmeal Raisin, Sugar):					
1 oz	125	5	100	20	1CHO+1FAT
2 oz	250	10	200	40	2CHO+2FAT
3 oz	375	16	300	58	3CHO+3FAT
Cream Puff, w/out filling	160	11	160	15	¾ST+2FAT
Cream Puff, w/ filling	300	18	380	35	1¾CHO+3½FAT
Crème Brûlée, ½ c	405	36	40	20	1CHO+1MT+6FAT
Crème Fraische or Heavy Cream, 2T	104	11	12	1	2FAT
Crepe, 1 w/out filling	135	7	na	18	1ST+1½FAT
w/ fruit filling, 1	270	11	na	40	1ST+1¼CHO+2FAT
Crepe Suzette, 3	600	30	na	83	4CHO+6FAT
Custard, Baked or Stirred, ½ c	150	4	70	15	½CHO+½Mlk+½MT
Doughnut, 2 oz cake	270	15	na	34	1¾ST+3FAT
2 oz yeast raised	200	8	na	32	1¾ST+1½FAT
Flan, 1c	220	2	140	43	3CHO
Funnel Cake, 7" diameter circle, 1" high w/confectioner's sugar	1440	85	na	165	9CHO+17FAT
Gelatin, ½ c	80	0	25	20	1CHO
Marzipan or Almond Paste, 1 oz (1½T)	150	5	70	23	1½CHO+1FAT
Pies from 9" pan, unless noted (slices from 10" pies are larger & deeper – estimate at least 50% more calories & fat):					
Apple, $^1/_8$	270	13	240	34	1½ST+1FR+2½FAT
$^1/_6$	360	17	320	45	2ST+1FR+3½FAT
Banana Cream Pie, $^1/_8$	270	12	300	40	1½ST+1FR+2½FAT
$^1/_6$	360	16	400	45	2ST+1FR+3FAT
Black Bottom Pie, $^1/_8$ of 10"	380	16	na	45	3CHO+3FAT
$^1/_6$ of 10"	506	21	na	60	4CHO+4FAT
Blueberry Pie, $^1/_8$	290	13	320	38	1½ST+1FR+2½FAT
$^1/_6$	390	17	430	45	2ST+1FR+3½FAT
Brown Sugar Pie, $^1/_8$ of 10"	590	25	na	68	4½CHO+5FAT
$^1/_6$ of 10"	787	33	na	90	6CHO+6½FAT

*Carbs=Carbohydrate, na=not available **Exchanges:** ST=Starch, Mlk=Milk (skim) FR=Fruit, CHO=Other Carbohydrates, V=Vegetable, MT=Meat (medium fat), FAT=Fat

Desserts (continued)

Pies from 9" pan, unless noted (slices from 10" pies are larger & deeper – estimate to contain at least 50% more calories & fat):

	Calories	Fat (g)	Sodium (mg)	Carbs* (g)	Exchanges**
Cherry Pie, 1/8	350	17	410	40	1½ST+1FR+3½FAT
1/6	465	23	540	56	2½ST+1FR+4½FAT
Chocolate Cream Pie, 1/8	290	18	300	25	1½CHO+3½FAT
1/6	380	24	395	35	2CHO+5FAT
Coconut Cream Pie, 1/8	275	14	170	26	1½CHO+3FAT
1/6	365	19	220	40	2½CHO+4FAT
Key Lime Pie, 1/6	460	20	na	57	3½CHO+4FAT
Lemon Meringue Pie, 1/8	350	15	260	40	2½CHO+3FAT
1/6	465	20	345	57	3½CHO+4FAT
Meringue only for 1/8 pie	45	0	27	9	½CHO
1/6 pie	60	0	36	11	¾CHO
Pecan Pie, 1/8	430	24	230	40	2½CHO+5FAT
1/6	570	32	310	55	3½CHO+6½FAT
Strawberry w/Glaze & whipped topping, 1/8	450	28	na	39	1½CHO+1FR+5½FAT
Pudding:					
Bread Pudding, ½ c	235	7	290	31	2CHO+1FAT
Chocolate, ½ c	240	9	110	30	½Mlk+1½CHO+1FAT
Butterscotch, ½ c	200	4	130	26	½Mlk+1¼CHO+1FAT
Vanilla, ½ c	220	8	100	30	½Mlk+1½CHO+1FAT
Rice, ½ c	190	5	50	30	1ST+1FR+1FAT
Scones, triangular wedge (2"X2"X3" long)	330	17	372	45	3ST+3FAT
Snow Cone, 1c ice + syrup	120	0	10	25	1½CHO
Tiramisu, 1/8 of 9" pan	220	14	na	16	1CHO+3FAT
Turnover, Fruit	330	15	306	38	2CHO+½FR+3FAT
Trifle including ½ c pudding, fruit, & 1½ ladyfinger	300	15	60	32	1ST+1FR+3FAT
Truffles, 1 Chocolate ball	80	7	4	4	1½FAT
1 Chocolate Nut ball	105	10	4	4	2FAT
Zabaglione, (Italian frothy egg pudding), ½ c	108	6	10	12	¾CHO+1FAT

PART

4

Ethnic Cuisines

Cajun & Creole Restaurants

Chapter Contents:

- Appetizers
- Salads
- Entrees
- Sandwiches
- Accompaniments
- Desserts

Cajun foods are those originating from the Acadian French immigrants living in Louisiana. Creole foods can be broadened to those foods traditionally prepared by a person of European parentage born in the West Indies, Central America, or Gulf States. Most of us think of Cajun and Creole foods as being spicy and flavorful. Typical Cajun spices include filé, onions, celery, hot & bell peppers, green onions, garlic and hot peppers. Creole chefs use more marjoram, sage, fennel, leeks, and mustard. Here are some general guidelines for dining lean at Cajun/Creole restaurants.

Appetizers

✓ **Avoid the fried appetizers**, share them with a friend, or have them instead of an entrée. More appetizer suggestions and nutritional information can be found in the *Appetizers* chapter.

✓ **Boiled shrimp, boiled crawfish, and oysters on the half shell are low fat** choices. Any of these appetizers make a perfect entrée. Nutritional information for these choices (and the sauces) can be found in the seafood section of the *Entrees & Sauces* chapter.

✓ **Choose the red sauce** for dipping. This selection is much lower in calories than tartar sauce or the butter sauces. Compare the different sauces in the *Entrees & Sauces* chapter.

Salads

✓ **Always order vegetable salads with the dressing on the side**. Or use just vinegar or fresh lemon as a dressing.

✓ **Ask what's in the salad.** You may want to omit some of the high fat ingredients such as cheese, olives, and croutons especially if you don't care for them.

✓ **Seafood salads should be ordered "dry."** Unless specified as such, seafood salads come prepared with mayonnaise or other high fat salad dressings.

Entrees

Fish is the most common protein source served in Cajun and Creole restaurants. It is served as an entrée and added to salads, soups, and sauces. Detailed ordering suggestions and nutritional information can be found in the seafood section of the *Entrees & Sauces* chapter. Here are some general recommendations:

✓ **Request that the fish be prepared grilled or broiled**. Fish is also offered fried, stuffed, sauteed, blackened, or pan broiled. If sauteed, ask them to use as little oil as possible. Fried fish has about twice as many calories as grilled or broiled fish. This calorie difference makes a major impact because fish portions are generally about 8-12 oz portions. Stuffed fish are often prepared with additional fat and are best avoided.

✓ **Skip the butter and sauces or ask for them to be served on the side**. Cajun fish is often served with a high fat sauce on top. If you want the taste of the sauce, order it on the side and dip your fork into the sauce with each bite.

"On the Side, Please":	Calories	Fat (g)
6 oz Fish w/Butter & Crab Sauce	390	35
6 oz Fish w/out butter or sauce	180	12
Savings:	**210**	**23**

✓ **Be sure to ask that the fish be blackened in *very little* oil**. Blackened fish *can be* relatively low in fat although some restaurants add a great deal of oil. Blackened meats and fish can be prepared two different ways. Usually, it is dipped in oil and then in a spice mixture containing the hotter spices such as garlic, cayenne, and white pepper. Some restaurants put oil in the pan or brush on oil and then sprinkle the "meat" with the spices. The "meat" is cooked in a very hot skillet or on the grill so that the outer portion gets crusty and blackened while the inside stays moist and juicy. The meatier fish such as salmon and swordfish hold up best. Blackened chicken or fish is lower in fat than blackened beef.

✓ **Foods prepared with roux contain more fat than it appears**. Roux, a mixture of melted fat and flour, is frequently used for thickening sauces for meats, gravies (etouffeés), and soups such as gumbo. This fat may not be visible but it can increase the calories of a food item much higher than you would guess from appearances.

Entrees

	Calories	Fat (g)	Sodium (mg)	Carbos* (g)	Exchanges**
Crayfish Étouffeé, 1 c + ¾ c rice	445	21	610	44	2ST+3MT+2V+2½FAT
Gumbo, seafood & sausage, 2c	460	27	950	38	2ST+1V+4MT +1½FAT
Jambalaya, chicken & sausage w/rice, 1½ c	360	15	460	31	1¼ST+2V+2MT +1FAT

Sandwiches

The most common sandwich served in a Cajun restaurant is the Po Boy (or Peaux Boy). This sandwich consists of fried or sautéed fish served in a Hoagie roll (or French bread) with a sauce. The bread is low in fat, but the fish and sauce are not.

✓ **Request a Po Boy sandwich prepared with *broiled or grilled* fish**. Also request the red sauce rather than tartar or remoulade sauce.

Ask for Lower Calorie Sauces:	Calories	Fat (g)
Po Boy: Roll, *Fried* Shrimp+¼c ***Tartar Sauce***	890	54
Po Boy: Roll, *Grilled* Shrimp+¼c ***Cocktail Sauce***	535	11
Savings:	**355**	**43**

✓ **Ask for the dressing on the side**. The dressing is usually a cocktail sauce and tartar sauce mixture; request only cocktail sauce instead and save the difference. Lettuce, tomato, and pickles are also frequently added to Po Boys.

Accompaniments

At Cajun and Creole restaurants, standard accompaniments are red beans & rice, so-called "Dirty" rice (prepared with sausage), and baked potatoes.

✓ **Ask for vegetables to be served without sauce or butter**. Many restaurants offer one vegetable and it is typically prepared steamed.

✓ **Ask for vegetables to be served without sauce or butter**. Many restaurants offer one vegetable and it is typically prepared steamed.

✓ **Red beans and rice *may* be a low fat choice** depending on the individual recipe used. When meat is added the calories increase greatly.

✓ **Request plain rice instead of dirty rice**. Dirty rice is not low fat or low cholesterol because it is prepared with a variety of meats including chicken liver, gizzards, sausage, and pork.

✓ **Baked potatoes are often very large but can be prepared with minimal toppings**. Keep in mind that a 1 pound baked potato (without any toppings!) contains 400 calories. Check out the *Accompaniments* chapter for more detail.

Accompaniments

	Calories	Fat (g)	Sodium (mg)	Carbos* (g)	Exchanges**
Red Beans & Rice, no meat, ½ c	160	1	na	20	2ST
Red Beans & Rice, w/meat, ½ c	280	10	na	20	2ST+2FAT
Dirty Rice (w/sausage), ½ c	195	9	500	22	1¼ST+1MT+½FAT
Hominy, ½ c	130	2	700	29	1¾ST
Cornbread, 2½"X2"	135	5	720	22	1¼ST+1FAT

Dessert

✓ **Fresh fruit is the leanest choice for dessert**. It is often available even if it's not mentioned on the menu.

✓ **Share high calorie desserts with your friends**. Bread pudding, pecan pie, pralines, and other rice desserts are best shared with many friends.

For nutritional information on your favorite dessert, see the *Desserts* chapter.

Chinese Restaurants

Chapter Contents:

■ General Recommendations
■ Estimating the Calories & Fat in your Stir Fry
■ Nutritional Information for Chinese Foods

Traditional Chinese cooking is considered healthy because small portions of meat are often combined with large amounts of low fat vegetables and rice or noodles. Unfortunately, many Chinese restaurants in this country use larger portions of meat than in traditional recipes. In addition, more oil is added than absolutely necessary when stir-frying. Fortunately, most dishes are made-to-order so you can ask the cook to prepare your dish according to your dietary specifications.

There are four main regions of China each with their own unique cuisine. Dishes are typically served with rice as is common in southern China; northern China is better known for their wheat products such as noodles. Cantonese style, from southern China, offers mild flavored food that is often steamed or stir-fried and served with rice. Beijing/Peking in northern China is noted for the sweet and sour sauces, plum, or hoisin sauces. Szechwan and Hunan cooking is from western China. This style is noted by the hot and spicy food flavored with chilies, garlic, and hot red peppers and tends to be higher in fat than the others. The last is Shanghai cooking, found in Eastern China. Shanghai uses a combination of soy sauces, wine, and sugar. Braising of foods, with these ingredients, is often referred to as "red" cooking. The following are some recommendations for dining lean that apply in any Chinese restaurant:

✓ **Avoid fried foods** indicated by the words "fried" or "crispy." The frying process alone may double the calories of any meat or vegetable. Check out the nutritional details in the Entrees & Sauces chapter.

✓ **Order "off the menu" rather than selecting the buffet.** Foods featured on the buffet table are prepared with more oil to prevent sticking and drying out.

Check out the shine – it's coming from the fat. If you can afford the extra time, order off the menu. No time? Consider calling in your order ahead of time.

✓ **Use chopsticks.** If you are inexperienced with using chopsticks, you will find it difficult to eat quickly which allows time for your stomach to signal when you're full.

✓ **Order steamed dumplings** instead of fried egg rolls. Or ask for double the steamed white rice.

✓ **Select non-fried foods.** Use caution at Dim Sum lunches; most of the items are fried.

✓ **Fill up on soup.** Most soups, although very high in sodium, are low in fat and calories. Select the Won Ton, Egg Drop (higher in cholesterol because of the egg), Hot & Sour, or Velvet Corn.

✓ **Request steamed rice or plain noodles rather than fried rice or fried noodles.** Even though steamed rice may not be listed on the menu or offered on the buffet, you can always request steamed rice or plain noodles at no additional charge.

✓ **Enjoy boiled noodles rather than the fried noodles.** The boiled noodles are similar to American wheat noodles.

✓ **Avoid restaurants that serve their food *too fast.*** For speed in serving, some restaurants will cut up the meat and poultry in advance and deep-fry them until the inside is cooked but the meat is not browned on the outside. When you order your meal, the individual orders are then stir-fried in the wok with even more oil. It is often difficult to determine whether the meat has been fried prior to being stir-fried because the color of the meat is the same. Be sure to ask how the meat is prepared.

✓ **Order dishes that contain more vegetables than meat.** Beef, poultry, and seafood contain in the range of 120-520 calories per cup. Most vegetables have only about 50 or less! Since most dishes are made to order, you can always request more vegetables than meat. Or ask them to add vegetables to a typical meat-only dish which helps to lower the calories and fat grams in the dish.

✓ **Avoid sweet and sour entrees.** Sweet and sour chicken, beef, and shrimp are typically all deep fat fried before the sugar-laden sauce is added.

✓ **"House Specialties" should be avoided,** as a rule. These higher priced items are usually dishes consisting of large portions of meat and little or no vegetables. Therefor, they are usually high in both fat and calories.

✓ **Avoid dishes with nuts.** Just a handful of nuts (about ¼ c) will add an extra 200 calories & 20 grams of fat. Your dish could have even more nuts! Water chestnuts (at just 20 calories per ¼ c) are a great crunchy, low calorie alternative.

✔ **Ask that your dish to be prepared with as "little oil as possible" in any stir-fried dish.** Usually 1-2 tablespoons of oil (and sometimes lard) is used to stir-fry an entree. That's 120-240 calories worth of fat. Some restaurants use even more!

✔ **Order steamed foods with sauce on the side.** Some restaurant goers are choosing to order their food steamed (cooking it over water or chicken broth). Please consider that steamed foods will taste bland without the zing of traditional Chinese flavors. As a remedy, mix the steamed foods with rice and Plum sauce. Or request a sauce to be made of only thickened broth - and no oil.

✔ **Order fewer meals than the number of people at your table.** It is common practice in Chinese restaurants to share your meal with others at your table. Consider ordering just three meals for a table of four.

✔ **Order Chop Suey instead of Chow Mein.** Chop Suey and Chow Mein are essentially the same mixture of meat and vegetables. Chow Mein is topped with *fried* noodles (fattening), Chop Suey is not.

✔ **Select tofu instead of meat.** Tofu is a soft cheese made from soybeans. It is high in protein and moderate in both calories and fat. Although tofu has little flavor by itself, it soaks up the flavor of the foods in which it was cooked. Avoid dishes prepared with *fried* tofu.

✔ **Ask for foods prepared without MSG** (Monosodium Glutamate, a flavor enhancer) **if you are sensitive to it's effects.** Some people are sensitive to MSG and report hot flashes, sweating, and headaches shortly after eating foods prepared with MSG. To reduce the symptoms, simply request that your food be prepared *without MSG*. Other components within the ingredients may still contain MSG, such as the chicken broth, which is used for making a sauce.

✔ **Most Chinese sauces are low in fat, but high in sugar and/or sodium.** If you are not restricting your sodium and sugar intake, these sauces are probably healthier for flavoring your meals than using oil.

■ **Black Bean Sauce** - a thick brown sauce commonly used in Cantonese cooking. It is made of fermented soy beans, wheat flour, and salt.

■ **Hoisin** - a thick sauce that is both sweet and spicy. It is made from soybeans, sugar, garlic, chili, and vinegar.

■ **Oyster sauce** - rich, thick sauce made from oysters and soy sauce. It is frequently used in Cantonese cooking.

■ **Plum sauce** - amber-colored, thick sauce made from plums, apricots, hot peppers, vinegar, and sugar. It has a spicy sweet-and-sour flavor.

■ **Sweet and Sour Sauce** - thick sauce made from sugar, vinegar, and soy sauce.

Estimating the Calories & Fat in Your Stir Fry

Every Chinese restaurant prepares their stir-fry dishes slightly different so it is difficult to list the *exact* calories per serving. On the average, a stir-fried dish contains approximately 2 cups of food. If we assume that each stir-fried dish contains 1 tablespoon (when you request "very little oil") or 2 tablespoons (for most Chinese meals) of oil we can estimate the calories and fat grams:

Chinese Food Calorimeter: Calories & fat (g) per serving

Calories & Fat (g) when stir-fried in 1T oil:				
2c Vegetables	1½c Vegetables ½c Beef *or* Pork	1c Vegetables 1c Beef *or* Pork	½c Vegetables 1½c Beef *or* Pork	2c Beef
220 14g	**335** 22g	**450** 30g	**565** 38g	**680** 44g
	1½c Vegetables ½c Chicken	1c Vegetables 1c Chicken	½c Vegetables 1½c Chicken	2c Chicken
	295 18g	**370** 22g	**445** 26g	**520** 30g
	1½c Vegetables ½c Seafood *or* Chicken Breast	1c Vegetables 1c Seafood *or* Chicken Breast	½c Vegetables 1½c Seafood *or* Chicken Breast	2c Seafood *or* Chicken Breast
	265 17g	**210** 20g	**355** 23g	**400** 26g

Calories & Fat (g) when stir-fried in 2T oil:				
2c Vegetables	1½c Vegetables ½c Beef *or* Pork	1c Vegetables 1c Beef *or* Pork	½c Vegetables 1½c Beef *or* Pork	2c Beef
440 28g	**455** 36g	**570** 44g	**685** 52g	**800** 58g
	1½c Vegetables ½c Chicken	1c Vegetables 1c Chicken	½c Vegetables 1½c Chicken	2c Chicken
	415 32g	**490** 36g	**565** 40g	**640** 44g
	1½c Vegetables ½c Seafood *or* Chicken Breast	1c Vegetables 1c Seafood *or* Chicken Breast	½c Vegetables 1½c Seafood *or* Chicken Breast	2c Seafood *or* Chicken Breast
	385 31g	**330** 34g	**475** 37g	**520** 40g

Some Chinese restaurants use as much as 4 tablespoons of oil per serving. Since each tablespoon of oil contains 120 calories and 14 grams of fat, the calories may be higher.

Nutritional Information for Chinese Foods

Chinese Foods

	Calories	Fat (g)	Sodium (mg)	Carbs* (g)	Exchanges**
Appetizers:					
Egg Foo Yong, 2 – 1oz patties	220	16	na	7	1V+1½MT+2FAT
Egg Roll, 1-4"	250	15	490	18	¾ST+1V+½MT+2½FAT
Fried Beef or Pork Dumplings, 6	490	27	na	36	2½ST+1½MT+4FAT
Fried Chicken Wing, 1	90	7	na	1	1MT+½FAT
Fried Pork & Shrimp Wonton, 1	45	2	100	3	¼ST+½FAT
Fried Won Ton, 4	340	25	na	16	1ST+1MT+4FAT
Shrimp Balls, 1	172	16	1462	2	1MT+2FAT
Shrimp Toast, 2 small pieces	250	24	220	8	½ST+1MT+4FAT
Spareribs, 3 oz	339	26	80	1	3MT+½FAT
Steamed Vegetable Dumplings, 6	230	5	na	37	2ST+1V+1FAT
Soups (1c):					
Chinese Noodle	210	9	1010	23	1½ST+2FAT
Egg Drop	50	3	1239	2	½MT
Hot and Sour	75	2	920	8	½ST+½FAT
Velvet Corn	165	5	1230	23	1½ST+1FAT
Won Ton w/ 4 won tons	180	8	1701	16	1ST+1MT+½FAT
Beef & Pork Entrees (1 c unless noted):					
Beef *or* Pork w/asparagus, broccoli, cabbage, *or* green peppers	360	28	na	8	1V+3MT+2½FAT
Beef *or* Pork w/cabbage *or* bok choy	395	30	na	7	1V+3MT+3FAT
Cashew Beef	580	49	na	3	4MT+6FAT
Chop Suey, Beef *or* Pork	220	12	na	18	3V+1MT+1½FAT
Chow Mein, Beef *or* Pork	345	17	na	32	1ST+3V+1MT+2½FAT
Mongolian Beef w/green onions & rice noodles	375	24	na	17	1ST+2MT+3FAT
Oriental Noodles w/beef *or* pork & sauce	385	25	na	18	1ST+2MT+3FAT
Pepper Steak, 4 oz	340	21	na	2	4MT
Pork in Hoisin Sauce	450	30	na	17	1CHO+4MT+2FAT
Shredded Pork w/Garlic or Peking Sauce	390	18	na	8	½CHO+4MT
Stir-fried Beef w/peppers, onions, mushrooms, & snow peas	315	24	na	12	2V+2MT+3FAT
Stir-fried Beef *or* Pork w/vegetables	315	24	na	13	2V+2MT+3FAT
Szechuan Beef *or* Pork	400	28	na	1	4MT+2FAT
Sweet & Sour Beef *or* Pork	525	35	na	17	4MT+1CHO+3FAT
Twice Cooked Pork	420	29	na	0	4MT+2FAT

*Carbs=Carbohydrate, na=not available   **Exchanges: ST=Starch, Mlk=Milk (skim)
FR=Fruit, CHO=Other Carbohydrates, V=Vegetable, MT=Meat (medium fat), FAT=Fat

Chinese Foods (continued)

Chicken Entrees (1 c unless noted):

	Calories	Fat (g)	Sodium (mg)	Carbs* (g)	Exchanges**
Almond *or* Cashew Chicken	495	40	na	5	4MT+4FAT
Chicken & Snow Peas	200	17	na	7	1V+2MT+1½FAT
Chicken Chop Suey	180	9	na	12	2V+1MT+1FAT
Chicken Chow Mein	290	14	na	18	½ST+2V+1MT+2FAT
Chicken Teriyaki, 1 quarter	335	16	na	6	½CHO+4MT
Kung Pao Chicken	520	45	na	5	4MT+5FAT
Lemon Chicken	675	44	na	19	1½CHO+4MT+5FAT
Moo Goo Gai Pan	190	9	na	9	2V+2MT
Noodles w/chicken & vegetables in Szechuan sauce	290	17	na	21	1ST+1V+1MT+2½FAT
Stir-fried Chicken w/vegetables	220	17	na	7	1V+2MT+1FAT
Sweet & Sour Chicken	550	39	na	16	1CHO+4MT+4FAT

Fish & Shellfish (1 c unless noted):

	Calories	Fat (g)	Sodium (mg)	Carbs* (g)	Exchanges**
Chinese Fried Shrimp, 6 oz	540	30	na	16	1ST+6MT
Shrimp Chop Suey	180	10	na	11	2V+1MT+1FAT
Shrimp Chow Mein	305	15	na	18	½ST+2V+1MT+2FAT
Shrimp w/cashews	460	38	na	5	4MT+3½FAT
Shrimp w/Snow Peas	165	17	na	7	1V+2MT+1½FAT
Sweet & Sour Shrimp	495	38	na	16	1CHO+4MT+4FAT
Szechuan noodles w/Chinese cabbage, snow peas & scallops	280	16	na	20	1ST+1V+1MT+2FAT

Vegetable (½ c):

	Calories	Fat (g)	Sodium (mg)	Carbs* (g)	Exchanges**
Bok Choy, oriental style	55	4	na	5	1V+1FAT
Chop Suey, vegetable	44	3	na	4	1V+½FAT
Snow Pea, Mushroom, & Bamboo	40	3	na	5	1V+½FAT
Snow Peas & Water Chestnuts	40	3	na	4	1V+½FAT
Stir-Fried Broccoli	70	5	na	6	1V+1FAT
Stir-Fried String Beans	70	5	na	6	1V+1FAT
Szechuan noodles w/Chinese cabbage & snow peas	195	11	na	19	1ST+½V+2FAT
Szechuan-Style Eggplant	135	11	na	6	1V+2FAT
Tofu, ½ c pieces raw firm	185	11	17	2	2½MT
Tofu, ½ c pieces fried	275	22	17	2	2½MT+2FAT
Water Chestnuts	50	0	6	9	½ST

Rice & Noodles:

	Calories	Fat (g)	Sodium (mg)	Carbs* (g)	Exchanges**
Steamed Rice, 1 c	240	0	400	50	3ST
Fried Rice, 1 c	370	12	900	48	3ST+2½FAT
Crispy Chow Mein Noodles, ½ c	250	11	440	38	2ST+2FAT
Oriental Noodles, ½ c	95	1	na	21	1ST

---

*Carbs=Carbohydrate, na=not available   **Exchanges: ST=Starch, Mlk=Milk (skim)
FR=Fruit, CHO=Other Carbohydrates, V=Vegetable, MT=Meat (medium fat), FAT=Fat

Chinese Foods (continued)

Sauces & Oils (2T unless noted):	Calories	Fat (g)	Sodium (mg)	Carbs* (g)	Exchanges**
Chinese BBQ Sauce	45	0	570	11	¾CHO
Mustard Sauce	60	6	na	0	1FAT
Oil, vegetable 1T	120	13	0	0	2½FAT
Plum or Duck Sauce	60	4	170	6	½CHO+1FAT
Sesame Oil, 1T	120	13	0	0	2½FAT
Sesame Soy Dip, 1T	30	2	na	1	½FAT
Soy Sauce, 1t	3	0	340	0	FREE
Soy Sauce, reduced sodium, 1t	3	0	170	0	FREE
Sweet and Sour Sauce	55	0	70	14	1CHO
Teriyaki Sauce, 1T	15	0	610	0	FREE
Teriyaki Sauce, reduced sodium, 1T	15	0	320	0	FREE
Worcestershire Sauce, 1T	10	0	235	0	FREE
Beverage:					
Tea, 1 c	0	0	0	0	FREE
Desserts:					
Fortune Cookie, 1	30	0	na	7	½CHO
Lychee, fruit/syrup, ½ c	60	0	na	15	1FR

Indian Restaurants

Chapter Contents:

■ Appetizers & Soups
■ Entrees
■ Breads
■ Accompaniments

Indian restaurants use some of the same ingredients as the Middle Eastern countries including rice, yogurt, onions, tomatoes, eggplant, legumes, and lamb. But Indian food more closely resembles the cuisine from Thailand because of the commonality of spices and curries. Spices used in Indian cooking includes: cardamon, cinnamon, clove, coriander, cumin, fennel, mint, saffron, and tumeric.

The many religions practiced in this country play a role in what is served in the particular regions of India. Many Buddhists practice vegetarianism. Moslems avoid pork and pork products while Hindus do not eat beef.

Restaurants in the United States serve food from all over India. South Indian cuisine is hotter than foods from the northern part of India. Chilies, peppers, and hot pickles are more common. Rice, seafood, and chutney are served frequently. The Northern region's food is milder and uses more wheat products.

Sesame oil and coconut oil are the fats commonly used in Indian cuisine. While sesame oil is an unsaturated fat, coconut oil is a highly saturated (unhealthy) fat. Ask which fat is being used before you make your selection.

Curries are often made with very high fat coconut milk but can also be prepared without. Yogurt is used in most recipes; typically whole milk is the norm, but low fat is becoming more popular.

Appetizers & Soups

✓ **Choose these lower fat starters to your meal:**

■ **Allu Chat** – appetizer of diced potatoes, chopped tomatoes, cucumber, and little or no oil

■ **Dahl Rasam** – pepper soup with lentils

■ **Mulligatawny** – lentil & vegetable soup

■ **Vegetable Salad** – usually dressing is on the side

✓ **Limit the amount of these fried appetizers:**

■ **Samosa** – vegetable turnover, stuffed & fried

■ **Papadum** – fried, crispy, thin lentil wafers served with dipping sauces

■ **Cheese** *or* **Chicken Pakoras** – deep fried, homemade cheese or chicken

Entrees

✓ **Ask for the meats to be sautéed in very little oil** or ghee (clarified butter).

✓ **Request curries to be prepared without coconut milk or cream**. Curry sauce is prepared by first sautéing onions in oil; yogurt and spices are then added. The addition of coconut milk or cream can be left off, if requested.

✓ **Split an entrée with a friend.** The tandori chicken is usually an 8 oz portion.

✓ **Plain rice comes with most entrées.** There's no need to order seperately.

✓ **Choose these lower fat entrées:**

■ **Aloo Chole** – chick peas cooked with tomatoes and potatoes

■ **Chicken** *or* **Shrimp Tandoori** – chicken or shrimp marinated in spices & yogurt and roasted in a tandoor (clay oven)

■ **Chicken** *or* **Fish Tikka** – roasted in an oven with mild spices

■ **Chicken, Fish,** *or* **Beef Vandaloo** – cooked with potatoes and hot spices

■ **Chicken** *or* **Fish Masala** – cooked with spices and a thick curry sauce made of yogurt

■ **Kebobs** – chunks of meat (preferably chicken) and vegetables cooked on a skewer. Request without the butter for basting.

■ **Shrimp** *or* **Lamb Bhuna** – cooked with onions and tomatoes

■ **Chicken** *or* **Lamb Saag** – cooked with spinach in a spicy curry sauce. Ask for without coconut milk or cream

- **Vegetable Curry** – ask for it without coconut milk or cream
- **Paneer** – homemade "cottage cheese." Ask for the high fat sauces to be served on the side.

✓ **Limit these higher fat entrees:**

- **Chicken Kandhari** – cooked with cream sauce and cashews
- **Shrimp Mali** - cooked with cream and coconut
- **Beef or Vegetable Korma** – curry cooked with cream

Breads

✓ **Ask for these low fat breads:**

- **Chapati** – thin, dry whole wheat bread
- **Nan** – leavened baked bread
- **Tandori roti** – unleavened bread similar to pita bread

✓ **Limit these higher fat breads:**

- **Poori** – light, puffed bread
- **Paratha** – fried bread, may be stuffed with potatoes or meats

Accompaniments

✓ **Select these low fat accompaniments:**

- **Biryani** – rice dish that contains chicken, shrimp, or beef, along with vegetables and dried fruit
- **Chutney** – usually mango or onion chutney
- **Dahi** – plain, unflavored yogurt
- **Pullao** – basmati rice, an aromatic long grain rice. Pullao is low fat when cooked plain; the fat content increases when cooked along with meat, nuts, paneer, or vegetables such as peas.
- **Raita** – yogurt with grated cucumbers, onions, and spices

✓ **Limit these higher fat accompaniments:**

- **Dahl** – lentil-based, spicy sauce

Italian Restaurants

Chapter Contents:

■ Appetizers, Antipasto, & Salads
■ Pasta
■ Meats & Cheese
■ Sauces
■ Nutritional Information for Italian Foods

When we think of Italian foods, the foods that often come to mind are pizza and pasta. For more information on how to order a leaner pizza refer to the *Pizza* chapter.

A moderate portion of pasta, by itself, is low in fat and relatively low in calories. Additions such as sauce, cheese, meats, and oil determine if a meal remains low fat.

Olive oil is one of the most common staples in Italian cooking. It is often considered a healthy fat because it contains no cholesterol and is high in monounsaturated fats. Keep in mind that, like other oils, it still has 120 calories per tablespoon. To eat lean in an Italian restaurant, avoid excessive amounts of meat, cheese, fried foods or those foods that have liberal amounts of oil added.

Appetizers, Antipasto, & Salads

✓ **Consider squid, mussels, or clams in a herb wine sauce.** Stay away from fried appetizers such as fried eggplant and fried cheese.

✓ **Inquire as to what comes with appetizers of Carpaccio or Prosciutto ham**. These thin slices of beef, fish, or ham are very high in fat but are often served in small portions. Refer to the *Entrees & Sauces* chapter for nutritional information. If these offerings are a must, enjoy them instead of a meat entrée and ask for the Carpaccio or Prosciutto to be served with vegetables or fruit such as melon. Often drizzled with olive oil or served with mayonnaise, this plate is lower in fat if eaten plain or with lemon juice.

✓ **Minestrone and Bean Soups are often prepared low fat** and are a good way to fill up prior to a meal.

Soups Satisfy:	Calories	Fat (g)
Minestrone Soup, 8 oz *or*	95	3
Bean Soup, 8 oz	180	6

✓ **Request Bruschetta to be prepared with very little oil.** This oil-ladened toast is best enjoyed in small quantities. The same advice is appropriate when restaurants offer you bread with a dish of oil for dipping - use little or no oil and keep your bread portion minimal.

Bruschetta can be Modified:	Calories	Fat (g)
1 oz Bread + 1T oil	198	15
1 oz Bread + 1t oil	118	6
Savings:	80	9

✓ **Order a vegetable salad with balsamic vinegar** or with the salad dressing on the side. Caesar salad is best avoided because of its high fat ingredients including eggs, Parmesan cheese, and Italian dressing.

✓ **Watch the high fat additions of olives, pine nuts, cheese, and oil.** Whenever possible, ask for your meal to be prepared without these ingredients or in limited amounts.

These Foods can Quickly Add Calories to Your Meal:	Calories	Fat (g)
Parmesan or Romano Cheese, 2T	46	3
Olive Oil, 1T	120	14
Pine Nuts, 1 oz *or* small handful	161	17
Olives, 6 super Colossal ripe	78	7

Pasta

✓ **Pasta noodles, made of mostly flour and water, are very low in fat**. Freshly prepared pasta noodles may have eggs as an added ingredient. This will add about 50 mg of cholesterol per cup and a few grams of fat. Some restaurants offer dried pastas, made without egg, for patrons who are closely monitoring their cholesterol.

✓ **Each half cup portion of pasta has only 100 calories** but serving sizes are often 2 cups. Frequently, appetizer portions can be ordered instead of a large entree portion; or you can request a doggie bag. This is what a half cup portion of spaghetti looks like.

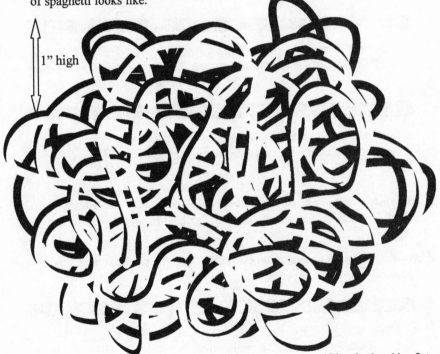

1" high

½ c plain pasta = 100 calories, ½ g fat

✓ **Here's a description of the most common pastas:**

■ **Straight (thinnest to widest):** Capellini (Angel hair), Vermicelli, Spaghetti, Linguine, Fettuccine, Lasagna

■ **Tubular:** Mostaccioli, Penne, Rigatoni, Ziti, Cannelloni (stuffed), Manicotti (stuffed)

■ **Other Shapes:** Capellitti (little hats), Farfalle (bowties), Fusilli (long pasta which is spiral shaped), Gnocchi (little dumplings), Ravioli (stuffed & usually square), Rotelle (corkscrew spirals), Shells

Meats & Cheese

✓ **Chicken, seafood, and veal are the leanest "meats" as long as they are not fried.** Pancetta (Italian bacon) and sausage are best avoided due to their high fat content.

✓ **Request for the meat to be steamed or grilled** instead of sautéed or fried even if the menu suggests otherwise. Nutritional information for a variety of meats can be found in the *Entrees & Sauces* chapter.

✓ **Choose "pasta with meat" rather than an entrée serving of meat.** In addition, choose a low fat sauce such as a tomato sauce.

Go with the Pasta:	Calories	Fat (g)
8 oz Beef Entrée + 1 c pasta w/tomato sauce	1090	71
2 c Pasta w/ 2 oz beef in tomato sauce	780	30
Savings:	**310**	**41**

But Don't Blow It with a High Fat Sauce:	Calories	Fat (g)
2 c Pasta w/ 2 oz beef in Alfredo sauce	1380	91
2 c Pasta w/ 2 oz beef in tomato sauce	780	30
Savings:	**600**	**61**

✓ **Also, ask that "no oil" be added to the preparation of the "meats"**; wine or broth can often be substituted. Request that the skin be removed from the poultry dishes.

✓ **Avoid dishes with excessive cheese.** Instead of pasta stuffed with cheese, choose pasta with a sprinkling of cheese.

Cheese is as Fattening as Fried Chicken:	Calories	Fat (g)
Manicotti, 2 stuffed	695	42
1½ c Pasta Primavera w/3T grated cheese	360	10
Savings:	**335**	**32**

✓ **Look for partially skimmed cheeses.** Occasionally, you may find dishes prepared with partially skimmed cheeses. While lower in fat, they are not fat-free.

Partially Skimmed Cheeses are a Better Choice:	Calories	Fat (g)
Ricotta Cheese, ½ c	215	16
Ricotta Cheese, part skim, ½ c	170	10
Savings:	**45**	**6**

✓ **Avoid Parmigiana meals.** Parmigiana refers to food that is floured, fried, and topped with a marinara sauce and cheese. These dishes are very high in fat whether made from chicken, veal, or eggplant. Instead, you can request the meat to be *grilled* and topped with a marinara sauce and cheese. Or consider ordering an appetizer (or luncheon) portion of your favorite parmigiana instead of the entrée portion. This option is often available even if it is not suggested on the menu.

Sauces

✓ **Ask for a lower calorie/fat sauce.** Even if the menu states a particular sauce you can always substitute a healthier sauce.

✓ **If you want the higher fat sauce, ask them to put on less or request the sauce to be served on the side.**

✓ **Order Pasta Primavera (pasta with vegetables) prepared with a tomato sauce or *very little* oil** instead of the typical butter or Alfredo sauce.

✓ **When ordering a side order of pasta, consider asking for no sauce to be added.** Use the sauce from the meat entrée to mix with the pasta instead.

✓ **Know your sauces:**

■ **Alfredo Sauce** - a very high fat cream sauce prepared with butter, heavy cream and parmesan cheese.

■ **Bolognese Sauce** - a cream or tomato-based sauce with a variety of meats, vegetables, and wine added.

■ **Carbonara Sauce** - made with butter, eggs, bacon, sausage, parmesan cheese, and cream.

■ **Meat Sauce** - a tomato sauce with added ground beef or sausage. Calories and fat grams are dependent upon the amount of meat added; sausage is higher in calories and fat than ground beef.

■ **Pesto Sauce** - a very high fat sauce prepared from fresh basil, pine nuts, parmesan cheese, and oil. If you want a dish prepared with pesto – request that it be prepared with "just a little."

■ **Red Clam Sauce** - consists of oil, tomatoes, and clams.

■ **Tomato Sauces** (such as marinara, spicy marinara, and pomodori) are typically the lowest fat sauces. Caution: creamy tomato sauce is much higher in fat and calories.

■ **White Clam Sauce** (Vongole) - made of butter, oil, white wine and clams.

✓ **Hold the oil**. Upscale Italian restaurants offer dishes of pasta combined with a variety of meat, chicken, seafood, and/or vegetables. These combinations are generally mixed with a creamy sauce or lots of oil - and loaded in calories. To make the dish lighter, ask for two things. Request the chef to use broth instead of oil to saute the mixings. Then, ask for a tomato sauce, "very little oil", or just half the usual amount of creamy sauce.

Consider the Difference:

	Calories	Fat (g)
2 c Pasta combined w/shrimp, prosciutto, peas, & tomatoes, in a cream sauce	1470	87
Above prepared with a tomato sauce instead	850	22
Savings:	**620**	**65**

Pasta Calorimeter: Calories & Fat per serving

Pasta with:	Calories & Fat (g) per serving		
	¾ c side dish	1½ c luncheon	2 c dinner
Tomato sauce	220 5g	435 9g	580 12g
Red Clam sauce	240 7g	480 14g	640 18g
Bolognese sauce	250 5g	495 11g	660 14g
White Clam sauce	285 8g	570 15g	760 20g
Meat sauce	355 14g	710 27g	945 36g
Pesto sauce	370 21g	743 42g	990 56g
Creamy Tomato sauce	390 20g	775 41g	1030 54g
Alfredo sauce	450 29g	900 58g	1200 77g
Carbonara sauce	480 29g	965 58g	1280 77g

Nutritional Information for Italian Foods

Italian Food

	Calories	Fat (g)	Sodium (mg)	Carbos* (g)	Exchanges**
Entrees:					
Cannelloni Florentine (4 noodles stuffed w/veal, spinach, beef)	450	27	na	33	2ST+2MT+3FAT
Chicken Cacciatore (6 *oz w/out skin*), w/sauce	585	33	na	26	4V+6MT+1FAT
Chicken Parmesan, 6 oz w/sauce	675	43	na	28	1ST+2V+6MT+2FAT
Chicken Saltimbocca (5 oz chicken + 1 oz prosciutto)	747	52	585	4	6MT+4FAT
Chicken Scaloppini, 6 oz	582	34	250	1	6MT+1FAT
w/ 3T Lemon Butter Sauce	845	63	625	5	6MT+6FAT
Chicken Tetrazzini, 1 c	425	21	na	31	1½ST+1V+2MT+2FAT
Eggplant Parmesan, 3" X 4"	340	22	1180	29	1ST+2V+1MT+2FAT
Fettuccine Alfredo, 1½ c	900	58	370	48	5ST+10FAT
Lasagna, traditional, 3"X3" square	390	16	1020	37	2ST+2V+2MT+1FAT
w/meat & cream sauce, 3"X4" sq	685	45	538	32	2ST+3MT+6FAT
Manicotti, 2 stuffed	695	42	1835	36	2ST+1V+5MT+3FAT
Ravioli, Cheese, 1 c	340	10	220	37	2½ST+1MT+1FAT
w/red sauce	430	15	490	43	2½ST+1V+1MT+2FAT
w/Alfredo sauce	740	48	1180	63	4ST+2½MT+7FAT
Ravioli, Beef or Chicken, 1 c	280	9	350	38	2½ST+1MT
w/red sauce	370	14	620	44	2½ST+1V+1MT+1FAT
w/Alfredo sauce	680	47	1310	61	3½ST+2½MT+7FAT
Tortellini, meat & cheese, 1 c	450	11	560	53	3½ST+1½MT
w/red sauce	540	16	830	57	3½ST+1V+1½MT+ 1FAT
w/Alfredo sauce	840	48	1520	77	5ST+3MT+5FAT
Veal Scaloppini, 6 oz cooked	700	50	300	2	6MT+4FAT
w/ 3T Lemon Butter Sauce	964	79	675	3	6MT+10FAT
Veal Saltimbocca, 5 oz veal + 1 oz prosciutto	650	42	600	2	6MT+2½FAT
Sauces for Entrees (2T):					
Butter Wine Sauce	140	14	140	0	3FAT
Cream Sauce, thin	50	4	180	1	1FAT
Cream Sauce, thick	108	12	50	1	2½FAT
Lemon Butter Sauce	175	19	250	2	4FAT
Meuneire Sauce	130	14	510	2	3FAT
Tomato Sauce	23	1	190	4	1V
Pasta:					
Pasta, no sauce or oil, ½ c	100	0.⁵	2	19	1¼ST
Pasta, no sauce or oil, 1 c	200	1	4	39	2½ST
Pasta Primavera, 1 c pasta + vegetables in very light oil	290	5	50	36	2ST+1V+1FAT
Pasta Primavera, 1 c pasta + vegetables in tomato sauce	300	6	270	41	2ST+2V+1FAT

*Carbs=Carbohydrate, na=not available   **Exchanges: ST=Starch, Mlk=Milk (skim) FR=Fruit, CHO=Other Carbohydrates, V=Vegetable, MT=Meat (medium fat), FAT=Fat

Italian Food (continued)

Pasta continued:	Calories	Fat (g)	Sodium (mg)	Carbos* (g)	Exchanges**
Pasta Primavera, 1 c pasta + vegetables in Alfredo sauce	530	32	1080	55	3ST+1V+1MT+5FAT
Pasta Puttanesca, 1 c pasta + sauce	388	16	910	37	2½ST+1V+3FAT

Accompaniments:

	Calories	Fat (g)	Sodium (mg)	Carbos* (g)	Exchanges**
Gnocchi Dumplings, 2 small	80	1	na	17	1ST
Meatballs, 1 @ 2" diameter	80	6	na	3	1MT
Polenta, 2½" X 4" piece	120	0	180	33	2ST
Fried Polenta, 2" X 2½" X ½"	90	4	130	18	1ST+1FAT
Polenta Pasticciata, w/sauce	375	23	470	32	2ST+4FAT
Prosciutto, Italian ham, 1 oz	80	6	na	0	1MT
Risotto w/ butter, ½ c	170	5	280	24	1½ST+1FAT
Roasted Potatoes, ½ c	155	7	na	16	1ST+1½FAT

Cheeses:

	Calories	Fat (g)	Sodium (mg)	Carbos* (g)	Exchanges**
Ricotta Cheese, ½ c	215	16	104	4	2MT+1FAT
Ricotta Cheese, part skim, ½ c	170	10	155	6	2MT
Parmesan or Romano Cheese, 1T	23	1.⁵	93	0	¼MT
Mozzarella, 1 oz	90	7	106	0	1MT+½FAT
Part skim, 1 oz	72	4.⁵	132	0	1MT
Feta Cheese, 1 oz	75	6	316	1	1MT
Cream Cheese, 1 oz (2T)	100	10	84	0	2FAT
Light, 1 oz (2T)	62	4.⁷	160	1	1FAT

Sauces (½ c):

	Calories	Fat (g)	Sodium (mg)	Carbos* (g)	Exchanges**
Alfredo Sauce	300	28	720	16	1ST+1MT+4FAT
Bolognese Sauce, cream-based	200	14	180	6	1V+1½MT+1½FAT
Bolognese Sauce, tomato-based	130	6	585	12	2V+1MT
Carbonara Sauce	330	28	770	0	2MT+2½FAT
Creamy Tomato Sauce	210	17	313	5	1V+1MT+2FAT
Marinara Sauce	85	4	750	8	1V+1FAT
Meat Sauce (little meat)	160	10	290	4	1V+½MT+1½FAT
Meat Sauce (chunky w/meat)	250	16	300	4	1V+1MT+2FAT
Pesto Sauce	600	60	880	0	1MT+10FAT
Pomodoro (Tomato Sauce)	90	5	270	11	2V+1FAT
Puttanesca (tomatoes & anchovies)	126	10	605	10	2V+2FAT
Red Clam Sauce	110	8	240	6	1V+½MT+1FAT
Spinach, Mushrooms, & Cream	190	19	160	5	1V+4FAT
White Clam Sauce	180	9	510	5	¼ST+1MT+1FAT

Desserts:

	Calories	Fat (g)	Sodium (mg)	Carbos* (g)	Exchanges**
Stuffed Cannoli, 1, 4"	315	19	70	32	2CHO+4FAT
Pirouline, 3 thin rolled cookies	150	7	25	23	1½CHO+1½FAT
Fruit Sorbet, ½ c	120	0	0	31	2CHO

---

*Carbs=Carbohydrate, na=not available   **Exchanges: ST=Starch, Mlk=Milk (skim)
FR=Fruit, CHO=Other Carbohydrates, V=Vegetable, MT=Meat (medium fat), FAT=Fat

Mexican Restaurants

Chapter Contents:

■ Appetizers
■ Soups
■ Salads
■ Entrees
■ Accompaniments
■ Dessert
■ Nutritional Information for Mexican Foods

If you like hot, spicy foods, Mexican restaurants may top your list of favorite ethnic cuisines. Common foods served in Mexican restaurants include beans, rice, tortillas as well as tomatoes, onions, salsa, and jalapeño peppers. Most people think that Mexican restaurants are definitely off the list when watching their fat intake. However, there are lean choices available.

Appetizers

✓ **Ask for baked chips**. Few restaurants serve baked chips when you are seated, but may prepare them upon request.

Baked is Better:		Calories	Fat (g)
Restaurant Style Tortilla Chips, 20		460	20
Baked Tortilla Chips, 20		240	2.5
	Savings:	**220**	**17.5**

✓ **Move the fried chips**. Count out the chips you have allotted yourself and then ask the server to remove the rest. Or move the chips out of your reach.

✓ **Ask for regular corn tortillas.** Some patrons ask for regular corn tortillas for dipping into the salsa. Try it! There's no crunch but plenty of flavor.

✓ **Enjoy the salsa.** Salsa and pico de gallo are made with little or no fat added and can be used freely.

✓ **Share the nachos with everyone.** Don't make nachos your meal. Instead, have just a few. Chips are high in fats and calories; so are all the nacho toppings.

Nachos are High Calorie – Even Just Six:	Calories	Fat (g)
Tortilla Chips, 6 large	130	6
Cheese, 2T	120	10
Refried Beans, ¼ c	125	7
Guacamole, 2T	55	3
Sour Cream, 2T	50	5
TOTAL:	**480**	**31**

✓ **Enjoy ceviche as an entrée.** Ceviche is fish "cooked" with lemons or limes and onions and jalapeno – not with heat. It's low fat and low calorie.

Soups

✓ **Ask about the tortilla soup.** Tortilla soup is often prepared from a simple low fat vegetable soup. The added bacon, cheese, avocado, and strips of fried tortilla is what contributes most of the calories and fat; some or all of these components can often be omitted.

Tortilla Soup:	Calories	Fat (g)
Vegetables in a broth	70	2
Cheese, 1T	60	5
Chicken, ½ oz	30	1
Avocado, 1/8	40	4
Tortilla Strips	40	2
TOTAL:	**240**	**14**

✓ **Have Black Bean soup.** This is often prepared with less fat than pinto beans.

✓ **Enjoy chili (made with beans)** rather than chili con carne (beans with meat). Ask what toppings are added such as sour cream and cheese; you can ask for them to be omitted.

Salads

✓ **Ask what's in the salad.** While lettuce and tomato are low in fat, most other additions are not. Ask yourself what components (such as cheese, sour cream, or avocado) you can do without.

✓ **Select the chicken fajita salad** over the beef fajita salad. These are both healthier options than the taco salad, which is prepared with ground beef.

✓ **Use the picante sauce or pico de gallo for a low calorie and spicy dressing**. If you want to tone down the spiciness, try mixing sour cream and picante sauce for a dressing with less than 20 calories per tablespoon.

✓ **Don't eat the shell**. Taco salads and fajita salads are often served in a fried flour tortilla shell. It's tempting to nibble away at the shell. Request that the salad be served on a plate for a savings of hundreds of calories.

On a Plate, Please:	Calories	Fat (g)
Taco Salad	930	69
Taco Salad without the Shell	<u>510</u>	<u>39</u>
Savings:	**420**	**30**

Entrees

✓ **Order ala carte**. Instead of ordering a complete meal, order only the items that you really want. Chicken fajitas or chicken tacos al carbon can be ordered individually in most restaurants as a lean entrée. Both selections will have 1-2 oz of meat in each taco. Request lettuce, tomatoes, and onions for a filling meal.

✓ **Ask for high calorie items to be left off the plate** – especially if you tend to eat them just because they are there, rather than because you like them. The higher calorie accompaniments include refried beans, Mexican rice, guacamole, sour cream, and cheese. Keep to lettuce, tomato, onion, salsa, and pico de gallo.

Eat it Plain:	Calories	Fat (g)
Beef Fajita: 2-6½" flour tortillas, 3 oz meat, ¼ avocado, 2T sour cream & 2T shredded cheese	600	36
Beef Fajita: 2-6½" flour tortillas, 3 oz meat, shredded, lettuce, tomato, onion	<u>415</u>	<u>19</u>
Savings:	**185**	**17**

✓ **Trim the meat.** This extra step will save at least 20 calories an ounce. That's more than 100 calories in a typical serving!

✓ **Choose chicken or fish over beef, beef over cheese.** Beef steak or strips are twice as fattening as chicken pieces, shrimp, or fish. Cheese or ground beef is three times more fatting.

✓ **Choose menu items prepared with soft tortillas rather than crispy.** Crispy tortillas have been fried and are, therefore, higher in fat and calories than the plain corn or flour tortilla.

✓ **Ask that the fajitas be prepared with very little oil.** Fajitas are often brushed with oil prior to serving and served with sautéed (oil) green peppers and onions. Now you know why it sizzles on your way to the table! Ask for the fajitas without the usual brushing. Also, try your fajitas with *raw* peppers and onions instead - very flavorful and crunchy!

✓ **Request these lower calorie entrees (preferably with chicken, fish, or shrimp):**

- **Fajitas** – marinated and grilled beef, chicken, or shrimp.

- **Tacos al carbon** *or* **Soft Taco**– Chicken or beef fajita strips wrapped in a flour tortilla.

- **Soft Burritos** – Non-fried large flour tortilla wrapped around chicken or beef fajitas.

- **Chicken Enchiladas**, corn tortillas dipped in hot oil, filled with chicken, and then rolled. Baked with a red or green tomato-based enchilada sauce. These can be requested without the cheese sauce topping.

- **Camarones de Hacha** – shrimp sautéed in red or green tomato sauce.

- **Arroz con Pollo** – boneless chicken breast served with Mexican rice.

✓ **Limit the higher calorie entrees:**

- **Chalupas** *or* **Tostadas** - flat, fried corn tortilla topped with beans, meat, and/or cheese.

- **Chimichanga or Fried Burrito** - flour tortilla filled with beef, chicken, cheese and/or beans and then deep-fried. This is often covered with a picante or cheese sauce.

- **Beef or Cheese Enchiladas** - corn tortillas dipped in hot oil and then rolled with cheese, or beef. These are generally served with a red or green tomato-based enchilada sauce.

- **Flauta con crema** – crisp tortillas stuffed with beef or chicken and covered with a cream sauce.

- **Chicken or Beef Mole** – chicken or beef cooked with mole (a high fat, high calorie sauce).

- **Tacos** - fried corn tortillas filled with chicken, beef, beans, and/or cheese.

- **Tamale** – corn husks spread with maize and covered with shredded beef, chicken, or pork. These are rolled up and cooked.

- **Chili Rellenos** – peppers that are stuffed, breaded, and then fried.

Accompaniments

✓ **Choose corn tortillas over flour tortillas**. Tortillas are great tasting when they are freshly made. While many restaurants make their own flour tortillas, few restaurants prepare corn tortillas fresh. If you think you don't like the taste of corn tortillas, find a restaurant that makes their own. You just might like them better than the higher calorie flour tortillas.

Corn Tortillas are lower in Fat & Calories:	Calories	Fat (g)
Flour Tortilla	110	3
Corn Tortilla	70	$0.^5$
Savings:	40	$2.^5$

✓ **Decide how many tortillas fit into your calorie and fat budget**. Plan ahead and you won't blow it!

✓ **Be selective with the accompaniments**. Many of us eat chips, rice, beans, *and* tortillas. This can add up to a very high fat and high caloric meal. Which of these accompaniments do you really enjoy and which do you eat simply because they are there?

✓ **Ask for cooked pinto or black beans instead of refried beans**. You may see the cooked beans listed on the menu as bean soup, Beans ala charra, or borracho beans. These are usually prepared with bacon or other fat. For that reason, it is best to eat the beans and leave the broth and added fat in the bowl. Every restaurant prepares their refried beans differently. They can be prepared with little fat or quite a bit of fat. You can't tell the difference by simply looking at it. Since most restaurants use lard, it is best to avoid the refried beans.

Dessert

✓ **Flan is a healthier choice than sopappillas**. Flan, a baked custard made with egg and whole milk, is usually served in a small portion. Sopapillas, fried flour dough sprinkled with sugar and cinnamon, are best shared with friends.

Nutritional Information for Mexican Foods

Mexican Foods	Calories	Fat (g)	Sodium (mg)	Carbos* (g)	Exchanges**
Appetizers:					
Tortilla Chip, 1 large	23	1	15	4	¼ST
5 Tortilla Chips	125	5.^{8}	65	18	1ST+1FAT
5 Baked Chips	75	1	65	17	1ST
Tortilla Chip, 1 regular size	18	0.^{8}	8	3	¼ST
5 Tortilla Chips	90	4	40	14	¾ST+1FAT
5 Baked Chips	60	0.^{6}	40	14	¾ST
Nacho w/Cheese only, 1 chip	42	2.^{5}	35	3	¼ST+¼MT+¼FAT
w/Bean & Cheese, 1 chip	80	5	105	4	¼ST+¼MT+¾FAT
w/Bean, Meat & Cheese, 1 chip	115	8	200	4	¼ST+½MT+1FAT
Ceviche, 4 oz	150	5	na	0	4MT(lean)
Soups (1c):					
Tortilla Soup	240	14	840	10	1V+¾ST+½MT+2FAT
Gazpacho Soup	90	2	475	12	2V+½FAT
Black Bean Soup	180	4	1000	25	1½ST+1MT
Chili (beans only)	190	6	860	26	1½ST+1MT
Chili con Carne	300	13	1080	3	1ST+1V+2MT+½FAT
Salads w/ 2 oz meat (w/out fried bowl *or* dressing):					
Taco Salad, w/chili meat	510	39	na	12	2V+3MT+5FAT
Chicken Taco Salad	400	29	850	11	2V+3MT+ 2½FAT
Chicken Fajita Salad	350	22	na	11	2V+3MT+1½FAT
Beef Fajita Salad	440	31	na	12	2V+3MT+3FAT
Fried Taco Shell Bowl only	420	30	250	32	2ST+6FAT

To estimate tortilla size, note this book is 5½" wide by 8½" high.

Corn Tortillas:	Calories	Fat (g)	Sodium (mg)	Carbos* (g)	Exchanges**
Corn Tortilla, 5" diameter	50	0.^{5}	30	12	¾ST
Tostada Chip, crispy, 4½" diameter	50	1	50	10	½ST
Taco Shell, crispy, small	50	2	70	10	½ST+½FAT
Taco Shell, crispy, large	100	6	130	13	1ST+1FAT
Flour Tortillas:					
Flour Tortilla, 6½" diameter	100	3	200	15	1ST+½FAT
Flour Tortilla, 8"	150	5	350	22	1½ST+1FAT
Flour Tortilla, 10"	250	8	450	32	2ST+1½FAT
Fried Flour Tortilla, 8"	220	11	350	22	1½ST+2FAT
Fried Flour Tortilla, 10"	325	16	450	32	2ST+3FAT
Rice & Beans (½ c):					
Mexican Rice	150	4	550	24	1½ST+1FAT
Refried Beans	250	13	325	27	1ST+2½FAT

*Carbs=Carbohydrate, na=not available **Exchanges: ST=Starch, Mlk=Milk (skim) FR=Fruit, CHO=Other Carbohydrates, V=Vegetable, MT=Meat (medium fat), FAT=Fat

Mexican Foods (continued)

	Calories	Fat (g)	Sodium (mg)	Carbos* (g)	Exchanges**
Rice & Beans (½ c) continued:					
Beans, cooked whole, drained	120	3	350	20	1ST+½FAT
Black Beans, whole	120	2	250	20	1ST+½FAT
Toppings:					
Avocado, ¼	78	8	5	3	1½FAT
Avocado, ⅛ slice	40	4	3	1	1FAT
Avocado + Salsa Verde, 2T	35	3	180	4	½V+½FAT
Cheddar Cheese, ¼ c	120	10	176	0	2MT
Cheddar Cheese, 2T not packed	57	5	88	0	1MT
Enchilada Sauce (red or green), 2T	15	0.8	130	3	FREE
Cheese Sauce (Queso), 2T	100	8	580	1	½MT+1FAT
Guacamole, ¼ c	110	10	420	3	2FAT
Hot Sauce, 1t	0	0	20	0	FREE
Jalapeño, 1	20	0	3	3	FREE
Mole Sauce, 2T	200	13	480	16	1CHO+2½FAT
Olives, ea	5	0	30	<1	FREE
Picante Sauce, 2T	10	0	220	2	2T=FREE or ½V
Pico de Gallo, 2T	15	1	150	3	2T=FREE or ½V
Salsa Verde (Green Sauce), 2T	10	0	150	2	2T=FREE or ½V
Salsa, 2T	10	0	150	2	2T=FREE or ½V
Sour Cream, 2 T	52	5	12	<1	1FAT

To estimate meat portions, note that 3 oz meat is the size of a deck of cards.

	Calories	Fat (g)	Sodium (mg)	Carbos* (g)	Exchanges**
Lean Meats (1 oz):					
Chicken Fajita Meat, white	35	2	250	0	1MT(lean)
Chicken Fajita Meat, dark	55	3.5	250	0	1MT
Chicken Breast, marinated & grilled	35	2	150	0	1MT(lean)
Shrimp, marinated & grilled (3)	35	1	200	2	1MT(very lean)
Medium Fat Meats (1 oz):					
Beef Fajita Meat, trimmed	70	4.3	250	0	1MT
High Fat Meats (1 oz):					
Beef Fajita Meat, untrimmed	90	7	250	0	1MT+½FAT
Beef Taco Meat, about ¼ c	90	7	275	0	1MT+½FAT
Cheddar or Jack Cheese, ¼ c loosely packed	110	9	175	0	1MT+1FAT
Chorizo (Mexican sausage)	105	10	250	3	1MT+1FAT

Carbs=Carbohydrate, na=not available   **Exchanges:** ST=Starch, Mlk=Milk (skim) FR=Fruit, CHO=Other Carbohydrates, V=Vegetable, MT=Meat (medium fat), FAT=Fat

Mexican Foods (continued)

Entrees:

	Calories	Fat (g)	Sodium (mg)	Carbos* (g)	Exchanges**
Arroz Con Pollo, 2 c	485	14	1600	46	3ST+1V+3MT
Soft Burritos: Bean & Cheese, 6½"	300	12	850	30	2ST+1MT+1FAT
Bean & Beef Burritos, 1	280	10	820	35	2ST+1MT+1FAT
Chicken Burritos, 1	260	7	730	31	2ST+1MT+½FAT
Chicken Enchiladas, 2	260	11	1110	24	1½ST+3MT
Cheese Enchiladas, 2	480	32	900	24	1½ST+3MT+3FAT
Spinach Enchiladas in cream sauce, 2	806	61	848	51	2½ST+2V+2MT+10FAT
Beef Fajita – 1½ oz trimmed meat in a 6½" flour tortilla	205	9	575	15	1ST+1½MT
Beef Fajita – 2 oz trimmed meat in a 8" flour tortilla	290	14	850	22	1½ST+2MT+1FAT
Chicken Fajita – 1½ oz white meat in a 6½" flour tortilla	160	6	575	15	1ST+1½MT
Chicken Fajita – 2 oz white meat in a 8" flour tortilla	220	9	850	22	1½ST+2MT
Shrimp Fajita – 5 marinated shrimp in a 6½" flour tortilla	160	5	500	15	1ST+1½MT
Shrimp Fajita – 7 marinated shrimp in a 8" flour tortilla	220	7	750	22	1½ST+2MT
Quesadilla, 6½"	430	24	760	30	2ST+2MT+2½FAT
Chicken Quesadilla, 6½"	465	26	1010	30	2ST+3MT+2FAT
Quesadilla, 10"	940	52	1620	64	4ST+4MT+6FAT
Chicken Quesadilla, 10"	950	56	2120	64	4ST+6MT+4FAT
Taco w/beef & cheese, 2 small	395	27	870	20	1ST+3MT+2FAT
Tamales, 4	350	17	500	33	2ST+1MT+2FAT
Taquito filled w/shredded beef, 5	350	12	460	37	2½ST+1MT+1½FAT
Bean & Cheese Tostada, 3 @ 4½"	465	23	630	37	2ST+3MT+1½FAT

Desserts:

	Calories	Fat (g)	Sodium (mg)	Carbos* (g)	Exchanges**
Flan, ½ c w/caramel topping	290	8	110	39	2½CHO+1MT+½FAT
Soppapilla, 1-3" piece	190	10	100	32	1ST+1CHO+2FAT
Honey, 1T	64	0	0	17	1CHO
Fruit Filled Chimichanga fried w/ caramel topping	690	29	600	86	4½CHO+1FR+6FAT

Middle Eastern Restaurants

Chapter Contents:

■ Appetizers & Salads
■ Entrees
■ Accompaniments
■ Desserts
■ Nutritional Information for Middle Eastern Foods

Middle Eastern cuisine includes foods which are native to Greece, Syria, Lebanon, Iran, Iraq, Turkey, Armenia, and surrounding areas. Some of the staples common to this region include eggplant, olives, olive oil, wheat, rice, legumes, yogurt, dates, figs, and lamb. Plain yogurt, a frequent ingredient in sauces and salads, is most commonly homemade with whole milk. Tahini or sesame seed butter (made of crushed sesame seeds, lemon juice, and spices) is a high fat ingredient added to a variety of dishes. Rice is served with most meats.

Frequently used spices are parsley, mint, cilantro, and oregano. The common Indian spices such as cinnamon, coriander, cumin, and ginger are also used. Middle Eastern food is generally healthy food with a few exceptions. Below are some general guidelines for dining lean in Middle Eastern restaurants.

✓ **Avoid fried foods** such as falafel.

✓ **Request "no oil" to be added on top of the dishes.** You may not be able to avoid the olive oil that is frequently used in the preparation of Middle Eastern dishes. But, you can ask for "no oil to be added" on top of the dishes prior to serving.

No Oil, Please:		Calories	Fat (g)
¼ c Hummus with 1T oil		220	18
¼ c Hummus		100	5
	Savings:	**120**	**13**

✓ **Request tomato sauce rather than lemon & butter sauce or cream sauce.**

Appetizers & Salads

✓ **Choose these lower fat starters to your meal:**

- ■ **Hummus** - mashed chick peas. Served with olive oil but can be omitted.

- ■ **Baba Ghanoush** – smoked and mashed eggplant mixed with tahini and spices. Often served with pita bread.

- ■ **Dolma** – Cold, stuffed grape leaves

- ■ **Greek Salad** – Ask to have dressing "on the side"

- ■ **Tabooli** – cracked wheat mixed with parsley, tomatoes, and spicy dressing

- ■ **Lentil Soup** – Soup made with lentils and vegetables

✓ **Limit these higher fat appetizers and salads:**

- ■ **Avgolemono soup** - traditional Greek soup made with chicken broth, rice, vegetables, lemon, and eggs. Enjoy this high fat soup only if lower fat vegetarian (rather than meat) dishes are chosen for the rest of the meal.

- ■ **Falafel** - fried patty consisting of mashed fava beans and chick peas.

- ■ **Fried Calamari** - fried squid

- ■ **Fish Roe Dip**

- ■ **Kasseri Casserole** - fried Kasseri cheese served with lemon & butter sauce

- ■ **Spanikopita** - spinach & feta cheese pie layered with phyllo dough

- ■ **Taramolsalata** - caviar blended with olive oil and lemon juice. Served with pita bread.

Entrees

✓ **Choose chicken rather than beef or lamb** (such as a chicken pita sandwich rather than gyros made with beef and lamb)

✓ **Meat dishes rather than casseroles.** Casseroles are typically prepared with ground meat and have added sauces.

✓ **Ask for the sauces on the side** including the commonly served tzateki sauce. Casseroles are made in advance and, therefore, sauces can't be substituted. Tomato sauces are leaner than the cream sauces.

✓ **Choose these lower fat entrees:**

■ **Chicken in pita bread**

■ **Dolma** - boiled stuffed grape leaves (green leaves of a grape vine stuffed with a rice, meat, and spice mixture).

■ **Lah Me June** - Armenian pizza topped with ground meat, tomatoes, and spices

■ **Kafta** - grilled ground beef with spices

■ **Kibbeh** - cracked wheat, meat, sautéed onions, and pine nuts

■ **Sheik el Mahski** - baked eggplant stuffed with ground lamb, pine nuts, onions, spices, and tomato sauce

■ **Shish Kebobs** - chunks of meat and vegetables cooked on a skewer. Chicken kabobs would be the leanest meat choice. Request without the butter for basting.

■ **Souvlaki** - marinated and grilled fish or chicken. Often served with tzateki sauce

✓ **Limit these higher fat entrees:**

■ **Falafel** - fried patty consisting of mashed fava beans and chick peas

■ **Gyros** - beef and lamb cut thin and stuffed into a pita pocket or other bread. Ask for the tzateki dressing, a spicy yogurt-based sauce, to be served on the side.

■ **Moussaka** - a casserole of layered eggplant, lamb, and cheese topped with a white sauce

■ **Spanikopita** - spinach and feta cheese pie made with phyllo dough

■ **Pasticchio** - baked macaroni with ground beef and eggs, topped with a creamy sauce

■ **Fried Kalamari** - squid

■ **Omelets** - 3 eggs combined with feta cheese, sausage and/or other meat

■ **Loukanika** - sausage

Accompaniments

✓ **Choose these low fat accompaniments:**

■ **Pita bread** - a flat round bread with a hollow center that is low in fat. It is eaten as an accompaniment to a meat or stuffed as a sandwich. Be aware, pita bread is sometimes served buttered and grilled; this would be much higher in fat.

■ **Couscous** - cooked cracked wheat

■ **Steamed rice**

■ **Rice pilaf** - a cooked rice dish made with sautéed vegetables and seasoned with butter and saffron. Although higher in fat than steamed rice, it is still relatively lean.

■ **Steamed vegetables**

Desserts

✓ **Choose fresh fruit or rice pudding** (rizogalo).

✓ **Share baklava**. This sweet, rich dessert is made up of layers of phyllo dough, butter, honey, and nuts. If you must order it, share your dessert with others.

Nutritional Information for Middle Eastern Foods

Middle Eastern Foods

	Calories	Fat (g)	Sodium (mg)	Carbos* (g)	Exchanges**
Appetizers & Salads:					
Falafel Patties, 3 oz fried	155	10	na	16	1ST+2FAT
Fattoush, 1½ c w/out dressing	95	1	na	11	2V+½ST
1T dressing	85	9	145	0	2FAT
Greek Salad - 1 c of lettuce only	25	0	5	5	1V
Kalamata olives	39	3	435	<1	¾FAT
1 oz feta cheese	75	6	315	0	1MT
2T lemon/herb dressing	170	18	290	1	3½FAT
Greek Salad w/olives, cheese, & dressing	309	27	1045	7	1V+1MT+4½FAT
Hummus, ¼ c	100	5	300	12	1ST+1FAT
Humus, ¼ c+1T oil	220	18	300	12	1ST+3½FAT

*Carbs=Carbohydrate, na=not available   **Exchanges: ST=Starch, Mlk=Milk (skim) FR=Fruit, CHO=Other Carbohydrates, V=Vegetable, MT=Meat (medium fat), FAT=Fat

Middle Eastern Foods (continued)

	Calories	Fat (g)	Sodium (mg)	Carbos* (g)	Exchanges**
Appetizers & Salads continued:					
Lentil Soup, 8 oz	190	5	1300	24	1½ST+1MT+1FAT
Pine Nuts, 1 oz or ¼ c	161	17	20	5	1MT+2½FAT
Stuffed Eggplant, 1 slice	270	23	na	8	1V+1MT+3½FAT
Tabouli Salad, ½ c	140	6	na	22	1ST+½V+1FAT
Tahini (sesame butter), 1T	90	8	17	3	2FAT
Yogurt & Cucumber Salad, ½ c	110	7	na	9	1V+¼Mlk+1½FAT
Entrees:					
Dolmades, 3	220	9	na	21	1V+1ST+1MT+1FAT
2 T lemon & egg sauce	175	19	250	2	4FAT
Moussaka, 4" X 4"	420	24	730	20	½ST+2V+3MT+2FAT
Gyro, 4 oz beef & lamb on pita bread w/out sauce	505	21	na	43	2½ST+4MT
Tzatziki sauce, 2T	45	3.⁵	na	0	½FAT
Gyro, 4 oz beef & lamb on pita bread w/4T tzatziki sauce	595	28	na	43	2½ST+4MT+1FAT
Chicken on Pita, 4 oz chicken breast on pita bread	310	3	na	43	2½ST+4MT(very lean)
w/1 oz feta cheese & 1T olive oil	535	22	na	43	2½ST+4MT
Greek-style Lamb w/orzo, 4 oz lamb +2 oz orzo	505	25	na	33	2ST+4MT+½FAT
Shish Kebab, 1 skewer w/2 oz beef & vegetables basted	240	14	na	7	1V+2MT+1FAT
Shish Kebab, 1 skewer w/2 oz chicken & vegetables basted	190	11	na	7	1V+2MT+½FAT
Lamb & artichoke w/lemon sauce	370	30	na	10	1V+2MT+4FAT
Baked Chicken Quarter, Greek Style w/potatoes, onions, lemon sauce	550	35	na	29	1½ST+1V+3MT +4FAT
Sheik el Mahshi, 1 c	175	10	na	12	2V+1MT+1FAT
Kibbeh, 1 c	225	10	na	23	1ST+1V+1MT+1FAT
Accompaniments:					
Rice, plain, ½ c	120	0	4	25	1½ST
Rice Pilaf, ½ c	160	4	520	28	1½ST+¼V+1FAT
Couscous, plain, ½ c	170	0	4	31	2ST
Couscous, buttered, ½ c	210	5	na	31	2ST+1FAT
Pita Bread, 6½" round diameter	190	1.⁵	510	42	2½ST
Hummus, 2T	50	2.⁵	150	9	½ST+½FAT
Desserts:					
Yogurt, plain whole, ¼ c	35	2	30	3	½Mlk+½FAT
Baklava, 2" X 2"	440	30	na	33	2CHO+6FAT

---

*Carbs=Carbohydrate, na=not available   **Exchanges:** ST=Starch, Mlk=Milk (skim)
FR=Fruit, CHO=Other Carbohydrates, V=Vegetable, MT=Meat (medium fat), FAT=Fat

PART
5

Favorite Restaurants

1 POTATO 2®

	Calories	Fat (g)	Sodium (mg)	Carbs* (g)	Exchanges**
Ultra Lites™ & Lite Potato® Baked Potatoes (assumes skin not eaten):					
Chicken Fajita Lite	272	2	556	50	3ST+1MT(lean)
Chicken, Mushroom & Roasted Peppers Lite	242	2	716	45	2½ST+1V+1MT(lean)
Crab & Broccoli DeLite	335	3	738	55	3ST+1V+1MT(lean)
Chicken Stir-Fry Lite	330	3	1289	62	3½ST+1V+1MT(lean)
Vegie & Herb Cheese Lite	237	2	423	44	2ST+1V+1MT(lean)
Chicken Caesar and Broccoli Lite	372	12	845	50	3ST+1V+1MT+1½FAT
Fresh Mex Chicken Lite	328	9	833	46	3ST+1MT+½FAT
Herb Roasted Vegetable Lite	259	6	210	47	2½ST+1V+1FAT
Spinach Soufflé Lite	310	9	569	44	2½ST+1V+1MT+1FAT
Gourmet Potato Entrees (assumes skin not eaten):					
Ham & Cheese Supreme	697	47	1617	43	2½ST+2½MT+7FAT
Broccoli & Cheese Supreme	641	43	875	46	2½ST+1V+2MT+6½FAT
Chicken Caesar & Broccoli	706	51	1374	50	2½ST+1V+1MT+9FAT
Crab, Broccoli, & Cheese	593	35	1229	46	2ST+1V+2½MT+4½FAT
Chicken, Broccoli, & Cheddar	591	37	816	43	2½ST+1V+2MT+5½FAT
Mexican	669	46	1071	48	3ST+1MT+8FAT
Broccoli & Cheese	545	36	575	42	2½ST+1V+1MT+6FAT
Bacon & Cheese	657	47	921	39	2½ST+1½MT+8FAT
3 Cheese	582	39	753	40	2½ST+1½MT+6FAT

Tip: If you request broth instead of margarine on Gourmet Potato Entrees, you will reduce calories by 202, fat by 23 g, and sodium by 304 mg. No-Fat Sour Cream is available on all entrees.

	Calories	Fat (g)	Sodium (mg)	Carbs* (g)	Exchanges**
Gourmet Wraps:					
Asian Chicken	969	44	2275	124	7ST+1V+1MT+8FAT
Broccoli, Ranch & Cheddar	1168	71	1684	114	6ST+1V+1MT+13FAT
Fresh Bread Bowl Soups (includes bread bowl):					
Baked Potato Soup	640	26	1630	81	5ST+1MT+4FAT
Broccoli and Cheese Potato Soup	662	29	1433	80	5ST+1MT+5FAT
Potato Skins:					
Bacon n'Cheddar w/sour cream	972	53	1337	100	6ST+1½MT+9FAT
Southwestern with sour cream	907	46	1423	105	6ST+1MT+8FAT
Country Skillet Combos:					
BBQ Chicken Cheddar & Bacon	890	57	759	74	4½ST+1½MT+10FAT
Bacon, Ranch & Cheddar	1090	74	937	87	5ST+1MT+14FAT
Idaho "Nachos"	1009	61	838	89	5ST+2MT+10FAT
Fresh Cut Fries:					
Small	612	39	321	63	3½ST+7½FAT
Medium	765	49	401	79	4½ST+9½FAT
Large	1224	78	642	126	7½ST+15½FAT
Fresh Fries'n Chicken Tenders	917	50	893	93	5½ST+1½MT+8½FAT
Nacho Cheese Fries	838	54	622	81	5ST+11FAT

Source: 1 Potato 2® Nutrition Guide. Current as of 12/99. All ® in this section are trademarks of 1 Potato 2®

*Carbs=Carbohydrate, na=not available **Exchanges: ST=Starch, Mlk=Milk (skim)
FR=Fruit, CHO=Other Carbohydrates, V=Vegetable, MT=Meat (medium fat), FAT=Fat

APPLEBEE'S®

Low Fat (LF) Menu Items:

	Calories	Fat (g)	Sodium (mg)	Carbs* (g)	Exchanges**
LF Veggie Quesadilla	344	8	1138	46	2½ST+1V+2½MT(lean)
LF Chicken Fajita Quesadilla	517	11	2244	63	4ST+4MT(lean)
LF Lemon Chicken Pasta	528	11	2438	78	4½ST+3MT(lean)
LF Blackened Chicken Salad, full	411	5	2188	39	1ST+2V+6MT(very lean)
medium size	287	3	1763	27	1ST+1V+4MT(very lean)
LF Asian Chicken Salad, full	623	9	2487	107	6ST+2V+2MT
medium size	370	6	1431	64	3½ST+1V+1MT
LF Garlic Chicken Pasta	587	8	1551	89	5ST+3½MT(lean)
Bikini Banana LF Strawberry Shortcake	248	2	223	48	1FR+2CHO+½FAT
LF & Fabulous Brownie Sundae	415	2	417	82	5CHO+½FAT
LF Marble Cheesecake	261	2	378	50	3CHO+½FAT

Source: Applebee's® International Inc. Current as of 12/99

ARBY'S®

Breakfast:

	Calories	Fat (g)	Sodium (mg)	Carbs* (g)	Exchanges**
Bacon, 2 strips	90	7	220	0	1MT+½FAT
Biscuit w/margarine	270	16	750	26	1½ST+3FAT
Croissant	260	16	300	28	2ST+3FAT
Scrambled Egg	70	5	70	0	1MT
French Toastix, 6 w/out powdered sugar or syrup	370	17	440	48	3ST+3½FAT
Ham	50	3	830	1	1MT(lean)
Maple Syrup, 1 ½ oz	220	0	50	54	3½CHO
Sausage Patty	200	19	290	1	1MT+1½FAT
Swiss Cheese Slice	45	3	220	0	½MT

Roast Beef Sandwiches:

	Calories	Fat (g)	Sodium (mg)	Carbs* (g)	Exchanges**
Arby's Melt w/Cheddar	380	19	960	38	2½ST+2MT+2FAT
Arby Q®	380	15	990	42	2½ST+2MT+1FAT
Beef'N Cheddar	510	28	1250	45	2½ST+3MT+2½FAT
Big Montana®	720	40	2270	44	2½ST+6MT+2FAT
Giant Roast Beef	550	28	1560	43	2½ST+4MT+1½FAT
Junior Roast Beef	340	16	790	36	2ST+1½MT+1½FAT
Regular Roast Beef	400	20	1030	36	2ST+2½MT+1½FAT
Super Roast Beef	530	27	1190	50	3ST+2½MT+3FAT

Other Sandwiches:

	Calories	Fat (g)	Sodium (mg)	Carbs* (g)	Exchanges**
Chicken Bacon'N Swiss	610	30	1620	52	3ST+4MT+2FAT
Chicken Breast Fillet	560	28	1080	49	3ST+3MT+2½FAT
Chicken Cordon Bleu	650	34	2120	50	3ST+4½MT+2FAT
Fish Fillet	540	27	880	51	3ST+2MT+3½FAT
Grilled Chicken Deluxe	420	16	930	42	2½ST+3MT
Roast Chicken Club	540	29	1590	39	2½ST+4MT+1½FAT

*Carbs=Carbohydrate, na=not available   **Exchanges:** ST=Starch, Mlk=Milk (skim) FR=Fruit, CHO=Other Carbohydrates, V=Vegetable, MT=Meat (medium fat), FAT=Fat

ARBY'S® (continued)

Sub Roll Sandwiches:	Calories	Fat (g)	Sodium (mg)	Carbs* (g)	Exchanges**
French Dip	490	22	1440	43	2½ST+3MT+1½FAT
Hot Ham'N Swiss	570	31	2660	47	3ST+3MT+3FAT
Italian	800	54	2610	49	3ST+3MT+8FAT
Philly Beef'N Swiss	780	48	2140	52	3ST+4MT+5½FAT
Roast Beef	770	49	2170	48	3ST+3MT+7FAT
Turkey	670	39	2130	49	3ST+3MT+5FAT
Light Menu:					
Garden Salad	110	3	150	16	½ST+1V+½MT
Light Grilled Chicken Salad	190	4	530	16	½ST+1V+3MT(very lean)
Light Grilled Chicken	280	5	920	33	2ST+3½MT(very lean)
Light Roast Chicken Deluxe	260	5	950	32	2ST+3MT(lean)
Light Roast Chicken Salad	200	5	800	16	½ST+1V+3MT(lean)
Light Roast Turkey Deluxe	230	5	870	33	2ST+2MT(lean)
Side Salad	90	3	130	12	½ST+1V+½MT
Potatoes:					
Cheddar Curly Fries	450	25	1420	52	3½ST+5FAT
Curly Fries, small	320	16	910	40	2½ST+3FAT
medium	380	19	1100	49	3ST+4FAT
large	600	30	1710	75	5ST+6FAT
Homestyle Fries, small	340	15	660	46	3ST+3FAT
medium	420	19	830	57	3½ST+4FAT
large	630	29	1240	86	5ST+6FAT
Potato Cakes	220	14	460	21	1½ST+2½FAT
Jalapeno Bites ™	330	21	670	29	2ST+4FAT
Mozzarella Sticks	470	29	1330	34	2ST+2MT+4FAT
Onion Petals	410	24	300	43	2½ST+5FAT
Chicken Fingers Snack	610	32	1610	62	4ST+1½MT+5FAT
Chicken Fingers Meal	880	47	2240	81	5ST+2½MT+7FAT
Baked Potato w/butter & s cream	500	24	170	65	4ST+5FAT
Broccoli'N Cheddar Bked Potato	550	25	730	71	4ST+1V+5FAT
Chicken Broccoli Baked Potato	830	47	970	68	4ST+3MT+6½FAT
Cool Ranch Baked Potato	500	23	150	67	4ST+4½FAT
Deluxe Baked Potato	610	31	860	68	4ST+1MT+5FAT
Jalapeno Baked Potato	660	36	930	72	4ST+1MT+6FAT
Philly Chicken Baked Potato	880	53	1020	75	4½ST+2½MT+8FAT
Shakes (10.3 oz):					
Vanilla Shake	380	9	270	67	4½CHO+1½FAT
Chocolate Shake	390	9	270	69	4½CHO+1½FAT
Strawberry Shake	380	9	270	67	4½CHO+1½FAT
Jamocha Shake	380	9	270	66	4½CHO+1½FAT
Desserts:					
Apple Turnover, iced	360	14	180	54	3CHO+3FAT
Cherry Turnover, iced	350	14	190	53	3CHO+3FAT

*Carbs=Carbohydrate, na=not available   **Exchanges: ST=Starch, Mlk=Milk (skim)
FR=Fruit, CHO=Other Carbohydrates, V=Vegetable, MT=Meat (medium fat), FAT=Fat

ARBY'S® (continued)

Sauces and Dressings:

	Calories	Fat (g)	Sodium (mg)	Carbs* (g)	Exchanges**
Arby's Sauce packet, ½ oz	15	0	110	3	FREE
BBQ Dipping Sauce, 1 oz	40	0	350	10	½CHO
Beef Stock Au Jus, 2 oz	10	0	440	0	FREE
Bleu Cheese Dressing, 2 ½ oz	390	39	770	3	8FAT
Bronco Berry Sauce™, 1 ½ oz	90	0	35	23	1½CHO
Buttermilk Ranch Drs'g, red cal, 2 oz	50	0	710	12	¾CHO
German Mustard packet	5	0	60	0	FREE
Honey French Dressing, 2 oz	350	27	530	24	1½CHO+5½FAT
Honey Mustard, 1 oz	130	12	170	5	¼CHO+2½FAT
Horsey Sauce® packet	60	5	100	3	1FAT
Italian Dressing, Red. Cal. 2 oz	20	1	1110	4	FREE or ¼FAT
Ketchup packet	10	0	90	3	1=FREE or ¼CHO
Mayonnaise packet	86	10	65	0	2FAT
Mayonnaise pkt, Light Chol. Free	20	2	110	1	1=FREE or ¼FAT
Marinara Sauce, 1 ½ oz	35	2	260	4	½V+½FAT
Tangy Southwest Sauce ™	250	25	280	3	5FAT
Thousand Island Dressing, 2 oz	350	33	580	11	¾CHO+6½FAT

Source: Arby's® Comprehensive Guide of Quality Ingredients© 1999.   Current as of 12/99.

AU BON PAIN®

Spreads (2 oz):

	Calories	Fat (g)	Sodium (mg)	Carbs* (g)	Exchanges**
Veggie Lite Cream Cheese	130	11	230	4	¾MT+1½FAT
Lite Honey Walnut Cream Cheese	150	11	190	9	½CHO+½MT+2FAT
Lite Vanilla Hazelnut Spread	140	11	210	6	½CHO+½MT+2FAT
Lite Cream Cheese	100	8	280	4	¾MT+1FAT
Lite Sun-dried Tomato Cream Cheese	120	8	320	6	½CHO+½MT+1FAT
Plain Cream Cheese	180	18	150	2	¾MT+3FAT

Sourdough Bagels:

	Calories	Fat (g)	Sodium (mg)	Carbs* (g)	Exchanges**
Sesame	380	4	540	71	4½ST+½FAT
Honey 9 Grain	360	2	580	72	4½ST+½FAT
Wild Blueberry	380	2	570	80	5ST+½FAT
Plain	350	2	660	72	4½ST+½FAT
Cinnamon Raisin	360	2	540	77	5ST+½FAT
Onion	370	2	660	78	5ST+½FAT
Everything	360	3	710	72	4½ST+½FAT
Asiago Cheese	380	6	690	66	4ST+1FAT
Cranberry Walnut	460	4	590	93	5½ST+½FAT
Dutch Apple w/walnut streusel	350	5	480	77	5ST+1FAT

Hot Croissants:

	Calories	Fat (g)	Sodium (mg)	Carbs* (g)	Exchanges**
Ham & Cheese	380	20	690	36	2ST+1½MT+2½FAT
Spinach & Cheese	270	16	330	27	1½ST+1MT+2FAT

*Carbs=Carbohydrate, na=not available   **Exchanges: ST=Starch, Mlk=Milk (skim)
FR=Fruit, CHO=Other Carbohydrates, V=Vegetable, MT=Meat (medium fat), FAT=Fat

AU BON PAIN® (continued)

	Calories	Fat (g)	Sodium (mg)	Carbs* (g)	Exchanges**
Dessert Croissants:					
Plain	270	15	240	30	2ST+3FAT
Almond	560	37	260	50	3CHO+7½FAT
Apple	280	10	180	46	3CHO+2FAT
Chocolate	440	23	230	53	3½CHO+4½FAT
Cinnamon Raisin	380	13	290	61	4CHO+2½FAT
Raspberry Cheese	380	19	300	47	3CHO+4FAT
Gourmet Muffins:					
Blueberry	410	15	380	64	4CHO+ 3FAT
Carrot Pecan	480	23	650	61	4CHO+4½FAT
Chocolate Chip	490	20	560	70	4½CHO+4FAT
Corn	470	18	570	70	4½CHO+3½FAT
Pumpkin with Streusel Topping	470	18	550	74	5CHO+3½FAT
Raisin Bran	390	11	1030	66	4CHO+2FAT
Low Fat Muffins:					
Triple Berry	270	3	560	60	4CHO+½FAT
Chocolate Cake	290	3	630	68	4½CHO+½FAT
Streudel Desserts:					
Apple Streudel	440	26	780	48	3CHO+5FAT
Cherry Streudel	450	29	730	45	3CHO+5½FAT
Sandwiches:					
Grilled Chic'n & Mozzarella Focaccia	910	20	267	83	4½ST+1V +10MT(lean)
Chicken Foco-cha-cha	870	29	2280	80	4ST+1V+9MT(lean)
Wraps Sandwiches:					
Fields & Feta	560	17	850	89	4½ST+1V+1MT+2½FAT
Chicken Caesar w/out dressing	440	12	880	43	3ST+4MT(lean)
Sandwich Fillings:					
Country Ham	150	7	1370	1	3MT(lean)
Turkey Breast	120	1	1110	1	3½MT(very lean)
Roast Beef	140	4.⁵	550	1	3MT(lean)
Tuna Salad	360	29	520	3	3MT+3FAT
Swiss Cheese, ½ portion	160	12	110	1	1½MT+1FAT
Cheddar Cheese, ½ portion	170	14	260	1	1½MT+1½FAT
Provolone, ½ portion	150	11	370	1	1½MT+½FAT

(½ portion cheese used when adding to meat sandwich)

	Calories	Fat (g)	Sodium (mg)	Carbs* (g)	Exchanges**
Chef's Creation Sandwiches:					
Fresh Mozzarello, Tomato, & Pesto	650	30	1090	69	4ST+1V+2MT+4FAT
Thai Chicken Sandwich	420	6	1320	72	4ST+1V+1MT
Hot Roasted Turkey Club SW	950	50	2240	80	4½ST+1V+5MT+5FAT
Honey Dijon Chicken Sandwich	730	18	1990	85	5ST+1V+6MT(lean)

*Carbs=Carbohydrate, na=not available **Exchanges:** ST=Starch, Mlk=Milk (skim)
FR=Fruit, CHO=Other Carbohydrates, V=Vegetable, MT=Meat (medium fat), FAT=Fat

AU BON PAIN® (continued)

	Calories	Fat (g)	Sodium (mg)	Carbs* (g)	Exchanges**
Fresh Sandwich Breads:					
Multigrain Loaf, 1 slice	130	1	340	26	1½ST
French Sandwich, 1 roll	240	1	640	50	3ST
Tomato Herb Loaf, 1 slice	130	1	310	27	1½ST
Fresh Loaf Breads (1 slice):					
Sun Dried Tomato Pepper Batard	110	0	270	22	1½ST
Multigrain Batard	110	1	310	22	1½ST
French Parisienne Baguette	110	2	260	22	1½ST+½FAT
Parisienne	120	0.^{5}	300	25	1½ST+½FAT
Baguette	140	0.^{5}	350	29	2ST
Rosemary Garlic Breadstick, 1	180	3	550	34	2ST+½FAT
Hot Soups per 8 oz (8 oz served w/½ sandwich only, 12 oz served in bread bowl):					
Tomato Florentine	61	1	1030	13	½ST+1V
Garden Vegetable	29	0	820	8	1V
Clam Chowder	270	19	730	16	1ST+1MT+3FAT
Chicken Noodle	80	1.^{5}	670	10	½ST+½MT
Cream of Broccoli	220	18	770	14	1ST+3½FAT
Beef Barley	75	2	660	11	½ST+½MT
Vegetarian Chili	139	2.^{5}	1070	27	1ST+2V+½FAT
Curry Chicken	110	5	1080	17	1ST+1FAT
Summer Asparagus	160	11	880	16	½ST+1V+2FAT
Hot & Sour Soup	70	2.^{5}	1180	10	2V+½FAT
Asiago Cheese Bisque	230	16	660	16	1ST+3FAT
Mushroom Orzo	60	1.^{5}	870	11	½ST+1V
Fresh Rolls (1 roll):					
Petit Pain	200	1	570	41	2½ST
Hearth	220	1.^{5}	410	43	2ST+½FAT
Fresh Salads:					
Field Green, Gorg & Roasted Walnut	400	34	800	9	1V+2½MT+4½FAT
Mozzarella & Roasted Red Pepper	340	18	135	26	3V+1MT+2½FAT
Large Garden Salad	160	1.^{5}	290	34	3V+1ST+½FAT
Small Garden Salad	100	1	150	20	2V+½ST
Oriental Chicken Salad	270	4	700	17	½FR+1V+5MT(very lean)
Tuna Salad	490	27	750	40	2ST+2V+2MT+3½FAT
Chicken Caesar Salad	360	11	910	28	1ST+2V+4MT(lean)
Salad Dressings (3 oz serving):					
Caesar	380	39	410	3	½MT+7FAT
Lite Italian	230	20	570	15	1CHO+4FAT
Blue Cheese	410	41	910	8	½ST+8FAT
Fat Free Tomato Basil	70	0	650	17	1CHO
Lemon Basil Vinaigrette	330	32	460	15	1CHO+6FAT

*Carbs=Carbohydrate, na=not available **Exchanges:** ST=Starch, Mlk=Milk (skim)
FR=Fruit, CHO=Other Carbohydrates, V=Vegetable, MT=Meat (medium fat), FAT=Fat

AU BON PAIN® (continued)

	Calories	Fat (g)	Sodium (mg)	Carbs* (g)	Exchanges**
Salad Dressings, continued (3 oz serving):					
Lite Honey Mustard	280	17	560	30	2CHO+3½FAT
Buttermilk Ranch	310	32	270	4	6½FAT
Mandarin Orange	380	33	310	23	1½CHO+6½FAT
Caribbean Balsamic Lime	170	16	630	5	¼CHO+ 3FAT
Sesame French	370	30	1010	26	1½CHO+6FAT
Greek	440	50	820	2	10FAT
Cookies:					
Shortbread	390	25	190	39	2½CHO+5FAT
Almond Biscotti	200	10	45	24	1½CHO+2FAT
Chocolate Almond Biscotti	240	13	50	28	1½CHO+2½FAT
Chocolate Chip	280	13	85	40	2½CHO+2½FAT
Oatmeal Raisin	250	10	240	40	2½CHO+2FAT
English Toffee Cookie	220	12	110	28	1½CHO+2½FAT
Holiday Tree Cookie	200	6	50	36	2½CHO+1FAT
Gingerbread Man Cookie	280	8	270	49	3CHO+1½FAT
Other Baked Goods:					
Cinnamon Roll	340	15	320	48	3CHO+3FAT
Cheese Swirl Danish	450	28	410	46	3CHO+5½FAT
Lemon Swirl Danish	450	24	410	53	3½CHO+5FAT
Walnut Coffee Cake Danish	480	28	290	50	3CHO+5½FAT
Pecan Roll	900	48	480	111	7CHO+9½FAT
Oreo Cookie Bar	550	29	190	58	4CHO+6FAT
Mochaccino Bar	404	24	294	44	3CHO+5FAT
Walnut Fudge Brownie	380	18	150	56	4CHO+3½FAT
Flavored Specialty Drinks (16 oz):					
Hot Strawberry Chocolate Blast	330	6	180	57	1Mlk+3CHO+1FAT
Hot Hazelnut Blast	310	6	180	57	1Mlk+3CHO+1FAT
Hot Vanilla Chocolate Blast	310	6	180	57	1Mlk+3CHO+1FAT
Hot Caramel Mocha Blast	330	6	180	57	1Mlk+3CHO+1FAT
Hot Raspberry Mocha Blast	310	6	180	57	1Mlk+3CHO+1FAT
Iced & Frozen Specialty Drinks:					
Peach Iced Tea, small, 8 oz	90	0	15	22	1½CHO
medium, 12 oz	130	0	20	33	2CHO
large, 16 oz	170	0	30	44	3CHO
Iced Cappuccino, small, 9 oz	110	4	110	10	½Mlk+¼CHO+1FAT
medium, 12 oz	150	6	150	15	¾Mlk+½CHO+1FAT
large, 20½ oz	270	10	270	26	1Mlk+1CHO+2FAT
Frozen Mocha Blast, 16 oz	320	3	150	64	1Mlk+3CHO+½FAT

*Carbs=Carbohydrate, na=not available   **Exchanges:** ST=Starch, Mlk=Milk (skim)
FR=Fruit, CHO=Other Carbohydrates, V=Vegetable, MT=Meat (medium fat), FAT=Fat

AU BON PAIN® (continued)

	Calories	Fat (g)	Sodium (mg)	Carbs* (g)	Exchanges**
Wilch Drinks (16 oz):					
Original Frozen Mocha Blast	350	7	240	56	1Mlk+3CHO+1½FAT
Blender Drinks (16 oz):					
Original Frozen Mocha Blast	320	3	150	64	4CHO+½FAT
Yogurt:					
Plain Yogurt w/fresh berries	210	3	115	38	1Mlk+1FR+½CHO+½FAT
Plain Yogurt w/granola	230	4	120	41	1Mlk+1FR+¾CHO+½FAT
Strawb'y Yogurt w/fresh berries	210	3	100	42	1Mlk+1FR+¾CHO+½FAT
Strawberry Yogurt w/granola	230	4	100	45	1Mlk+1FR+¾CHO+½FAT
Blueberry Yogurt w/fresh berries	210	3	100	42	1Mlk+1FR+¾CHO+½FAT
Blueberry Yogurt w/granola	230	4	100	45	1Mlk+1FR+¾CHO+½FAT

Source: Au Bon Pain® Nutritional Information. Current as of 12/99.

BASKIN 31 ROBBINS®

	Calories	Fat (g)	Sodium (mg)	Carbs* (g)	Exchanges**
Regular Deluxe Ice Cream, permanent flavors (1/2 cup):					
Chocolate	150	9	60	18	1CHO+2FAT
Chocolate Chip or Mint Choc Ch	150	10	45	15	1CHO+2FAT
Choc. Chip Cookie Dough	170	9	70	20	1¼CHO+2FAT
Choc Fudge or Pralines'N Cream	160	9	80-85	19-21	1¼CHO+2FAT
Cookies'N Cream	170	11	80	16	1CHO+2FAT
French Vanilla	160	10	45	14	1CHO+2FAT
Gold Medal Ribbon	150	8	95	20	1¼CHO+1½FAT
Jamoca or Vanilla	140	8-9	40-45	14	1CHO+2FAT
Jamoca Almond Fudge	160	9	40	17	1CHO+2FAT
Old Fashioned Butter Pecan	160	11	50	13	1CHO+2FAT
Peanut Butter'N Chocolate	180	12	95	15	1CHO+2FAT
Pistachio Almond	170	12	45	13	1CHO+2FAT
Rocky Road	170	10	60	19	1¼CHO+2FAT
Very Berry Strawberry	130	7	40	16	1CHO+1½FAT
World Class Chocolate	160	9	55	18	1CHO+2FAT
Regular Deluxe Ice Cream, rotating flavors (1/2 cup):					
Banana Strawberry or Pumpkin Pie	130	7	40-50	16-17	1CHO+1½FAT
Baseball Nut	160	9	55	18	1CHO+2FAT
Black Walnut	160	11	45	13	1CHO+2FAT
Blueberry Cheesecake	150	8	70	15	1CHO+1½FAT
Cherries Jubilee or Rum Raisin	140	7	40	16-18	1CHO+1½FAT
Chocolate Almond	180	11	55	17	1CHO+2FAT
Chocolate Mousse Royale	170	10	60	20	1¼CHO+2FAT
Choc. Raspberry Truffle	180	9	60	23	1½CHO+2FAT
Chunky Heath Bar	170	10	70	19	1¼CHO+2FAT

*Carbs=Carbohydrate, na=not available   **Exchanges: ST=Starch, Mlk=Milk (skim)
FR=Fruit, CHO=Other Carbohydrates, V=Vegetable, MT=Meat (medium fat), FAT=Fat

BASKIN 31 ROBBINS® (continued)

	Calories	Fat (g)	Sodium (mg)	Carbs* (g)	Exchanges**
Regular Deluxe Ice Cream, rotating flavors (1/2 cup):					
Egg Nog or Lemon Custard	150	8	45-55	16	1CHO+1½FAT
English Toffee or Strawb Shortcake	160	9	70	18-19	1¼CHO+2FAT
Everybody's Favorite Candy Bar	170	9	90	20	1¼CHO+2FAT
Fudge Brownie	170	11	75	19	1¼CHO+2FAT
German Chocolate Cake	180	10	75	20	1¼CHO+2FAT
Mississippi Mud	160	8	85	22	1½CHO+1½FAT
Oregon Blackberry	140	8	50	16	1CHO+1½FAT
Quarterback Crunch	160	10	75	18	1CHO+2FAT
Reeses® Peanut Butter	180	11	70	17	1CHO+2FAT
Triple Chocolate Passion	180	11	70	21	1¼CHO+2FAT
Winter White Chocolate	150	9	50	18	1CHO+2FAT
FroZone Kids Flavors (½ cup):					
Dirt'N Worms	160	8	80	22	1½CHO+1½FAT
Eerrie I Scream or Pink Bubblegum	150	8	40-45	18-19	1CHO+1½FAT
Neon Sour Apple or Watermelon Ice	110	0	10	27-28	1½CHO
Polar Paws	160	10	45	17	1CHO+2FAT
Skullicious	170	10	55	18	1CHO+2FAT
Sherbet (½ cup):	120	1-1.⁵	25-30	22-26	1½CHO
Sorbet (½ cup):	110-120	0	10-15	28-31	2CHO
Ices (½ cup):	110-120	0	10	27-29	1½CHO
Non-Fat Ice Cream (½ c):	100-110	0	90-105	21-24	1½CHO
Low Fat (½ c):	100	2.⁵	60	18	1CHO+½FAT
Yogurt Gone Crazy (½ c):	130-140	3	80-105	24-26	1½CHO+½FAT
No Sugar Added (½ c):					
Call Me Nuts	110	2	55	21	1½CHO+½FAT
Cherry Cordial or Mad About Chocolate	100	2	40-55	18-19	1CHO+½FAT
Pineapple Coconut	90	1.5	60	16	1CHO+¼FAT
Thin Mint	100	2.5	65	16	1CHO+½FAT
Blasts (8 oz):					
Cappucino w/whipped cream	160	7	60	22	1½CHO+1FAT
NF Cappucino	90	0	60	20	1½CHO
Chocolate w/whipped cream	250	7	120	46	3CHO+1FAT
NF Chocolate	170	0	105	40	2½CHO
Mocha Cappy w/whipped cream	180	6	70	28	1½CHO+1FAT
NF Mocha Cappucino	120	0	75	26	1½CHO
Smoothies (8 oz):					
Aloha Berry Banana w/soft serve	180	0	80	40	2½CHO
Aloha Berry Banana w/hard scoop	210	0	85	46	3CHO
Bora Berry Bora w/soft serve	170	0	75	38	2½CHO
Bora Berry Bora w/hard scoop	190	0	75	44	3CHO

*Carbs=Carbohydrate, na=not available **Exchanges:** ST=Starch, Mlk=Milk (skim)
FR=Fruit, CHO=Other Carbohydrates, V=Vegetable, MT=Meat (medium fat), FAT=Fat

BASKIN 31 ROBBINS® (continued)

Smoothies (8 oz):	Calories	Fat (g)	Sodium (mg)	Carbs* (g)	Exchanges**
Calypso Berry w/soft *or* hard	160	0	75	35	2½CHO
Copa Banana w/soft serve	140	0	65	30	2CHO
Copa Banana w/hard scoop	170	0	70	38	2½CHO
Sunset Orange w/soft serve	150	0	70	32	2CHO
Sunset Orange w/hard scoop	170	0	75	38	2½CHO
Tropical Tango w/soft serve	160	0	65	36	2½CHO
Tropical Tango w/hard scoop	190	0	70	43	3CHO

Source: Baskin 31 Robbins® Nutritional information. Current as of 12/99.

BLIMPIE®

6" White Bread Subs (Nutritional info does *not* include toppings & condiments):	Calories	Fat (g)	Sodium (mg)	Carbs* (g)	Exchanges**
Blimpie® Best Sub	410	13	1480	47	3ST+2½MT
Turkey Sub	320	5	890	51	3ST+2MT(lean)
Roast Beef Sub	340	5	870	47	3ST+2MT(lean)
Cheese Trio Sub	510	23	1060	51	3ST+2½MT+2FAT
Club Sub	450	13	1350	53	3ST+2½MT
Ham & Swiss Sub	400	13	970	47	3ST+2½MT
Ham, Salami, Provolone Sub	590	28	1880	52	3ST+3MT+2½FAT
Tuna Sub	570	32	790	50	3ST+1½MT+5FAT
Steak & Cheese Sub	550	26	1080	51	3ST+2MT+3FAT
Grilled Chicken Sub	400	9	950	52	3½ST+2MT
5 Meatball Sub	500	22	970	52	3½ST+1½MT+3FAT
Grilled Chicken Salad	350	12	1190	13	1ST+5MT(lean)

Source: Blimpie® Nutritional Facts. Current as of 12/99.

BOB'S BIG BOY®

Pitas (includes Ranch dressing):	Calories	Fat (g)	Sodium (mg)	Carbs* (g)	Exchanges**
Turkey Pita	245	6	936	23	1ST+1V+3MT(lean)
Breast of Chicken & Mozzarella	361	11	369	23	1ST+1V+5MT(lean)

Soups & Salads (salads noted with * includes 1 roll and Promise® margarine):

Tossed Salad	35	2	71	7	1½V
Cabbage Soup, bowl	40	0.5	347	7	1 ½ V
*Oriental Chicken Breast Salad	660	20	855	73	4ST+1V+5MT(lean)+1FAT
*Chicken Breast Salad	523	16	654	50	3ST+1V+4MT(lean)+1FAT

Dinners (nutritional info includes tossed salad w/out dressing, roll, & Promise® margarine):

Chicken'n Veg Stir Fry + baked potato	795	18	845	109	6ST+2V+4MT(lean)+1FAT
Vegetable Stir-Fry + baked potato	616	14	774	109	6ST+2V+2FAT
Br Chicken w/Mozz'lla + baked potato	697	20	613	80	4½ST+1V+5MT(lean)+½FAT
Baked Cod + baked potato	744	21	655	82	4½ST+1V+6MT(lean)+½FAT
Cajun Cod + baked potato	736	21	745	80	4½ST+1V+6MT(lean)+½FAT
Spaghetti Marinara	589	11	784	105	5½ST+3V+1FAT

*Carbs=Carbohydrate, na=not available   ****Exchanges:** ST=Starch, Mlk=Milk (skim)
FR=Fruit, CHO=Other Carbohydrates, V=Vegetable, MT=Meat (medium fat), FAT=Fat

BOB'S BIG BOY® (continued)

	Calories	Fat (g)	Sodium (mg)	Carbs* (g)	Exchanges**
Breakfast (includes 2 slices of whole wheat bread and Promise® margarine):					
Scrambled Egg Beaters®	305	10	603	36	2ST+2MT(lean)+1FAT
Plain Egg Beaters® Omelette	305	10	603	36	2ST+2MT(lean)+1FAT
Vegetarian Egg Beaters® Omelette	330	10	613	40	2ST+1V+2MT(lean)+1FAT
Sides:					
Rice Pilaf	145	3	225	26	1½ST+½FAT
Baked Potato	163	2	7	37	2½ST
Promise® Margarine	25	2.5	35	0	½FAT
Reduced Calorie Ranch Dressing, 1 oz	41	3	151	3	½FAT
Italian Dressing, fat-free, 1 oz	11	0	191	3	FREE
Fat-free Oriental Dressing, 1 oz	20	0.2	189	4	¼CHO
Dinner Roll	210	5	340	36	2½ST
Desserts:					
Frozen Yogurt, fat-free	118	0	60	27	1½CHO
Frozen Yogurt Shake	158	0.1	120	33	2CHO

Source: Bob's Big Boy®. Current as of 12/99

BOJANGLE'S®

	Calories	Fat (g)	Sodium (mg)	Carbs* (g)	Exchanges**
Cajun Spiced Chicken, breast	278	17	565	12	¾ST+2MT+1½FAT
leg	264	16	530	11	¾ST+2MT+1FAT
thigh	310	23	465	11	¾ST+2MT+2½FAT
wing	355	25	630	11	¾ST+2½MT+2½FAT
Cajun Roast Ch'n breast, skinfree	143	5	562	<1	3½MT(lean)
leg, skinfree	161	8	566	<1	3½MT(lean)
thigh, skinfree	215	15	428	<1	3MT
wing	231	15	617	3	3MT
Southern Style Chicken, breast	261	16	702	12	¾ST+2MT+1FAT
leg	254	15	446	11	¾ST+2½MT+½FAT
thigh	308	21	630	14	1ST+2MT+2FAT
wing	337	21	684	19	1ST+2MT+2FAT
Sweet Biscuits, BoBerry™	220	10	410	29	2CHO+2FAT
Cinnamon	320	18	560	37	2½CHO+3½FAT
Sandwiches:					
Cajun Filet, without mayo	337	11	401	41	2½ST+2MT
Grilled Filet, without mayo	235	5	540	25	1½ST+2½MT(lean)
Cajun Filet with mayo	437	22	506	41	2½ST+2MT+2FAT
Grilled Filet with mayo	335	16	645	25	1½ST+2½MT+1FAT
Cajun Steak SW w/horseradish & p'kles	434	26	985	39	2½ST+1½MT+3FAT
Biscuit, plain	243	12	663	29	2ST+2½FAT
Bacon Biscuit Sandwich	290	17	810	26	1½ST+½MT+3FAT
Bacon, Egg, & Cheese Biscuit SW	550	42	1250	27	1½ST+2MT+6FAT

*Carbs=Carbohydrate, na=not available   ****Exchanges:** ST=Starch, Mlk=Milk (skim)
FR=Fruit, CHO=Other Carbohydrates, V=Vegetable, MT=Meat (medium fat), FAT=Fat

BOJANGLES® (continued)

Sandwiches (continued):

	Calories	Fat (g)	Sodium (mg)	Carbs* (g)	Exchanges**
Cajun Filet Biscuit Sandwich	454	21	949	46	3ST+1½MT+2½FAT
Country Ham Biscuit Sandwich	270	15	1010	26	1½ST+1MT+2FAT
Egg Biscuit Sandwich	400	30	630	26	1½ST+1MT+5FAT
Sausage Biscuit Sandwich	350	23	810	26	1½ST+1MT+3½FAT
Smoked Sausage Biscuit SW	380	26	940	27	1½ST+1MT+4FAT
Steak Biscuit Sandwich	649	49	1126	37	2½ST+1½MT+8FAT

Individual Fixin':

	Calories	Fat (g)	Sodium (mg)	Carbs* (g)	Exchanges**
Bo Rounds	235	11	328	31	2ST+2FAT
Cajun Pintos	110	0	480	18	1ST+½MT(very lean)
Marinated Cole Slaw	136	3	454	26	1CHO+1½V
Corn on the Cob	140	2	20	34	2ST
Dirty Rice	166	6	762	24	1½ST+1FAT
Green Beans	25	0	710	5	1V
Macaroni & Cheese	198	14	418	12	¾ST+1MT+2FAT
Potatoes w/out Gravy	80	1	380	16	1ST
Seasoned Fries	344	19	480	39	2½ST+4FAT

Snacks:

	Calories	Fat (g)	Sodium (mg)	Carbs* (g)	Exchanges**
Chicken Supremes	337	16	629	26	1½ST+2½MT+1FAT
Buffalo Bites	180	5	720	5	¼ST+4MT(very lean)

Source: Bojangle's® Nutritional Factions 6/97. Current as of 12/99.

BOSTON MARKET®

Entrees:

	Calories	Fat (g)	Sodium (mg)	Carbs* (g)	Exchanges**
¼ White Mt Chicken no skin or wing	170	4	480	2	4½MT(very lean)
¼ White Mt Chicken w/skin & wing	280	12	510	2	5½MT(lean)
¼ Dark Meat Chicken, no skin	190	10	440	1	3MT(lean)
¼ Dark Meat Chicken with skin	320	21	500	2	4MT
½ Chicken with skin	590	33	1010	4	10MT(lean)
Skinless Rotisserie Turkey Breast	170	1	850	1	5MT(very lean)
Boston Hearth™ Ham	210	9	1490	9	½CHO+3MT(lean)
Meat Loaf & Chunky Tomato Sauce	370	18	1170	22	1ST+1V+4½MT+1FAT
Meat Loaf & Brown Gravy	390	22	1040	19	1ST+4½MT
Chicken Pot Pie	780	46	1480	61	3½ST+1V+3MT+6FAT
Chunky Chicken Salad	370	27	800	3	4MT+1½FAT
Teriyaki Chicken ¼ dark w/skin	380	21	870	17	1CHO+4MT
Teriyaki Chicken ¼ white w/skin	340	12	890	17	1CHO+5½MT(lean)
Tabasco BBQ Drumstick	130	6	190	4	2MT(lean)
Tabasco BBQ Wings	110	7	170	4	1MT+½FAT
Triple Topped Chicken	470	22	1350	20	1CHO+7MT(lean)
Southwest Savory Chicken	400	15	1670	26	1½ST+5MT(lean)
Caesar Side Salad	200	17	450	7	¼ST+1V+1MT+2½FAT

*Carbs=Carbohydrate, na=not available   **Exchanges: ST=Starch, Mlk=Milk (skim)
FR=Fruit, CHO=Other Carbohydrates, V=Vegetable, MT=Meat (medium fat), FAT=Fat

BOSTON MARKET® (continued)

	Calories	Fat (g)	Sodium (mg)	Carbs* (g)	Exchanges**
Soups, Salads, and Sandwiches:					
Caesar Salad Entrée	510	42	1130	17	½ST+2V+2MT+6½FAT
Caesar Salad without Dressing	230	12	500	14	½ST+1V+2MT+½FAT
Chicken Caesar Salad	650	45	1580	17	½ST+1V+6MT+3FAT
Tossed Salad w/Fat Free Ranch	160	2.⁵	940	29	1½ST+1V+½FAT
Tossed Salad w/Old Venice Drsg	340	27	1110	20	1ST+1V+5½FAT
Tossed Salad w/Caesar Dressing	380	31	810	18	1ST+1V+6FAT
Chicken Noodle Soup	130	4.⁵	1310	12	1ST+1MT
Chicken Tortilla Soup	220	11	1410	19	1ST+1MT+1FAT
Potato Soup	270	16	1020	24	1½ST+½MT+2½FAT
Tomato Bisque	280	23	1280	16	½ST+1V+4½FAT
Chicken Chili	220	7	1000	21	1ST+2MT(lean)
Chicken SW w/Cheese & Sauce	750	33	1860	72	4½ST+5MT+1½FAT
Chicken SW, no Sauce or Cheese	430	4.⁵	910	62	4ST+4MT(very lean)
Chicken Salad Sandwich	680	30	1360	63	4ST+4MT+2FAT
Turkey SW w/Cheese & Sauce	710	28	1390	68	4½ST+5MT
Turkey SW, no Cheese or Sauce	400	3.⁵	1070	61	4ST+4MT(very lean)
Ham SW w/Cheese & Sauce	750	34	1730	72	4½ST+3½MT+3FAT
Ham SW, no Cheese or Sauce	440	8	1450	66	4ST+2MT
Meat Loaf Sandwich w/Cheese	860	33	2270	95	6ST+4MT+2FAT
Meat Loaf Sandwich, no Cheese	690	21	1610	86	5½ST+3MT
Turkey Club Sandwich	650	26	1590	64	4ST+4MT+1FAT
Open Faced Turkey Sandwich	500	12	2170	61	4ST+3½MT
Open Faced Meat Loaf Sandwich	760	35	2110	71	4½ST+3½MT+3FAT
BBQ Chicken Sandwich	540	9	1690	84	5½ST+2MT
Pastry SW – Broc, Chick, Ch'dar	690	47	1050	45	3ST+2MT+7FAT
Pastry SW – Ham & Cheddar	640	41	1560	47	3ST+2MT+6FAT
Pastry SW – Italian Chicken	630	41	910	43	3ST+2MT+6FAT
Pastry Sandwich – BBQ Chicken	640	39	1260	56	3½ST+1MT+6FAT
Hot & Cold Side Dishes (¾ cup unless noted):					
Baked Sweet Potato, 1	460	7	510	94	3ST+2½CHO+1FAT
BBQ Baked Beans	270	5	540	48	2½ST+1FAT
Black Beans and Rice, 1 c	300	10	1050	45	2½ST+2FAT
Broccoli Cauliflower Au Gratin	200	11	600	14	2V+1MT+1FAT
Broccoli with Red Peppers	60	3.⁵	130	5	1V+1FAT
Broccoli Rice Casserole	240	12	800	26	1ST+1V+2½FAT
Butternut Squash	160	6	580	25	1½ST+1FAT
Chicken Gravy, 2Tbs	15	1	170	2	FREE
Creamed Spinach	260	20	740	11	¼ST+1V+1MT+3FAT
Green Beans	80	6	200	5	1V+1FAT
Green Bean Casserole	130	9	440	10	¼ST+1V+2FAT
Homestyle Mashed Potatoes, ²/₃ c	190	9	570	24	1½ST+1½FAT
with gravy	210	10	740	26	1½ST+2FAT
Honey Glazed Carrots	280	15	80	35	1¾CHO+1V+3FAT
Hot Cinnamon Apples	250	4.⁵	45	56	2½ST+1FR+1FAT

*Carbs=Carbohydrate, na=not available **Exchanges:** ST=Starch, Mlk=Milk (skim)
FR=Fruit, CHO=Other Carbohydrates, V=Vegetable, MT=Meat (medium fat), FAT=Fat

BOSTON MARKET® (continued)

Hot & Cold Side Dishes (¾ cup unless noted):

	Calories	Fat (g)	Sodium (mg)	Carbs* (g)	Exchanges**
Macaroni & Cheese	280	11	830	32	2ST+1MT+1FAT
New Potatoes	130	2.5	150	25	1½ST+½FAT
Oven Roasted Potato Planks, 5	180	5	370	32	2ST+1FAT
Red Beans & Rice, 1 c	260	5	1050	45	2½ST+1FAT
Rice Pilaf, ⅔ c	180	5	600	32	2ST+1FAT
Savory Stuffing	310	12	1140	44	3ST+2½FAT
Squash Casserole	330	24	1110	20	1ST+5FAT
Steamed Vegetables, ⅔ c	35	0.5	35	7	1½V
Sweet Potato Casserole	280	18	190	39	2½ST+3FAT
Whole Kernel Corn	180	4	170	30	2ST+1FAT
Zucchini Marinara	60	3	330	7	1½V+½FAT
Cranberry Relish	370	5	5	84	1FR+4CHO+1FAT
Cole Slaw	300	19	540	30	1V+1½CHO+4FAT
Chunky Cinnamon Applesauce	250	0	30	62	2FR+2CHO
Coyote Bean Salad	190	9	210	24	1ST+2FAT
Fruit Salad	70	0.5	10	15	1FR
Old Fashioned Potato Salad	340	24	870	30	2ST+5FAT

Baked Goods:

	Calories	Fat (g)	Sodium (mg)	Carbs* (g)	Exchanges**
Corn Bread, 1 loaf	200	6	390	33	2ST+1FAT
Cinnamon Apple Pie, 1/5 pie	390	23	250	46	2ST+1FR+4FAT
Chocolate Chip Cookie	340	17	240	48	3ST+3FAT
Brownie	450	27	190	47	3ST+5FAT

Source: Boston Chicken nutritional information ©1999. Current as of 12/99

BRUEGGER'S® BAGELS

Bagels (based on the 4.6 oz size):

	Calories	Fat (g)	Sodium (mg)	Carbs* (g)	Exchanges**
Blueberry	330	2	530	68	4ST
Cinnamon Raisin	320	2	510	68	4ST
Cranberry Orange	330	2	510	68	4ST
Egg	320	2.5	570	64	4ST
Everything	320	2	710	64	4ST
Garlic	320	2	540	65	4ST
Honey Grain	330	3	500	65	4ST
Onion	310	2	540	64	4ST
Plain	310	2	540	63	4ST
Poppy	320	2.5	540	64	4ST
Pumpernickel	320	2.5	600	65	4ST
Salt	310	2	1550	63	4ST
Sesame	330	2	540	63	4ST
Spinach Herb	310	2	610	63	4ST
Sun Dried Tomato	320	2	630	65	4ST
Wheat Bran	310	2	550	64	4ST

*Carbs=Carbohydrate, na=not available   **Exchanges: ST=Starch, Mlk=Milk (skim)
FR=Fruit, CHO=Other Carbohydrates, V=Vegetable, MT=Meat (medium fat), FAT=Fat

BRUEGGER'S® BAGELS

	Calories	Fat (g)	Sodium (mg)	Carbs* (g)	Exchanges**
Specialty Sandwiches:					
Chicken Fajita	500	12	970	74	4½ST+2½MT
Leonardo Da Veggie	460	11	740	69	4½ST+1MT+1FAT
Herby Turkey	530	14	1180	73	4½ST+2½MT
Hot Shot Turkey	430	6	1250	70	4½ST+2½MT(lean)
Santa Fe Turkey	480	10	1630	71	4½ST+2½MT
Garden Veggie	390	6	580	70	4½ST+1MT

Source: Bruegger's® Bagels nutritional information. Current as of 12/99.

BURGER KING®

Burgers:	Calories	Fat (g)	Sodium (mg)	Carbs* (g)	Exchanges**
Whopper® Sandwich	660	40	900	47	3ST+3MT+5FAT
w/out mayo	510	23	na	47	3ST+3MT+1½FAT
Whopper® w/Cheese Sandwich	760	48	1380	47	3ST+4MT+5½FAT
w/out mayo	600	31	na	47	3ST+4MT+2FAT
Double Whopper® Sandwich	920	59	980	47	3ST+5½MT+6½FAT
w/out mayo	760	42	na	47	3ST+5½MT+3FAT
Double Whopper® w/Cheese SW	1010	67	1460	47	3ST+6½MT+7FAT
w/out mayo	850	50	na	47	3ST+6½MT+3½FAT
Whopper Jr® Sandwich	400	24	530	28	2ST+2 MT+3FAT
w/out mayo	320	15	na	28	2ST+2 MT+1FAT
Whopper Jr® w/Cheese SW	450	28	770	28	2ST+2½ MT+3FAT
w/out mayo	370	19	na	28	2ST+2½MT+1½FAT
Big King® Sandwich	640	42	980	28	2ST+4½ MT+4FAT
Hamburger	320	15	520	27	2ST+2 MT+1FAT
Cheeseburger	360	19	760	27	2ST+2½ MT+1FAT
Bacon Cheeseburger	400	22	940	27	2ST+2½ MT+2FAT
Double Cheeseburger	580	36	1060	27	2ST+4½MT+2½FAT
Bacon Double Cheeseburger	620	38	1230	28	2ST+5 MT+2½FAT
Sandwiches/Side Orders:					
Chicken Tenders®, 4 pieces	180	11	470	9	½ST+1½MT+½FAT
5 pieces	230	14	590	11	¾ST+2MT+1FAT
8 pieces	350	22	940	17	1ST+3MT+1½FAT
BK Broiler® Sandwich	530	26	1060	45	3ST+2½MT+2½FAT
w/out mayo	370	9	na	45	3ST+2½MT
Chicken Sandwich	710	43	1400	54	3½ST+2MT+6½FAT
w/out mayo	500	20	na	54	3½ST+2MT+2FAT
Chick'N Crisp	460	27	890	37	2½ST+1MT+4½FAT
w/out mayo	360	16	na	37	2½ST+1MT+2FAT
BK Big Fish® Sandwich	720	43	1180	59	4ST+2MT+6½FAT
Onion Rings, medium	380	19	550	46	3ST+4FAT
king size	600	30	880	74	4½ST+6FAT

*Carbs=Carbohydrate, na=not available **Exchanges: ST=Starch, Mlk=Milk (skim)
FR=Fruit, CHO=Other Carbohydrates, V=Vegetable, MT=Meat (medium fat), FAT=Fat

BURGER KING® (continued)

	Calories	Fat (g)	Sodium (mg)	Carbs* (g)	Exchanges**
French Fries, small salted	250	13	550	32	2ST+2½FAT
not salted	250	13	480	32	2ST+2½FAT
French Fries, medium salted	400	21	820	50	3ST+4FAT
not salted	400	21	760	50	3ST+4FAT
French Fries, King size salted	590	30	1180	74	4½ST+6FAT
not salted	590	30	1110	74	4½ST+6FAT
Dutch Apple Pie	300	15	230	39	1ST+½CHO+1FR+3FAT

Dipping Sauces:

	Calories	Fat (g)	Sodium (mg)	Carbs* (g)	Exchanges**
Barbecue	35	0	400	9	½CHO
Honey Flavored	90	0	10	23	1½CHO
Honey Mustard	90	6	150	10	¾CHO+1FAT
Ranch	170	17	200	2	3½FAT
Sweet & Sour	45	0	50	11	¾CHO

Breakfast:

	Calories	Fat (g)	Sodium (mg)	Carbs* (g)	Exchanges**
Croissan'wich® w/Saus, Egg & Ch	530	41	1120	23	1½ST+2MT+6FAT
w/Sausage & Cheese	450	35	940	21	1½ST+1½MT+5½FAT
Biscuit	300	15	830	35	2½ST+3FAT
with Egg	380	21	1010	37	2½ST+1MT+3FAT
with Sausage	490	33	1240	36	2½ST+1MT+5½FAT
with Sausage, Egg, & Cheese	620	43	1650	37	2½ST+2MT+6½FAT
French Toast Sticks, 5 sticks	440	23	490	51	3½ST+4½FAT
Cini-minis, 4 rolls w/out icing	440	23	710	51	3½ST+4½FAT
Vanilla Icing	110	3	40	20	1CHO+½FAT
Hash Brown Rounds, small	240	15	440	25	1½ST+3FAT
Large	410	26	750	42	2½ST+5FAT
Bacon, 3 pieces	40	3	170	0	½MT
Ham	35	1	770	0	½MT(lean)
A.M. Express® Grape Jam	30	0	0	7	½CHO
A.M. Express® Strawb'ry Jam	30	0	0	8	½CHO
A.M. Express® Dip	80	0	20	21	1½CHO
Land O'Lakes® Wh. Classic Blend	65	7	75	0	1½FAT

Shakes:

	Calories	Fat (g)	Sodium (mg)	Carbs* (g)	Exchanges**
Vanilla, small	330	7	250	56	4CHO+1½FAT
medium	430	9	330	73	5CHO+2FAT
Chocolate, small	330	7	250	58	4CHO+1½FAT
Medium	440	10	330	75	5CHO+2FAT
Chocolate, small, w/syrup added	390	7	350	72	5CHO+1½FAT
Medium w/syrup added	570	10	520	105	7CHO+2FAT
Strawberry, small, w/syrup added	390	7	260	72	5CHO+1½FAT
Medium, w/syrup added	550	9	350	104	7CHO+2FAT

Source: Burger King® nutritional information used with permission of Burger King Corporation.
Current as of 12/99. All ® in this section are trademarks of Burger King®

*Carbs=Carbohydrate, na=not available   **Exchanges: ST=Starch, Mlk=Milk (skim)
FR=Fruit, CHO=Other Carbohydrates, V=Vegetable, MT=Meat (medium fat), FAT=Fat

CAPTAIN D'S® SEAFOOD

	Calories	Fat (g)	Sodium (mg)	Carbs* (g)	Exchanges**
Captain's Broilers (Lunch): includes rice w/vegetable medley & breadstick.					
Broiled Chicken Lunch	503	9	na	na	na
Broiled Fish Lunch	435	7	na	na	na
Broiled Shrimp Lunch	421	7	na	na	na
Broiled Fish & Chicken Lunch	478	8	na	na	na
Captain's Broilers (Platters): includes rice w/veg medley, plain baked potato, salad, & breadstick					
Broiled Shrimp Platter	720	8	na	na	na
Broiled Chicken Platter	802	10	na	na	na
Broiled Fish Platter	734	7	na	na	na
Baked Fish & Chicken Platter	777	10	na	na	na
Sandwiches & Accompaniments:					
Broiled Chicken Sandwich	451	19	858	29	2ST+4½LM+1FAT
Baked Potato	278	0	na	na	3½ST
Imitation Sour Cream	29	3	na	na	½FAT
Margarine	102	12	na	na	2½FAT
Salad	20	0	na	na	1V
Light Italian Dressing, 1 oz pkt	16	0.5	na	na	FREE
French Dressing, 1 oz pkt	111	11	187	4	2FAT+¼CHO
Blue Cheese Dressing, 1 oz pkt	105	12	101	0.2	2½FAT
Ranch Dressing, 1 oz pkt	92	10	230	0.4	2FAT
Cracklins, 1 oz (with dinner)	218	17	741	16	1ST+3½FAT
French Fried Potatoes, 1 portion	302	10	152	50	3ST+2FAT
Cole Slaw, 1 portion	158	12	246	12	1V+½CHO+2½FAT
Cob Corn	251	2	13	60	4ST+½FAT
Green Beans, seasoned, 1 portion	46	2	75	5	1V+½FAT
White Beans, 1 portion	126	0.5	99	22	1½ST
Rice, 1 portion	124	0	9	28	2ST
Fried Okra	300	16	445	34	2ST+1V+3FAT
Hushpuppy, 1	126	4	465	20	1ST+1FAT
Hushpuppies, 6	756	25	2790	119	8ST+5FAT
Crackers, 4	50	1	147	8	½ST+¼FAT
Slice of Cheese	54	5	206	0.2	½HFM
Cocktail Sauce, 1 oz side portion	34	0.4	252	8.4	½CHO
Tartar Sauce, 1 oz side portion	75	7	158	3	¼CHO+1½FAT
Sweet & Sour Sauce, side portion	52	0	5	13	1CHO
Desserts, one piece:					
Pecan Pie	458	20	373	64	4CHO+4FAT
Chocolate Cake	303	10	259	49	3CHO+2FAT
Cheesecake	420	31	480	30	2CHO+6FAT
Carrot Cake	434	23	414	49	3CHO+4½FAT

Source: Captain D's Nutritional Information 4/98. Current as of 12/99.

*Carbs=Carbohydrate, na=not available   **Exchanges: ST=Starch, Mlk=Milk (skim)
FR=Fruit, CHO=Other Carbohydrates, V=Vegetable, MT=Meat (medium fat), FAT=Fat

CARL'S JR.®

Sandwiches & Sides:	Calories	Fat (g)	Sodium (mg)	Carbs* (g)	Exchanges**
Carl's Famous Star™ Hamburger	580	32	910	49	3ST+2MT+4½FAT
Super Star® Hamburger	790	46	970	50	3ST+5MT+4FAT
Western Bacon Cheeseburger®	650	30	1430	63	4ST+3MT+3FAT
Double Western Bacon CB®	900	49	1770	64	4ST+5½MT+4½FAT
Jr. Hamburger	330	13	480	34	2ST+1½MT+1FAT
Charbr. BBQ Chicken SW™	280	3	830	37	2½ST+2½MT(lean)
Charbr. Chicken Club SW™	460	22	1110	33	2ST+3½MT+1FAT
Charb. Santa Fe Chicken SW™	510	31	1240	32	2ST+3MT+3FAT
Carl's Ranch Crispy Chicken SW	620	29	1220	65	4ST+2MT+4FAT
Carl's Bacon Sw Crispy Ch. SW	720	36	1610	66	4ST+2MT+5FAT
Charbroiled Sirloin Steak SW	580	26	1110	50	3ST+3½MT+1½FAT
Carl's Catch Fish Sandwich™	510	27	1030	50	3ST+1½MT+4FAT
American Cheese	60	5	280	0	½MT+½FAT
Swiss-style Cheese	50	4	250	0	½MT+½FAT
French Fries, reg.	290	14	170	37	2ST+3FAT
Onion Rings	430	21	700	53	3ST+4FAT
Zucchini	340	19	860	37	2ST+1V+4FAT
Hash Brown Nuggets	330	21	470	32	2ST+4FAT
CrissCut Fries®	410	24	950	43	3½ST+5FAT
Chicken Stars (6 piece)	280	19	330	15	1ST+1½MT+2½FAT
"Great Stuff"™ Potatoes:					
Broccoli & Cheese Potato	530	21	950	74	4ST+1V+4FAT
Bacon & Cheese Potato	630	29	1700	76	4ST+1MT+5FAT
Plain Potato w/out margarine	290	0	20	68	4ST
Sour Cream & Chives Potato	430	14	135	70	4ST+3FAT
Salads & Salad Dressings:					
Char. Chicken Salad-To-Go™	200	7	440	12	½ST+1V+3MT(lean)
Garden Salad-To-Go™	50	3	60	4	1V+½FAT
House Dressing, 2 oz	220	22	440	3	4½FAT
Blue Cheese Dressing, 2 oz	320	35	370	1	7FAT
1000 Island Dressing, 2 oz	230	23	420	5	4½FAT
Fat Free Italian Dressing, 2 oz	15	0	770	4	FREE
Fat Free French Dressing, 2 oz	60	0	660	16	1FR
Bakery/Desserts/Shakes:					
Blueberry Muffin	340	14	340	49	3ST+3FAT
Bran Raisin Muffin	370	13	410	61	3½ST+2½FAT
Chocolate Chip Cookie	370	19	350	49	3CHO+4FAT
Chocolate Cake	300	10	260	49	3CHO+2FAT
Cheese Danish	400	22	390	49	3CHO+4½FAT
Strawberry Swirl Cheesecake	290	17	230	30	2CHO+3½FAT
Vanilla Shake, small	330	8	250	54	4CHO+1½FAT
Chocolate Shake, small	390	7	280	74	5CHO+1½FAT
Strawberry Shake, small	400	7	240	77	5CHO+1½FAT

*Carbs=Carbohydrate, na=not available   **Exchanges: ST=Starch, Mlk=Milk (skim)
FR=Fruit, CHO=Other Carbohydrates, V=Vegetable, MT=Meat (medium fat), FAT=Fat

CARL'S JR.® (continued)

Breakfast:	Calories	Fat (g)	Sodium (mg)	Carbs* (g)	Exchanges**
French Toast Dips® w/out syrup	370	20	430	42	2½ST+4FAT
Sunrise SW®, bacon/sausage not includ	360	21	700	28	2ST+1MT+3FAT
Breakfast Burrito	480	30	750	26	1½ST+3MT+3FAT
Scrambled Eggs	160	11	125	1	2MT
English Muffin w/ margarine	210	9	300	27	1½ST+2FAT
Breakfast Quesadilla	310	16	670	27	1½ST+1½MT+1½FAT
Bacon, 2 strips	50	4	140	0	½MT+½FAT
Sausage, 1 patty	200	19	480	2	1MT+3FAT
Breads/Sauces:					
Croutons	35	1	65	5	½ST
Breadsticks	35	1	60	7	½ST
Table Syrup	90	0	0	21	1½CHO
Mustard Sauce	50	0	210	11	½CHO
Honey Sauce	90	0	0	22	1½CHO
BBQ Sauce	50	0	270	11	1CHO
Sweet n' Sour Sauce	50	0	80	12	1CHO

Source: Carl's Jr® Nutritional Guide ©1998. Current as of 12/99. All ® in this section are trademarks of Carl's Jr®

CARROWS® & COCO's®

	Calories	Fat (g)	Sodium (mg)	Carbs* (g)	Exchanges**
Oatmeal with 2oz skim milk	175	3	330	30	2ST
Oatmeal Combo w/fruit	428	6	716	82	4½ST+1MT+1FR
Oatmeal Combo w/juice	426	6	708	81	4½ST+1MT+1FR
Raisin Bran Combo w/fruit	388	4	639	80	4½ST+1FR
Raisin Bran Combo w/juice	386	4	631	79	4½ST+1FR
Bagel (average)	215	1	504	43	3ST
English Muffin	150	2	230	27	2ST
Poached Eggs, 2	148	10	280	1	2MFM
Granola with skim milk	588	30	242	70	4ST+½Mlk+6FAT
Granola without milk	545	30	179	64	4ST+6FAT
Omelette Primavera	576	38	968	38	2½ST+2½MT+5FAT
Egg White Omelette w/out feta	413	4	738	69	4ST+2½MT+1FR
Egg White Omelette w/1oz feta	497	11	1093	71	4ST+3MT+1FR
Turkey Burger	547	32	1381	31	2ST+4MT+2FAT
Garden Burger	565	25	1378	72	5ST+1MT+4FAT
Soup & Salad Combo	375	16	1810	43	3ST+1MT+1FAT
Pasta Marinara	643	14	929	108	6½ST+1V+2FAT
Fresh Fish w/spinach & rice	562	6	1828	78	4½ST+1V+5MT(very lean)
Baked Potato, 7 oz medium	220	0	16	51	3ST
Tomato Slices, 6	18	0	6	3	FREE

Source: Carrow's® & Coco's® nutritional information. Current as of 12/99.

---

*Carbs=Carbohydrate, na=not available   ****Exchanges:** ST=Starch, Mlk=Milk (skim)
FR=Fruit, CHO=Other Carbohydrates, V=Vegetable, MT=Meat (medium fat), FAT=Fat

Chick-fil-A®

Specialties:	Calories	Fat (g)	Sodium (mg)	Carbs* (g)	Exchanges**
Chick-fil-A® Chicken Sandwich	290	9	870	29	2ST+3MT(lean)
Chicken Deluxe Sandwich	300	9	870	31	2ST+3MT(lean)
Chicken, no bun, no pickles	160	8	690	1	3MT(lean)
Chick-fil-A Chargrilled Ch. SW®	280	3	640	36	2ST+3MT(very lean)
Chargrilled Chicken Deluxe SW	290	3	640	38	2ST+1V+3MT(very lean)
Char Chicken, no bun or pickles	130	3	630	0	3MT(very lean)
Chick-fil-A® Chicken Club SW no dressing	390	12	980	38	2ST+4MT(lean)+1V
Chick-fil-A® Chick-n-Strips®, 4	230	8	380	10	½ST+4MT(lean)
Chick-fil-A® Nuggets®, 8 pack	290	14	770	12	1ST+3½MT
Chick-fil-A® Chicken Salad SW on whole wheat	320	5	810	42	3ST+2MT(lean)
Hearty Breast Chick. Soup, cup	110	1	760	10	½ST+1V+2MT(very lean)
Chick-fil-A® Chargrilled Chicken Garden Salad	170	3	650	10	2V+2MT(very lean)
Chick-fil-A® Chick-n-Strips Salad	290	9	430	21	½ST+4MT+2V
Chick-fil-A ® Chicken Salad Plate	290	5	570	40	2ST+2V+ 2MT(lean)

Side Orders:

Tossed Salad	70	0	0	13	2½V
Cole Slaw, small	130	6	430	11	2½V+1FAT
Carrot & Raisin Salad, small	150	2	650	28	2V+1FR+½FAT
Chick-fil-A Waffle Potato Fries®, small, salted	290	10	960	49	3ST+2FAT
Chick-fil-A Waffle Potato Fries®, small unsalted by request	290	10	80	49	3ST+2FAT

Desserts/Beverages:

Icedream®, small cup	350	10	390	50	1½CHO+1Mlk+2FAT
Icedream®, small cone	140	4	240	16	¼CHO+1Mlk+1FAT
Lemon Pie, slice	320	16	280	40	½CHO+1FR+3FAT
Fudge Nut Brownie	350	16	650	41	2CHO+1FR+3FAT
Cheesecake, slice	270	21	510	23	1½CHO+1MT+3FAT
w/ Strawberry Topping	290	23	580	24	1½CHO+1MT+3FAT
w/ Blueberry Topping	290	23	550	25	1½CHO+1MT+3FAT
Chick-fil-A® Lemonade, 9 oz	90	0	4	23	1½CHO
Chick-fil-A® Diet Lemonade, 9 oz	5	0	4	2	FREE

Source: Chick-fil-A Ingredient and Nutrition Guide ©8/97. Current as of 12/99. All ® in this section are the trademarks of Chick-fil-A®.

*Carbs=Carbohydrate, na=not available   **Exchanges: ST=Starch, Mlk=Milk (skim)
FR=Fruit, CHO=Other Carbohydrates, V=Vegetable, MT=Meat (medium fat), FAT=Fat

CHI-CHI'S®

	Calories	Fat (g)	Sodium (mg)	Carbs* (g)	Exchanges**
Low Fat Chicken Soft Taco (two grilled soft tacos, served w/Spanish rice, Mexi-Veggies,& Salsa)	692	7.⁴	1379	na	5ST+3V+4MT(lean)
Low Fat Chicken Enchiladas (two soft flour tortillas filled w/chicken, served w/Spanish rice & Mexi-Veggies)	688	18.⁶	2325	na	5ST+3V+2MT(lean)+2½FAT

Source: Chi-Chi's® Low Fat Items Nutritional Information. Current as of 12/99.

CHILI'S®

	Calories	Fat (g)	Sodium (mg)	Carbs* (g)	Exchanges**
Guiltless Grill (GG) Menu Items:					
GG Veggie Pasta	632	13	na	na	na
GG Veggie Pasta with Chicken	717	15	na	na	na
GG Chicken Platter	652	9	na	na	na
GG Chicken Pita	425	9	na	na	na
GG Chicken Sandwich	553	8	na	na	na
GG Chicken Salad with Dressing	445	5	na	na	na

Source: Chili's Guiltless Nutritional Information. Current as of 12/99.

CHURCH'S CHICKEN®

	Calories	Fat (g)	Sodium (mg)	Carbs* (g)	Exchanges**
Fried Chicken ± Refers to edible portion (without bones, cob, etc.):					
Wing, 3.¹ oz±	250	16	540	8	½ST+2MT+1FAT
Leg, 2 oz±	140	9	160	2	2MT
Thigh, 2.⁸ oz±	230	16	520	5	½ST+2MT+1FAT
Breast, 2.⁸ oz±	200	12	510	4	½ST+2½MT
Tender Strip™, 1.¹ oz	80	4	140	5	1MT
Side Orders:					
Cajun Rice	130	7	260	16	1ST+1½FAT
Potatoes & Gravy	90	3	520	14	1ST+½FAT
Okra	210	16	520	19	1ST+3FAT
Biscuits	250	16	640	26	1½ST+3FAT
Corn on the Cob	139	3	15	24	1½ST+½FAT
Apple Pie	280	12	340	41	1½CHO+1FR+2½FAT
Cole Slaw	92	6	230	8	1½V+1FAT
French Fries	210	11	60	29	2ST+2FAT

Source: Churchs Chicken®. Current as of 12/99.

---

*Carbs=Carbohydrate, na=not available **Exchanges:** ST=Starch, Mlk=Milk (skim)
FR=Fruit, CHO=Other Carbohydrates, V=Vegetable, MT=Meat (medium fat), FAT=Fat

DAIRY QUEEN®/BRAZIER®

	Calories	Fat (g)	Sodium (mg)	Carbs* (g)	Exchanges**
DQ Homestyle® Hamburger	290	12	630	29	2ST+2MT
DQ Homestyle® Cheeseburger	340	17	850	29	2ST+2½MT+1FAT
DQ Homestyle® Double ChB	540	31	1130	30	2ST+4MT+2FAT
DQ Homestyle® Bacon Dble ChB	610	36	1380	31	2ST+5MT+2FAT
DQ Ultimate® Burger	670	43	1210	29	2ST+5MT+3FAT
Hot Dog	240	14	730	19	1ST+1MT+2FAT
Chili 'n' Cheese Dog	330	21	1090	22	1½ST+1½MT+2FAT
Chicken Breast Fillet Sandwich	430	20	760	37	2½ST+2½MT+1FAT
Grilled Chicken Sandwich	310	10	1040	30	2ST+2½MT
Chicken Strip Basket™ w/fries, Texas toast, & gravy	1000	50	2260	102	7ST+2½MT+6FAT
The Great Steakmelt™ Basket w/small fries	750	37	2000	70	4½ST+3MT+3½FAT
French Fries, small	350	18	630	42	3ST+3FAT
French Fries, medium	440	23	790	53	3½ST+4FAT
Onion Rings	320	16	180	39	2½ST+3FAT

DAIRY QUEEN®

	Calories	Fat (g)	Sodium (mg)	Carbs* (g)	Exchanges**
Cones:					
DQ® Vanilla Soft Serve, ½ c	140	5	70	22	1½CHO+½FAT
DQ® Chocolate Soft Serve, ½ c	150	5	75	22	1½CHO+½FAT
Small Vanilla Cone	230	7	115	38	2½CHO+1FAT
Medium Vanilla Cone	330	9	160	53	3½CHO+1FAT
Large Vanilla Cone	410	12	200	65	4CHO+2FAT
Small Chocolate Cone	240	8	115	37	2½CHO+1FAT
Medium Chocolate Cone	340	11	160	53	3½CHO+1½FAT
Small Dipped Cone	340	17	130	42	3CHO+3FAT
Medium Dipped Cone	490	24	190	59	4CHO+4FAT
Yogurt:					
DQ® Nonfat Frozen Yogurt, ½ c	100	0	70	21	1½CHO
Medium Yogurt Cone	260	1	160	56	4CHO
Medium Cup of Yogurt	230	0.5	150	48	3CHO
Med Yogurt Strawberry Sundae	280	0.5	160	61	4CHO
Small Strawberry Breeze®	320	0.5	190	68	4½CHO
Medium Strawberry Breeze®	460	1	270	99	6½CHO
Small Heath® Breeze®	470	10	380	85	5½CHO+1½FAT
Medium Heath® Breeze®	710	18	580	123	8CHO+2½FAT
Malts, Shakes, Smoothys, Misty® Slushes:					
Small Chocolate Malt	650	16	370	111	7½CHO+2FAT
Medium Chocolate Malt	880	22	500	153	10CHO+3½FAT
Small Chocolate Shake	560	15	310	94	6CHO+2½FAT

*Carbs=Carbohydrate, na=not available   **Exchanges: ST=Starch, Mlk=Milk (skim) FR=Fruit, CHO=Other Carbohydrates, V=Vegetable, MT=Meat (medium fat), FAT=Fat

DAIRY QUEEN®

	Calories	Fat (g)	Sodium (mg)	Carbs* (g)	Exchanges**
Malts, Shakes, Smoothys, Misty® Slushes, continued:					
Medium Chocolate Shake	770	20	420	130	8½CHO+3FAT
Straw Banana DQ Glacier Smoothy™	670	14	250	128	8½CHO+2FAT
Frozen Hot Chocolate	860	35	350	127	8½CHO+6FAT
Small Misty® Slush	220	0	20	56	4CHO
Medium Misty® Slush	290	0	30	74	5CHO
Sundaes:					
Small Chocolate Sundae	280	7	140	49	3CHO+1FAT
Medium Chocolate Sundae	400	10	210	71	5CHO+1FAT
Royal Treats®:					
Banana Split	510	12	180	96	3FR+3½CHO+1½FAT
Peanut Buster® Parfait	730	31	400	99	6½CHO+5FAT
Pecan Mudslide™ Treat	650	30	420	85	5½CHO+5FAT
Strawberry Shortcake	430	14	360	70	4½CHO+2FAT
Chocolate Rock™ Treat	730	38	280	87	6CHO+6FAT
Novelties:					
DQ® Sandwich	150	5	115	24	1½CHO+½FAT
Chocolate Dilly Bar®	210	13	75	21	1½CHO+2FAT
Buster Bar®	450	28	280	41	3CHO+5FAT
Starkiss®	80	0	10	21	1½FR
DQ® Fudge Bar, no sugar added	50	0	70	13	1CHO
DQ® Van Orange Bar, no sugar added	60	0	40	17	1CHO
Lemon DQ® Freez'r®, ½ c	80	0	10	20	1FR
Blizzard® Flavor Treats:					
Choc SW Cookie Blizzard®, sm	520	18	380	79	5CHO+3FAT
medium	640	23	500	97	6½CHO+4FAT
CC Cookie Dough Blizzard®, sm	660	24	440	99	6½CHO+4FAT
medium	950	36	660	143	9½CHO+6FAT
DQ Treatzza Pizza™ (¹/₈ of Pizza):					
Heath®	180	7	160	28	2CHO+1FAT
M&M®	190	7	160	29	2CHO+1FAT
DQ® Cake (undecorated, ¹/₈ of cake):					
DQ® Frozen 8" Round Cake	370	13	280	56	4CHO+2FAT
DQ® Layered 8" Round Cake	330	12	350	49	3CHO+2FAT

The ® items previously listed are the trademark of American Dairy Queen Corporation except: M&M is a registered trademark of Mars, Inc.; Heath® toffee bar is a registered trademark of Hershey's. The nutrient values & suggested exchanges are meant for general information purposes only. Although the information is based on our recommended product preparation procedures, variations may occur due to differences in product procedures between restaurants. Seasonal differences and slight variations among different manufacturers must also be expected. Menu items listed may not be available at all *Dairy Queen/Brazier* stores.

*Carbs=Carbohydrate, na=not available   ****Exchanges:** ST=Starch, Mlk=Milk (skim) FR=Fruit, CHO=Other Carbohydrates, V=Vegetable, MT=Meat (medium fat), FAT=Fat

D'ANGELO®

	Calories	Fat (g)	Sodium (mg)	Carbs* (g)	Exchanges**
D'Angelo D'Lites:					
Turkey D'Lite Pokket	330	2	490	na	2ST+1V+3MT(lean)
Small Sub	365	4	535	na	2½ST+1V+3MT(lean)
Roast Beef D'Lite Pokket	330	6	710	na	2ST+1V+3MT(lean)
Small Sub	365	7	755	na	2½ST+1V+3MT(lean)
Steak D'Lite Pokket	390	11	735	na	3ST+2V+2MT
Spicy Steak D'Lite Pokket	425	11	735	na	3ST+2V+2MT
Ginger StirFry Ch. D'Lite Pokket	400	5	1240	na	2½ST+1V+3MT(lean)
Stuffed Turkey D'Lite Pokket	510	8	880	na	3ST+1FR+1V+4MT(lean)
Small Sub	545	9	920	na	3½ST+1FR+1V+4MT(lean)
Classic Vegetable D'Lite Pokket	340	10	960	na	2ST++3V+1MT 1FAT
Crunchy Vegetable D'Lite Pokket	350	10	1000	na	2ST+3V+1MT+1FAT
Small Sub	385	11	1045	na	2½ST+3V+ 1MT+1FAT
Super Salads:					
Turkey D'Lite	355	2	714	na	2ST+1V+3MT(lean)
Roast Beef D'Lite	355	6	935	na	2ST+1V+3MT(lean)
Tuna D'Lite	295	2	853	na	2ST+1V+2MT(very lean)
Chicken D'Lite	345	4	980	na	2ST+1V+2MT(lean)

Source: D'Angelo®. Current as of 12/99.

DEL TACO

	Calories	Fat (g)	Sodium (mg)	Carbs* (g)	Exchanges**
Quesadillas:					
Chicken Quesadilla	580	31	1240	41	2½ST+3½MT+2½FAT
Spicy Jack Chicken Quesadilla	570	30	1300	40	2½ST+3½MT+2½FAT
Regular Quesadilla	500	27	660	39	2½ST+2MT+3½FAT
Spicy Jack Regular Quesadilla	490	26	920	38	2½ST+2MT+3FAT
Salads:					
Deluxe Taco Salad™	760	37	2010	76	4ST+1V+2½MT+5FAT
Tostada	210	9	640	24	1½ST+2FAT
Burgers:					
Double Del Cheeseburger™	560	35	960	35	2½ST+3MT+4FAT
Del Cheeseburger™	430	25	710	35	2½ST+1½MT+3½FAT
Cheeseburger	330	13	870	37	2½ST+1½MT+1FAT
Tacos:					
Big Fat Steak Taco™	390	19	960	38	2½ST+1½MT+2½FAT
Big Fat Chicken Taco™	340	13	840	38	2½ST+1½MT+1FAT
Big Fat Taco™	320	11	680	39	2½ST+1½MT+½FAT
Chicken Soft Taco	210	12	520	16	1ST+1MT+1½FAT
Taco	160	10	150	11	¾ST+1MT+1FAT
Soft Taco	160	8	330	16	1ST+1MT+½FAT

*Carbs=Carbohydrate, na=not available   **Exchanges: ST=Starch, Mlk=Milk (skim)
FR=Fruit, CHO=Other Carbohydrates, V=Vegetable, MT=Meat (medium fat), FAT=Fat

DEL TACO (continued)

Burritos:	Calories	Fat (g)	Sodium (mg)	Carbs* (g)	Exchanges**
Macho Beef Burrito™	1170	62	2190	89	5½ST+6MT+6½FAT
Macho Combo Burrito™	1050	44	2760	113	6½ST+4MT+5FAT
Deluxe Del Beef Burrito™	590	33	1110	45	2½ST+3½MT+3FAT
Del Beef Burrito™	550	30	1090	42	2½ST+3½MT+2½FAT
Deluxe Combo Burrito™	530	25	1390	56	3ST+2½MT+2½FAT
Combo Burrito	490	21	1380	53	3ST+2½MT+1½FAT
Del Classic Chicken Burrito™	580	38	1100	42	2½ST+2½MT+5FAT
Spicy Chicken Burrito	480	16	1620	65	3½ST+2MT+1FAT
The Works Burrito™	480	18	1500	69	4ST+1MT+2½FAT
Regular Red Burrito	390	12	1439	59	3ST+1MT+1½FAT
Regular Green Burrito	400	12	1450	59	3ST+1MT+1½FAT
Red Burrito	270	8	1020	38	2ST+1MT+½FAT
Green Burrito	280	8	1030	38	2ST+1MT+½FAT
Nachos:					
Macho Nachos®	1200	66	2720	130	7ST+2MT+ 11FAT
Nachos	380	24	630	40	2½ST+5FAT
Sides:					
Rice Cup	150	2	600	28	2ST+½FAT
Beans 'n Cheese Cup	260	3	1810	44	2½ST+1½MT(very lean)
Value Fries:					
Deluxe Chili Cheese Fries™	710	49	880	53	3ST+1MT+9FAT
Chili Cheese Fries	670	46	880	51	3ST+1MT+8FAT
Best Value Large Fries	490	32	380	47	3ST+6½FAT
Regular Fries	350	23	270	34	2ST+4½FAT
Small Fries	210	14	160	20	1ST+3FAT
Breakfast:					
Macho Bacon & Egg Burrito™	1030	60	1760	82	5ST+3½MT+8½FAT
Steak & Egg Burrito	580	34	1270	41	2½ST+3½MT+3½FAT
Egg & Cheese Burrito	450	24	740	39	2½ST+2MT+3FAT
Breakfast Burrito	250	11	520	24	1½ST+1MT+1FAT
Bacon & Egg Quesadilla	450	23	920	40	2½ST+2MT+2½FAT
Side of Bacon, 2 slices	50	4	170	0	1FAT
Shakes & Drinks:					
Orange Juice	140	0	0	34	2FR
Small Chocolate Shake	520	12	270	89	6CHO+2½FAT
Small Strawberry Shake	410	6	220	76	5CHO+1FAT
Small Vanilla Shake	420	7	250	75	5CHO+1½FAT
Large Chocolate Shake	680	16	350	117	7½CHO+3FAT
Large Strawberry Shake	540	8	280	100	6½CHO+1½FAT
Large Vanilla Shake	550	10	320	97	6½CHO+2FAT

Source: Del Taco Nutritional Information 9/98. Current as of 12/99. All ® in this section are
   trademarks of Del Taco.

*Carbs=Carbohydrate, na=not available   ****Exchanges:** ST=Starch, Mlk=Milk (skim)
FR=Fruit, CHO=Other Carbohydrates, V=Vegetable, MT=Meat (medium fat), FAT=Fat

DENNY'S®

Fit Fare™ Breakfast:	Calories	Fat (g)	Sodium (mg)	Carbs* (g)	Exchanges**
Slim Slam™ w/out syrup	495	12	1746	98	4ST+4MT(lean)
Blueberry Topping	106	0	15	26	2FR
Strawberry Topping	115	1	12	26	2FR
Cherry Topping	86	0	5	21	1½FR
Cereal Combo:					
Choice: Toast, dry, 1 sl	92	1	166	17	1ST
English Muffin, dry, whole	125	1	198	24	1½ST
Bagel, dry, whole	235	1	495	46	3ST
Choice: Oatmeal	100	2	175	18	1ST
Grits	80	0	520	18	1ST
Cereal (average)	100	0	276	23	1½ST
2% milk	87	5	70	7	½Mlk+1FAT
Choice: Applesauce	60	0	13	15	1FR
Cantaloupe	32	0	16	8	½FR
Grapefruit, ½	60	0	0	16	1FR
Grapes	55	1	0	15	1FR
Honeydew	31	0	22	8	½FR
Banana, 1	110	0	0	29	2FR
Choice: Apple Juice	126	0	24	33	2FR
Grapefruit Juice	115	0	0	29	2FR
Orange Juice	126	0	31	31	2FR
Tomato Juice	56	0	921	11	2V

Fit Fare™ Sandwiches, Salads, & Soups:	Calories	Fat (g)	Sodium (mg)	Carbs* (g)	Exchanges**
Garden Chicken Delite Salad, w/out dressing	277	5	785	30	1ST+3V +4MT(very lean)
Grilled Chicken Sandwich	434	9	1705	56	3½ST+1V+3MT(lean)
Side Garden Salad, w/out dressing	113	4	147	16	½ST+1V+1FAT
Fat Free Honey Mustard, 1 oz	38	0	121	9	½CHO
Reduced Calorie Italian, 1 oz	23	1	515	3	FREE
Vegetable Beef	79	1	820	11	1ST
Chicken Noodle	60	2	640	8	½ST+½FAT

Fit Fare™ Entrees (entrée only):	Calories	Fat (g)	Sodium (mg)	Carbs* (g)	Exchanges**
Grilled Chicken Breast	130	4	566	0	3½MT(very lean)
Grilled Alaskan Salmon	210	4	103	1	6MT(very lean)

Fit Fare™ Sides:	Calories	Fat (g)	Sodium (mg)	Carbs* (g)	Exchanges**
Baked Potato, plain	186	0	14	43	2½ST
Rice Pilaf	112	2	328	21	1½ST
Broccoli in butter sauce	50	2	280	7	1V+½FAT
Corn in butter sauce	120	4	260	19	1ST+1FAT
Carrots in honey glaze	80	3	220	12	½CHO+1V+½FAT
Green Beans with bacon	60	4	390	6	1V+1FAT
Green Peas in butter sauce	100	2	360	14	1ST+½FAT
Applesauce Musselman's®	60	0	13	15	1FR
Sliced Tomatoes, 3 slices	13	0	6	3	½ V

*Carbs=Carbohydrate, na=not available   **Exchanges: ST=Starch, Mlk=Milk (skim)
FR=Fruit, CHO=Other Carbohydrates, V=Vegetable, MT=Meat (medium fat), FAT=Fat

DENNY'S® (continued)

	Calories	Fat (g)	Sodium (mg)	Carbs* (g)	Exchanges**

Breakfast (nutritional information *doesn't* include syrup or margarine):

	Calories	Fat (g)	Sodium (mg)	Carbs* (g)	Exchanges**
Original Grand Slam	795	50	2237	65	4ST+3MT+7FAT
French Slam	1029	71	1428	58	4ST+4½MT+10FAT

Breakfast (nutritional information *doesn't* include bread choice, potatoes, or grits):

	Calories	Fat (g)	Sodium (mg)	Carbs* (g)	Exchanges**
Scram Slam	740	62	1293	14	1ST+5MT+7FAT
All American Slam	712	62	1281	9	½ST+5½MT+4FAT
Ultimate Omelette	564	47	939	9	½ST+3½MT+5½FAT
Veggie-Cheese Omelette	480	39	535	9	2ST+3MT+7½FAT
Ham'n'Cheddar Omelette	581	45	1180	4	5MT+4FAT
Farmer's Omelette®	650	51	1158	17	1ST+3½MT+6½FAT
Chicken Fried Steak & Eggs	430	36	861	9	½ST+3MT+4FAT
T-bone Steak & Eggs	991	77	1003	1	10½MT+5FAT
Sirloin Steak & Eggs	622	49	632	1	6MT+3½FAT

Breakfast (nutritional information *doesn't* include bread choice):

	Calories	Fat (g)	Sodium (mg)	Carbs* (g)	Exchanges**
Sausage Supreme Skillet	1054	83	1740	30	2ST+3MT+13FAT
Meat Lover's Skillet	1147	93	2507	24	1½ST+5MT+13FAT
Big TX Chicken Fajita Skillet®	1217	70	1817	25	2ST+6MT+8FAT

Other Breakfasts (nutritional information doesn't include margarine or toppings):

	Calories	Fat (g)	Sodium (mg)	Carbs* (g)	Exchanges**
Sausage Lover's Slam	960	68	1934	33	2ST+2½MT+11FAT
Farmer's Slam	1200	80	3204	82	5½ST+5MT+10FAT
Cinnamon Swirl Slam	1105	78	1374	68	4½ST+4MT+10½FAT
Play it Again Slam®	1192	75	3555	98	6½ST+4½MT+9½FAT
Cinn. Swirl French Toast, no meat	1030	49	675	124	8ST+10FAT

Other Breakfasts:

	Calories	Fat (g)	Sodium (mg)	Carbs* (g)	Exchanges**
Southern Slam	1065	84	2449	47	3ST+4MT+13FAT
Moons Over My Hammy® w/out potato	807	48	2247	46	3ST+5MT+4½FAT
Country Slam™	1000	66	2727	61	4ST+4MT+8½FAT
Eggs Benedict, w/out potato	695	46	1718	34	2ST+4MT+5FAT
Waffle, plain (w/out syrup or meat)	304	21	200	23	1½ST+4FAT
French Toast, 2 plain (w/out meat)	507	24	594	54	3½ST+5FAT
Buttermilk Hotcakes, 3 plain	491	7	1818	95	6ST+1½FAT
Potato Pancakes (w/out meat)	530	27	1125	59	4ST+5FAT
One Egg	134	12	61	1	1MT+2FAT
Egg Beaters™ Egg Substitute	71	5	138	1	1MT
Ham	94	3	761	2	2MT(lean)
Bacon, 4 slices	162	18	640	1	1½MT+2FAT
Sausage, 4 links	354	32	944	0	2½MT+4FAT
Sausage Patties, 2	300	28	466	1	1½MT+4FAT
Biscuit, buttered	272	11	790	39	2½ST+2FAT
Biscuit & Sausage Gravy	398	21	1267	45	3ST+4FAT
Sausage Gravy	126	10	477	6	2FAT
Country Fried Potatoes	515	35	805	23	1½ST+7FAT

***Carbs**=Carbohydrate, na=not available   ****Exchanges:** ST=Starch, Mlk=Milk (skim) FR=Fruit, CHO=Other Carbohydrates, V=Vegetable, MT=Meat (medium fat), FAT=Fat

DENNY'S® (continued)

	Calories	Fat (g)	Sodium (mg)	Carbs* (g)	Exchanges**
Hashed Browns	218	14	424	20	1½ST+3FAT
covered	318	23	604	21	1½ST+1MT+3FAT
covered & smothered	359	26	790	26	2ST+1MT+4FAT
double covered & smothered	460	26	1213	48	3ST+5FAT

Other tips: Egg substitutes may be requested instead of eggs in any of the egg dishes. You may substitute fresh fruit or tomato slices for either the breakfast meats or hash browns.

Salads (nutritional info doesn't include dressing & bread, unless noted):

Fried Chicken Salad	438	26	1030	26	1ST+3V+3MT+2FAT
Grilled Chicken Caesar w/dressing	600	41	1792	19	1ST+1V+5MT+3FAT
Buffalo Chicken Salad	516	35	1197	26	1ST+3V+3MT+3FAT
Garden Chicken De-lite	277	5	785	30	1ST+3V+4MT(lean)
Side Caesar, w/dressing	362	26	913	20	1ST+1V+½MT+4FAT
Side Garden Salad	113	4	147	16	½ST+1V+1FAT
California Grilled Chicken Salad	277	12	720	10	2V+4MT(lean)

Condiments (1 oz unless specified):

Bleu Cheese Dressing	124	12	405	4	2½FAT
Caesar Dressing	133	14	380	1	3FAT
French Dressing	106	10	274	3	2FAT
Fat Free Honey Mustard	38	0	121	9	½CHO
Reduced Calorie Italian	23	1	515	3	¼CHO
Ranch Dressing	101	11	215	1	2FAT
Thousand Island Dressing	104	10	208	2	2FAT
Sour Cream, 1.⁵ oz	91	9	23	2	2FAT
BBQ Sauce, 1.⁵ oz	47	1	595	11	1CHO

Sandwiches w/out condiments or french fries (you may substitute tomato slices or vegetables *instead* of french fries):

Club Sandwich	718	38	1666	62	4ST+3MT+4FAT
The Super Bird® Sandwich	620	32	1880	48	3ST+4MT+2½FAT
Classic Burger	673	40	1142	42	3ST+4½MT+3½FAT
Classic Burger w/cheese	836	53	1595	43	3ST+6MT+4½FAT
Charleston Chicken SW™	632	32	1967	53	3½ST+4MT+2FAT
Bacon Cheddar Burger	875	52	1672	58	3ST+7MT+6FAT
Bacon, Lettuce, & Tomato	634	46	1116	37	2½ST+1½MT+7FAT
Grilled Chicken Sandwich	520	14	1613	64	4½ST+3MT
Gardenburger®	665	33	1051	75	4½ST+1MT+5½FAT
Reuben	580	35	2726	37	2½ST+3MT+4FAT
Double Decker Burger	1247	80	2200	82	5½ST+5½MT+10½FAT
Garlic Mushroom Swiss	872	51	1529	58	4ST+5MT+5FAT
Buffalo Chicken Burger	803	45	2143	67	4½ST+3½MT+3FAT

Classic Combos (nutritional information doesn't include condiments, soup or salad):

Turkey Breast on multigrain	476	26	1107	39	2½ST+2½MT+2½FAT
Ham & Swiss on rye	533	31	1638	40	2½ST+2½MT+4FAT

*Carbs=Carbohydrate, na=not available **Exchanges: ST=Starch, Mlk=Milk (skim) FR=Fruit, CHO=Other Carbohydrates, V=Vegetable, MT=Meat (medium fat), FAT=Fat

DENNY'S® (continued)

Soup (8 oz):	Calories	Fat (g)	Sodium (mg)	Carbs* (g)	Exchanges**
Vegetable Beef	79	1	820	11	1ST
Chicken Noodle	60	2	640	8	½ST+½FAT
Cream of Potato	222	12	761	23	1½ST+2FAT
Cream of Broccoli	193	12	818	15	1ST+2FAT
Cheese	293	23	895	13	1ST+½MT+4FAT
Clam Chowder	214	11	903	22	1½ST+2FAT
Split Pea	146	6	819	18	1ST+1MT
Chili w/cheese topping	401	19	1039	21	1½ST+3MT+1FAT

Appetizers (nutritional information doesn't include condiments):

	Calories	Fat (g)	Sodium (mg)	Carbs* (g)	Exchanges**
Sampler™	1405	80	5305	124	8ST+4½MT+10FAT
Buffalo Wings, 12	856	54	5552	1	13MT
Mozzarella Sticks, 8 w/sauce	710	41	5220	49	3½ST+4MT+4FAT
Buffalo Chicken Strips, 5	734	42	1673	43	3ST+6MT+2FAT
Chicken Strips, 5	720	33	1666	56	4ST+5MT+1½FAT
Smothered Cheese Fries	767	48	875	69	4½ST+2MT+7FAT
Chili Cheese Fries	816	44	917	77	5ST+2MT+6FAT

Entrees (nutritional info doesn't include bread or side dishes):

	Calories	Fat (g)	Sodium (mg)	Carbs* (g)	Exchanges**
T-Bone Steak	642	50	719	1	6½MT+3½FAT
Sirloin Steak	271	21	273	0	3MT+1FAT
Grilled Chopped Steak	400	26	447	12	1ST+4MT+1FAT
Pot Roast, with gravy	265	11	1165	6	½CHO+6MT(lean)
Pork Chop, with gravy	386	24	844	0	5½MT
Fish Dinner	732	47	1335	48	3ST+3½MT+6FAT
Chicken Fried Steak, w/gravy	265	17	668	14	1ST+2MT+1½FAT
Grilled Alaskan Salmon	210	4	103	1	6MT(very lean)
Steak & Shrimp	645	42	1143	31	2ST+4½MT+3½FAT
Fried Shrimp	558	32	1114	49	3ST+2MT+4FAT
Roast Turkey, Stuffing & gravy	701	27	2346	63	4ST+5½MT
Grilled Chicken	130	4	560	0	3½MT(very lean)
Charleston Chicken Dinner, w/gravy	327	18	993	16	1ST+3MT+½FAT
Chicken Strip w/ Honey Mustard	635	25	1510	55	3½ST+5MT

Sides:

	Calories	Fat (g)	Sodium (mg)	Carbs* (g)	Exchanges**
French Fries, unsalted	323	14	130	44	3ST+3FAT
Seasoned Fries	261	12	556	35	2½ST+2½FAT
Onion Rings	381	23	1003	38	2½ST+4½FAT
Baked Potatoes, plain w/skin	220	0	16	51	3ST
Mashed Potatoes, plain	105	1	378	21	1½ST
Vegetable Rice Pilaf	85	1	325	16	1ST
Bread Stuffing, plain	100	1	405	19	1ST
Cottage Cheese	72	3	281	2	1MT(lean)
Applesauce Mussleman's®	60	0	13	15	1FR
Sliced Tomatoes, 3 slices	13	0	6	3	½V
Broccoli in butter sauce	50	2	280	7	1V+½FAT
Corn in butter sauce	120	4	260	19	1ST+1FAT

*Carbs=Carbohydrate, na=not available **Exchanges:** ST=Starch, Mlk=Milk (skim)
FR=Fruit, CHO=Other Carbohydrates, V=Vegetable, MT=Meat (medium fat), FAT=Fat

DENNY'S® (continued)

Sides (continued):	Calories	Fat (g)	Sodium (mg)	Carbs* (g)	Exchanges**
Carrots in honey glaze	80	3	220	12	1V+½CHO+½FAT
Green Beans with bacon	60	4	390	6	1V+1FAT
Green Peas in butter sauce	100	2	360	14	1ST+½FAT
Brown Gravy, 1 oz (2T)	13	0	184	2	1FREE
Chicken Gravy, 1 oz (2T)	14	0.5	139	2	1FREE
Country Gravy, 1 oz (2T)	17	1	93	2	1FREE
Grilled Mushrooms	14	0	0	2	1FREE
Herb Toast	170	11	325	15	1ST+2FAT
Pies ($^1/_6$ pie):					
Apple Pie	470	24	470	64	3CHO+1FR+4FAT
Cherry Pie	630	25	550	101	5½CHO+1FR+4FAT
Chocolate Peanut Butter Pie	653	39	319	64	4CHO+8FAT
Cheesecake Pie w/out topping	470	27	280	48	3CHO+5½FAT
3 oz Blueberry topping	106	0	15	26	1FR+½CHO
3 oz Strawberry topping	115	1	12	26	1FR+½CHO
3 oz Cherry topping	86	0	5	21	1FR+½CHO
Dutch Apple Pie	440	19	290	65	3CHO+1FR+4FAT
Chocolate Silk Pie	650	43	220	60	4CHO+8½FAT
Key Lime Pie	600	27	300	79	5CHO+5½FAT
Other Desserts:					
Chocolate Layer Cake	275	12	62	42	3CHO+2½FAT
Hot Fudge Cake	620	35	170	73	5CHO+7FAT
Oreo® Cookies & Cream Pie, $^1/_6$ pie	590	30	390	73	5CHO+6FAT
Banana Royale	548	25	184	80	3½CHO+2FR+5FAT
Banana Split Sundae	894	43	177	121	6CHO+2FR+8½FAT
Butterfinger® Hot Fudge Sundae	780	38	333	106	7CHO+7FAT
Dble Scoop Sundae w/out toppings	375	27	86	29	2CHO+5½FAT
Single Scoop Sundae w/out toppings	188	14	43	14	1CHO+3FAT
Butterfinger® Blender Blaster™	768	38	345	97	6½CHO+7FAT
Malted Milkshake, Van/Choc	583	26	278	82	5½CHO+5½FAT
Milkshake, Van/Choc	560	26	272	76	5CHO+5½FAT
Float (Cola or Rootbeer)	280	10	109	47	3CHO+2FAT
Lowfat Choc/Choc Chip Yogurt	110	2	60	19	1¼CHO+½FAT
Rainbow Sherbet	120	2.5	30	25	1½CHO+½FAT
Toppings (2 oz *or* 4 Tbsp):					
Chocolate Topping	317	25	83	27	1½CHO+5FAT
Blueberry Topping	71	0	10	17	1CHO
Cherry Topping	57	0	3	14	1CHO
Fudge Topping	201	10	96	30	2CHO+2FAT
Strawberry Topping	77	1	8	17	1CHO
Whipped Cream, 2 Tbsp	23	2	3	2	½FAT
Nut Topping, 1 tsp	42	4	0	1	1FAT

*Carbs=Carbohydrate, na=not available   **Exchanges: ST=Starch, Mlk=Milk (skim)
FR=Fruit, CHO=Other Carbohydrates, V=Vegetable, MT=Meat (medium fat), FAT=Fat

DENNY'S® (continued)

	Calories	Fat (g)	Sodium (mg)	Carbs* (g)	Exchanges**
Flavored Beverages:					
Hazelnut Coffee	66	1	4	14	1CHO
French Vanilla Coffee	76	1	4	16	1CHO
Irish Cream	73	1	4	16	1CHO
Raspberry Iced Tea w/ice	78	0	0	21	1½CHO
Orange Straw Banana Juice Drink	137	0	0	38	2½CHO

Source: Denny's® nutritional information 9/99. Current as of 12/99.

DOMINO'S PIZZA®

	Calories	Fat (g)	Sodium (mg)	Carbs* (g)	Exchanges**
2 Slices (¼) of a 12" Medium Pizza:					
Hand Tossed, Cheese only	374	11	776	55	3½ST+1MT+½FAT
Thin Crust, Cheese only	273	12	835	31	2ST+1MT+1FAT
Deep Dish, Cheese only	482	22	1123	56	3½ST+1½MT+3FAT
"Add A Topping" (Single toppings) to 2 Slices Med. Pizza:					
Green Pepper, Onion, Mushrooms, Banana Peppers, *or* Pineapple	3-10	0	0-92	0-3	FREE
Ripe Olives *or* Ham	14-18	1	71-162	0	1=FREE, 2=½FAT
Green Olives *or* Anchovies	12-23	1	225-395	0	1=FREE, 2=½FAT
Xtra Cheese, Bf, Cheddar, *or* Ital Saus	48-57	4-5	88-171	0-2	1=½MT+½FAT
Bacon *or* Pepperoni	62-82	6-7	199-226	0	½MT+½FAT
"Add A Topping" (Combination Pizzas) to 2 Slices Med. Pizza:					
Pepperoni	147	12	527	1.^{1}	1MT+1½FAT
Vegi	65	4.^{7}	211	2.^{6}	½MT+½FAT
America's Favorite	135	11	450	2.^{5}	1MT+1FAT
Hawaiian	76	4.^{6}	326	3.^{6}	¾MT
Meatzza	185	15	687	2.^{3}	1½MT+1½FAT
Deluxe	90	7	287	2.^{7}	½MT+1FAT
ExtravaganZZa	153	12	573	3.^{3}	1MT+1½FAT
2 Slices ($^1/_4$) of a 14" Large Pizza:					
Hand Tossed, Cheese only	516	15	1080	75	4½ST+1½MT+1FAT
Thin Crust, Cheese only	382	17	1172	43	2¾ST+1½MT+1½FAT
Deep Dish, Cheese only	677	30	1575	80	5ST+1½MT+3½FAT
"Add A Topping" (Single Toppings) to 2 Slices Large Pizza:					
Green Pepper, Onion, Mushrooms, Banana Peppers, *or* Pineapple	2-8	0	0-81	0	FREE
Ripe Olives *or* Ham	12-17	0-1	63-156	0	1=FREE, 2=½FAT
Green Olives *or* Anchovies	11-23	1	227-395	0	1=FREE, 2=½FAT
Extra Cheese, Beef, Cheddar, Pepperoni, *or* Italian Sausage	44-47	3-4	73-140	0-1	1=½MT
Bacon	75	6	207	0	1=½MT+½FAT

Carbs=Carbohydrate, na=not available   **Exchanges:** ST=Starch, Mlk=Milk (skim)
FR=Fruit, CHO=Other Carbohydrates, V=Vegetable, MT=Meat (medium fat), FAT=Fat

DOMINO'S PIZZA® (continued)

"Add A Topping" (Combination Pizzas) to 2 Slices Large Pizza:

	Calories	Fat (g)	Sodium (mg)	Carbs* (g)	Exchanges**
Pepperoni	204	17	729	1.5	1½MT+1FAT
Vegi	88	7	289	3.³	¾MT+½FAT
America's Favorite	175	14	580	3.³	1½MT+1½FAT
Hawaiian	107	6	463	5	1MT
Meatzza	237	19	867	3	2MT+2FAT
Deluxe	112	9	352	3.³	¾MT+1FAT
ExtravaganZZa	189	15	699	4.²	1½MT+1½FAT

6"Deep Dish Pizza:

	Calories	Fat (g)	Sodium (mg)	Carbs* (g)	Exchanges**
Cheese Only	598	28	1341	68	4ST+2MT+3½FAT

"Add A Topping" to 6" Deep Dish Pizza:

	Calories	Fat (g)	Sodium (mg)	Carbs* (g)	Exchanges**
Green Pepper, Onion, Mushrooms, Banana Peppers, or Pineapple	2-5	0	0-73	0-1	FREE
Ripe Olives	11	1	57	0	1=FREE, 2=½FAT
Green Olives or Ham	10-17	0-1	156-204	0	1=FREE, 2=½FAT
Anchovies	45	2	790	0	1MT(lean)
Xtra Cheese, Bf, Pepp, or Ital Sausage	44-59	3-5	123-159	0-1	1=½MT
Bacon	75	6	207	0	½MT+½FAT
Cheddar Cheese	86	7	132	0	1MT+½FAT

Domino's Buffalo Wings & Bread:

	Calories	Fat (g)	Sodium (mg)	Carbs* (g)	Exchanges**
Barbecue Wings, 1 wing	50	2.⁵	175	1.⁶	½MT
Hot Wings, 1 wing	45	2.⁵	354	0.⁵	½MT
Breadsticks, 1 piece	116	4	152	18	1ST+1FAT
Cheesy Bread, 1 piece	142	6	183	18	1ST+1FAT

Domino's Garden Salads:

	Calories	Fat (g)	Sodium (mg)	Carbs* (g)	Exchanges**
Small Salad, no dressing	22	0.³	14	4	1V
Large Salad, no dressing	39	0.⁵	26	8	1½V

Marzetti Dressings (43 g serving):

	Calories	Fat (g)	Sodium (mg)	Carbs* (g)	Exchanges**
Thousand Island Dressing	200	20	320	5	4FAT
Honey French Dressing	210	18	300	14	1CHO+3½FAT
Light Italian Dressing	20	1	780	2	FREE
House Italian Dressing	220	24	440	1	5FAT
Blue Cheese Dressing	220	24	440	2	5FAT
Ranch Dressing	260	29	380	1	6FAT
Fat Free Ranch Dressing	40	0	560	10	1FR
Creamy Caesar Dressing	200	22	470	2	4½FAT

Source: Domino's Pizza Nutritional Facts. Current as of 12/99.

*Carbs=Carbohydrate, na=not available   **Exchanges: ST=Starch, Mlk=Milk (skim)
FR=Fruit, CHO=Other Carbohydrates, V=Vegetable, MT=Meat (medium fat), FAT=Fat

DUNKIN' DONUTS®

	Calories	Fat (g)	Sodium (mg)	Carbs* (g)	Exchanges**
Regular Muffins:					
Blueberry, Cherry, Apple n' Spice	320-350	12	390-510	49-57	3½CHO+2FAT
Oat Bran, Lemon Poppy Seed	360-370	13	530-620	55-56	3½CHO+2FAT
Cranberry Orange Nut, Banana Nut, Corn	350-390	15	490-590	52-57	3½CHO+2½FAT
Honey Raisin Bran	390	12	620	60	4CHO+2FAT
Chocolate Chip	400	17	440	58	4CHO+3FAT
Lowfat Muffins, all flavors:	240-250	1.⁵-2.⁵	430-480	53-57	3½CHO
Bagels:					
Onion, Plain, Cinn Raisin, Wheat, Pumpernickel, Blueberry, Egg, Garlic, Everything	330-360	1-2	480-710	70-76	4½ST
Poppyseed, Sesame	360-380	2.⁵-4.⁵	710-720	74	4½ST
Salt	340	1	3030	73	4½ST
Cream Cheeses (1 packet):					
Lite	130	11	250	3	2FAT
Chive, Salmon, Garden Vegetable, Plain	180-200	17-19	150-310	2-3	3½FAT
Croissants:					
Plain	290	18	270	26	1¾ST+3½FAT
Almond	350	22	270	34	2CHO+4FAT
Chocolate	400	25	240	37	2½CHO+4½FAT
Cake Donuts:					
Jelly Stick	290	12	390	44	3CHO+2FAT
Old Fashioned (machine cut), Dunkin' Donuts	240-250	15	340-360	25-26	1½CHO+3FAT
Plain Cruller, Powdered Cruller, Sugar Cruller, Cinnamon, Powdered, Sugared	240-270	15	340-360	25-32	2CHO+3FAT
Glazed, Glazed Choc Cruller, Glazed Cruller, Choc Glazed, Blueberry, Butternut, Choc Frosted, Double Choc, Coconut, Toasted Coconut	270-310	15-17	350-400	33-38	2½CHO+3FAT
Whole Wheat Glazed, Chocolate Coconut	300-310	19	370-380	31-32	2CHO+4FAT
Yeast Donuts:					
Sugar Raised, Glazed	170-180	8	250	22-25	1½CHO+1½FAT
Frosted (marble, choc, maple, strawberry, vanilla)	200-210	9	260	29-30	2CHO+1½FAT

*Carbs=Carbohydrate, na=not available **Exchanges: ST=Starch, Mlk=Milk (skim) FR=Fruit, CHO=Other Carbohydrates, V=Vegetable, MT=Meat (medium fat), FAT=Fat

DUNKIN'DONUTS®

	Calories	Fat (g)	Sodium (mg)	Carbs* (g)	Exchanges**
Yeast Doughnuts (continued):					
Apple n' Spice, Lemon, Strawberry, Bavarian Kreme, Black Raspberry, Jelly Filled	200-210	8-9	260-280	28-32	2CHO+1½FAT
Apple Crumb, Boston Kreme, Blueberry Crumb	230-240	9-10	260-280	34-36	2½CHO+2FAT
Vanilla or Choc Kreme Filled	270	13	250-260	35-36	2½CHO+2½FAT
Cake Munchkins® (Donut Hole Treats):					
3 of Butternut, Coconut, Glazed Cake, Choc Cake, *or* Toasted Coconut	200	10-12	240-250	23-27	1½CHO+2FAT
4 of Plain, Cinnamon, Sugared,	220-250	14	310-330	22-30	2CHO+2½FAT
Yeast Munchkins® Donut Hole Treats:					
Glazed Raised, 4 or Jelly, 3	200-210	9	220-240	27-30	2CHO+1½FAT
Lemon, 3	170	8	190	23	1½CHO+1FAT
Sugar Raised, 6	220	12	290	26	1½CHO+2FAT
Fancies:					
Éclair	270	11	290	39	2½CHO+2½FAT
Bismark, Chocolate Iced	340	15	290	50	2½CHO+3FAT
Bow Tie	300	17	340	34	2CHO+2FAT
Coffee Roll; Van, Choc, or Maple Frosted Coffee Roll	270-290	14-15	340	33-36	2½CHO+2½FAT
Glazed Fritter	260	14	330	31	2CHO+2½FAT
Apple Fritter	300	14	360	41	2½CHO+2½FAT
Cookies (1):					
Choc Chunk, Choc Choc Chunk, Choc Chunk w/Nut, Choc White Choc. Chunk Oatmeal Raisin Pecan	210-230	10-12	105-120	26-29	1½CHO+2FAT
P'nut But w/nuts, P'nut Butter Choc Chunk w/nuts	240	14	125-150	24	1½CHO+2½FAT
Coolata™ (16 oz):					
Pink Lemonade, Strawberry Fruit, Orange Mango Fruit	350	0	30	86-88	5½CHO
Chocolate	370	4	115	77	5CHO
Coffee w/cream	410	22	65	51	3½CHO+4FAT
w/milk	260	4	75	52	3½CHO
w/skim milk	230	0	80	52	3½CHO

Source: Dunkin'Donuts® and dunkindonuts.com 12/99. All ® in this section are registered trademarks of Dunkin'Donuts®.

---

*Carbs=Carbohydrate, na=not available   **Exchanges: ST=Starch, Mlk=Milk (skim) FR=Fruit, CHO=Other Carbohydrates, V=Vegetable, MT=Meat (medium fat), FAT=Fat

EL POLLO LOCO®

	Calories	Fat (g)	Sodium (mg)	Carbs* (g)	Exchanges**
Tacos:					
Taco al Carbon	164	6	21	14	1ST+2MT
Chicken Soft Taco	237	12	629	15	1ST+2MT+½FAT
Bowls:					
Southwest Chicken Salad Bowl	529	31	1332	40	2½ST+2½MT+3FAT
Mexican Caesar Chicken Salad	491	30	1170	32	2ST+2½MT+3FAT
Flame Broiled Chicken Salad	357	13	1079	39	2½ST+3½MT(lean)
Pollo Bowl	469	11	1868	66	4½ST+2½MT(lean)
Smokey Black Bean Bowl	604	23	1955	75	5ST+2MT+3 FAT
Salads:					
Garden Salad, regular	105	7	99	7	1V+½MT+1FAT
Garden Salad, large	225	13	214	17	1ST+1V+1MT+1FAT
Tostado Salad w/out shell or sour cr	304	11	1175	28	1ST+1V+4MT(lean)
Tostaco Shell	440	27	610	42	3ST+5FAT
Sandwiches & Other:					
Crazy Chicken Sandwich	516	28	1375	44	3ST+2MT+4FAT
Chicken Taquito	370	17	690	43	3ST+1MT+2FAT
Chicken Strips, 6 pieces	557	25	1873	48	3ST+4MT
Kid's Chicken Strips, 2 pieces	186	8	624	16	1ST+2MT
Chicken:					
Breast	160	6	390	0	3½MT(lean)
Leg	90	5	150	0	1½MT(lean)
Thigh	180	12	230	0	2MT
Wing	110	6	220	0	2MT(lean)
Tortillas:					
4 ½" Corn Tortilla	32	0.5	21	6	½ST
6" Corn Tortilla	70	1	35	14	1ST
6" Flour Tortilla	90	3	224	13	1ST
11" Flour Tortilla	260	7	583	42	3ST+1FAT
Spicy Tomato	254	6	577	42	3ST+1FAT
Burritos:					
BRC Burrito	440	14	1105	64	4ST+3FAT
Classic Chicken Burrito	580	22	1595	66	4ST+3MT+½FAT
Smokey Black Bean Burrito	515	20	1197	71	5ST+3FAT
Classic Chicken Grande Burrito	648	26	1705	72	5ST+2½MT+1FAT
Southwest Chicken Burrito	627	27	1795	69	4½ST+2½MT+3FAT
Chicken Lovers Burrito	476	19	1373	47	3ST+3MT+1FAT

Carbs=Carbohydrate, na=not available **Exchanges:** ST=Starch, Mlk=Milk (skim)
FR=Fruit, CHO=Other Carbohydrates, V=Vegetable, MT=Meat (medium fat), FAT=Fat

EL POLLO LOCO® (continued)

	Calories	Fat (g)	Sodium (mg)	Carbs* (g)	Exchanges**
Side Dishes:					
Cole Slaw	206	16	358	12	2V+3FAT
Corn-on-Cob, 3"	80	1	10	18	1ST
French Fries	444	19	605	61	4ST+4FAT
Mashed Potatoes	97	1	369	21	1½ST
Gravy	14	0	139	2	FREE
Pinto Beans	185	4	744	29	2ST+1MT
Potato Salad	256	14	527	30	2ST+3FAT
Smokey Black Beans	255	13	609	29	2ST+3FAT
Spanish Rice	130	3	397	24	1½ST
Tortilla Chips, unsalted	760	42	22	86	6ST+7FAT
Condiments:					
Guacamole, 1.^{75} oz	52	3	280	5	1V+½FAT
Jalapeño Hot Sauce, 1 pkt	5	0	110	1	FREE
Light Sour Cream, 1 oz	45	3	25	2	1FAT
House Salsa, 1 oz	6	0	96	1	FREE
Pico de Gallo Salsa, 1 oz	11	0.5	131	2	FREE
Fire Roasted Salsa, 1 oz	7	0	100	1	FREE
Avocado Salsa, 1 oz	12	1	204	1	FREE
Desserts:					
Cheesecake	310	18	228	30	2CHO+3½FAT
Churro, 1¼ oz	179	11	221	18	1ST+2FAT
Foster's Freeze, w/out toppings	180	5	100	30	2CHO+1FAT
Strawberry Banana Smoothie	367	7	136	68	2CHO+2FR+1FAT
Kiwi Strawberry Smoothie	357	7	141	66	3½CHO+1FR+1FAT
Banana Split	717	28	310	107	4CHO+1Mlk+2FR +4FAT

Source: Advantiga Restaurant Group, updated 1/99. Current as of 12/99.

EL TORITO

Lite Specialties:	Calories	Fat (g)	Sodium (mg)	Carbs* (g)	Exchanges**
Sonoro Burrito	625	20	1598	na	na
Chicken Quesadilla Lite	530	19	800	na	na

Source: El Torito. Current as of 12/99.

FAZOLI'S®

Pasta:	Calories	Fat (g)	Sodium (mg)	Carbs* (g)	Exchanges**
Spaghetti w/Tomato Sauce	343	7	175	62	3ST+2V+1½FAT
Spaghetti w/Meat Sauce	372	8	161	60	3ST+2V+1MT+½FAT
Spaghetti w/Meat Balls	582	25	864	67	3½ST+2V+2MT+3FAT

*Carbs=Carbohydrate, na=not available **Exchanges: ST=Starch, Mlk=Milk (skim) FR=Fruit, CHO=Other Carbohydrates, V=Vegetable, MT=Meat (medium fat), FAT=Fat

FAZOLI'S® (continued)

	Calories	Fat (g)	Sodium (mg)	Carbs* (g)	Exchanges**
Large Spaghetti w/Tomato Sauce	509	10	244	93	4½ST+3V+2FAT
Large Spaghetti w/Meat Sauce	553	12	223	90	4½ST+3V+1½MT+1FAT
Large Spaghetti w/Meat Balls	829	34	1163	100	5ST+3V+2½MT+4FAT
Fettuccine Alfredo	400	13	711	58	3½ST+2½FAT
Large Fettuccine Alfredo	596	20	1048	87	5½ST+1MT+3FAT
Broccoli Fettuccine	424	13	731	62	3½ST+1V+1MT+1½FAT
Large Broccoli Fettuccine	619	20	1068	91	5ST+1V+1½MT+2½FAT
Baked Ziti	331	13	347	38	2ST+1V+1½MT+1FAT
Large Baked Ziti	573	21	519	68	3½ST+2V+2½MT+2FAT

Specialty Items:

	Calories	Fat (g)	Sodium (mg)	Carbs* (g)	Exchanges**
Cheese Ravioli w/Tomato Sauce	562	25	1214	62	3½ST+1V+2MT+3FAT
Cheese Ravioli w/Meat Sauce	591	26	1200	60	3½ST+1V+3MT+2FAT
Chicken Parmesan	481	14	368	34	2ST+6MT(lean)
Lasagna	533	24	1148	47	2½ST+1V+4MT+1FAT
Broccoli Lasagna	571	27	1443	50	2½ST+1V+4MT+1½FAT
Meat Ball Sub	650	30	1534	62	3½ST+1V+3MT+3FAT
Sampler Platter	607	20	904	80	4½ST+2V+2MT+2FAT
Shrimp & Scallop Fettucine	522	14	1093	63	3½ST+4MT
Baked Spaghetti Parmesan	563	21	589	65	3½ST+1V+3MT+1FAT

Soup, Salad, Bread:

	Calories	Fat (g)	Sodium (mg)	Carbs* (g)	Exchanges**
Breadstick	131	4	330	20	1¼ST+1FAT
Breadstick, dry	99	0.8	204	20	1¼ST
Minestrone Soup	90	1	1038	16	1ST
Bean & Pasta Soup	174	7	1079	20	1ST+1MT+½FAT
Italian Chef Salad	391	30	1307	10	½ST+1V+3MT+3FAT
Pasta Salad	397	20	1030	46	3ST+4FAT
Garden Salad	28	0.3	17	5	1V
House Italian Dressing, 1oz	138	15	224	3	3FAT
Reduced Cal Italian Dressing 1oz	69	4	112	2	1FAT
Honey French Dressing, 1 oz	160	14	230	11	½ST+3FAT
Thousand Island Dressing, 1 oz	140	14	230	4	3FAT
Ranch Dressing, 1 oz	180	20	250	1	4FAT

Pizza:

	Calories	Fat (g)	Sodium (mg)	Carbs* (g)	Exchanges**
Cheese Pizza, double slice	360	11	622	45	3ST+2MT
Pepperoni Pizza, double slice	430	17	908	45	3ST+2½MT+1FAT
Combination Pizza, double slice	484	21	1042	47	3ST+3MT+1FAT

Desserts:

	Calories	Fat (g)	Sodium (mg)	Carbs* (g)	Exchanges**
Lemon Italian Ice, 12 oz	142	0	9	36	2½CHO
Cheesecake, plain	270	21	208	16	1CHO+4FAT
Chocolate Cheesecake	298	22	201	22	1½CHO+4½FAT
Strawberry Topping, 1 oz	40	0	1	10	½CHO

Source: Fazoli's/Seed Restaurant Group Inc. Current as of 12/99.

*Carbs=Carbohydrate, na=not available **Exchanges: ST=Starch, Mlk=Milk (skim)
FR=Fruit, CHO=Other Carbohydrates, V=Vegetable, MT=Meat (medium fat), FAT=Fat

FURR'S CAFETERIA®

Most Furr's cafeteria offers the choice of the All-You-Can-Eat concept, By-The-Item pricing, *or* Delight Plate. Some restaurants offer just the All-You-Can-Eat concept. The Delight Plate includes a full portion of an entrée with 2 vegetables. The leanest are the Baked Fish (remove bread topping), Roast Beef, and Baked Chicken (remove skin). Portion sizes are about 3 oz cooked. Sugar-free Jello is always available. Light salad dressings are offered; all salad dressings may also be requested *on the side*. Fresh strawberries (without the syrup) are available, just ask.

Salads (approximately ½ cup):	Calories	Fat (g)	Sodium (mg)	Carbs* (g)	Exchanges**
Furr's Fruit Salad	120	2	7	26	1½FR+½FAT
Five Cup Fruit Salad	181	9	57	26	1½FR+2FAT
German Potato Salad	304	12	762	41	2½ST+2½FAT
Cauliflower Salad	205	16	670	13	2V+3FAT
Broccoli & Cauliflower Salad	206	16	672	13	2V+3FAT
Crunchy Vegetable Salad	144	10	349	12	2V+2FAT
Sweet Slaw with Nutrasweet	62	4	225	6	1V+1FAT
Three Bean Salad	145	6	381	21	1ST+1V+1FAT
Sweet Slaw	141	8	331	19	½FR+1V+1½FAT
Spanish Slaw	63	3	635	10	1½V+½FAT
Apple Cabbage Slaw	179	17	126	8	½FR+½V+3FAT
Carrot Cabbage Slaw	129	10	95	11	½FR+1V+2FAT
Coleslaw with Sour Cream	64	4	104	5	1V+1FAT
Colorado Coleslaw	163	13	312	12	½FR+1V+2½FAT
Country Corn Coleslaw	107	6	320	14	½ST+1V+1FAT
Cream Slaw w/Raisins Pineapple	153	12	93	13	½FR+1V+2½FAT
Health Slaw	108	8	68	9	1½V+1½FAT
Old Fashioned Coleslaw	53	3	450	7	1V+½FAT
Red Coleslaw	114	11	147	5	1V+2FAT
Sweet and Sour Slaw	221	10	697	34	1½FR+1½V+2FAT
Carrot Coconut Pineapple Salad	189	16	133	12	½FR+1V+3FAT
Carrot and Raisin Salad	127	7	171	16	½FR+1V+1½FAT
Cauliflower and Olive Salad	171	18	533	3	½V+3½FAT
Copper Carrot Salad	229	9	448	35	1½FR+2V+2FAT
Country Style Cucumbers	137	12	559	9	½FR+½V+2½FAT
Cucumber Salad	42	1	538	7	1½V
Cucumber in sour cream & mayo	261	25	299	10	½FR+½V+5FAT
Avocado & Diced Tomato Salad	277	22	653	21	3V+4½FAT
Carrot Ambrosia	201	8	57	33	1½FR+1½V+1½FAT

Entrees:

	Calories	Fat (g)	Sodium (mg)	Carbs* (g)	Exchanges**
Mexican Chicken Casserole, 8 oz	517	31	1415	28	1½ST+4MT+2FAT
Barbecued Pork Tips, 6oz pork +1c rice	447	19	524	46	3ST+2MT+2FAT
Apple Pork Oriental, 6oz pork+6oz rice	550	21	529	64	4ST+2MT+2FAT
Beef & Green Chili Casserole, 8 oz	621	47	1112	16	1ST+4½MT+5FAT
Liver and Onions	562	35	576	34	2ST+3MT+4FAT
Peppery Beef Stir Fry	471	8	597	72	4ST+1V+2MT
Chicken Fried Steak w/ Gravy	626	44	1181	31	2ST+3MT+6FAT
Chicken Fry w/Pan Fry Potato	789	51	1387	55	3½ST+3MT+7FAT

*Carbs=Carbohydrate, na=not available   **Exchanges: ST=Starch, Mlk=Milk (skim) FR=Fruit, CHO=Other Carbohydrates, V=Vegetable, MT=Meat (medium fat), FAT=Fat

FURR'S CAFETERIA® (continued)

	Calories	Fat (g)	Sodium (mg)	Carbs* (g)	Exchanges**
Side Dishes (approximately ½ cup):					
Lemon Celery Rice Pilaf	241	10	699	34	2ST+2FAT
Almond Rice Pilaf	232	10	603	32	2ST+2FAT
Cranberry Orange Relish	232	0	1	61	2FR+2CHO
Cranberry Cream	216	7	10	40	1½FR+1CHO+1½FAT
Sweet Potato Soufflé	395	17	379	58	2ST+1½CHO+3½FAT
Almond Rice	211	10	445	27	1½ST+2FAT
Fruited Rice	250	7	39	48	2ST+1FR+1½FAT
Carrots, Asparagus, Squash	77	3	423	12	1½V+½FAT
Broccoli w/ Lemon Butter	119	11	377	5	1V+2FAT
Steamed Broccoli	56	4	283	5	1V+1FAT
Brussel Sprouts Almondine	111	7	338	10	1V+1½FAT
Steamed Brussel Sprouts	70	4	284	8	1V+1FAT
Steamed Cabbage	42	3	315	4	½V+½FAT
German Boiled Cabbage	90	3	365	13	2V+½FAT
Scalloped Cabbage	151	9	575	13	2V+2FAT
Bacon Fried Carrots	106	4	427	14	2V+1FAT
Braised Carrots and Onion	86	4	354	13	1½V+1FAT
Carrots and Green Onions	74	2	415	13	2V+½FAT
Carrots Supreme	121	5	504	15	2V+1FAT
Glazed Carrots and Celery	128	5	393	20	1FR+1V+1FAT
Scalloped Corn	272	11	781	39	2½ST+2FAT
Whole Kernel Corn	152	4	281	29	2ST+1FAT
Sautéed Mushrooms	148	15	563	3	1V+3FAT
Green Beans	125	9	820	6	1V+2FAT
Blackeyed Peas	106	5	468	9	1V+1MT
Harlequin Rice	168	4	596	29	1½ST+1FAT
Seasoned Spinach	63	4	305	6	1V+½MT
Breads:					
Jalapeno Cornbread, 3.^{3} oz	213	9	298	28	1½ST+2FAT
Cornbread Muffins, 1	176	5	229	27	1½ST+1FAT
Hard Rolls, 3.^{8} oz	272	5	529	47	3ST+1FAT
Applesauce Spice Muffins, 1	267	13	76	36	2½CHO+2½FAT
Brown Sugar Muffins, 1	316	6	245	61	4CHO+1FAT
Desserts (1/7 pie, unless noted):					
Pumpkin Cake Roll, 1 slice	359	18	273	45	3CHO+3½FAT
Texas Sheet Cake w/icing, 3"X4"	577	28	448	81	5CHO+5½FAT
Oatmeal Cake, 3"X4"	492	24	297	68	4CHO+5FAT
Rocky Road Cake, 3"X4"	431	20	323	63	4CHO+4FAT
Lemon Chess Pie	481	21	270	71	4½CHO+4FAT
Millionaire Pie	427	26	277	44	3CHO+5FAT
Pecan Pie	584	23	287	90	6CHO+4½FAT
Pumpkin Pie	333	16	200	44	3CHO+3FAT

*Carbs=Carbohydrate, na=not available **Exchanges: ST=Starch, Mlk=Milk (skim)
FR=Fruit, CHO=Other Carbohydrates, V=Vegetable, MT=Meat (medium fat), FAT=Fat

FURR'S CAFETERIA® (continued)

Desserts, continued (1/7 pie, unless noted):	Calories	Fat (g)	Sodium (mg)	Carbs* (g)	Exchanges**
German Chocolate Pie	425	21	446	56	3½CHO+4FAT
Cool Lime Pie	436	19	278	66	4½CHO+4FAT
Holiday Billionaire Pie	371	16	286	55	3 ½CHO+3FAT
Raspberry Ribbon Pie	359	20	205	35	2CHO+4FAT
Sour Cream Cheese Cake w/out topping	334	21	204	32	2CHO+4FAT
Butter Chess Pie	486	23	302	67	4½CHO+4½FAT
Buttermilk Pie	587	36	363	58	4CHO+7FAT
French Pineapple Pie	463	26	383	54	3½CHO+5FAT
Surprise Pecan Pie	349	18	148	45	3CHO+3½FAT
Coconut Custard Pie	420	19	257	56	3½CHO+4FAT
Strawberry Ambrosia Pie	438	25	305	51	3½CHO+5FAT
No Sugar Added Pies (1/7 pie):					
Strawberry	194	12	204	18	1CHO+2½FAT
Cherry Cream	338	20	249	31	2CHO+4FAT
Peach Cream	319	18	260	32	2CHO+3½FAT
Pineapple Cream	322	18	224	33	2CHO+3½FAT
Banana Cream	312	17	207	34	2CHO+2½FAT
Strawberry Cream	307	18	224	29	2CHO+3½FAT
Lemon Ice Box	245	16	194	23	1½CHO+3FAT

Source: Furr's Cafeteria. Current as of 12/99.

GODFATHERS™ PIZZA

	Calories	Fat (g)	Sodium (mg)	Carbo* (g)	Exchanges**
Original Crust, Cheese Pizza, per slice:					
Mini, ¼ of whole pizza	131	3	183	19	1¼ST+½MT
Medium, 1/8 of whole pizza	231	5	338	34	2ST+½MT+½FAT
Large, 1/10 of whole pizza	258	6	396	36	2¼ST+1MT
Jumbo, 1/10 of whole pizza	382	9	580	53	3ST+2MT
Original Crust, Combo Pizza, per slice:					
Mini, ¼ of whole pizza	176	7	382	21	1¼ST+1MT+½MT
Medium, 1/8 of whole pizza	306	11	660	36	2ST+1½MT+½FAT
Large, 1/10 of whole pizza	338	12	740	38	2¼ST+1½MT+1FAT
Jumbo, 1/10 of whole pizza	503	18	1096	56	3½ST+2½MT+1FAT
Golden Crust, Cheese Pizza, per slice:					
Medium, 1/8 of whole pizza	212	8	311	26	1½ST+1MT+½FAT
Large, 1/10 of whole pizza	242	9	363	28	1¾ST+1¼MT+½FAT
Golden Crust, Combo Pizza, per slice:					
Medium, 1/8 of whole pizza	271	12	562	28	1½ST+1½MT+1FAT
Large, 1/10 of whole pizza	305	14	674	31	2ST+1¾MT+1FAT

Source: Godfather's Pizza Nutritional Info. Current as of 12/99.

*Carbs=Carbohydrate, na=not available   **Exchanges: ST=Starch, Mlk=Milk (skim)
FR=Fruit, CHO=Other Carbohydrates, V=Vegetable, MT=Meat (medium fat), FAT=Fat

GOLDEN CORRAL®

Golden Corral has started a "Wise Choice" labeling program in all of their restaurants. This program uses the Wise Choice Owl to label individual products on the buffet that are healthier choices. In some cases the label will state "fat free" or list the fat grams. Golden Corral offers an abundance of fresh vegetables and fruits, fat-free salad dressings, fresh carved meats (including roast turkey, steamed fish and/or baked chicken), fat free and low fat soft serves, and fresh baked bread that all fit into a healthy diet.

Source: Golden Corral®. Current as of 12/99.

GRANDY'S®

Breakfast:	Calories	Fat (g)	Sodium (mg)	Carbs* (g)	Exchanges**
Biscuit	250	9	615	36	2ST+2FAT
Breakfast Steak, 2.^{3} oz	209	15	415	8	½ST+1½MT+1½FAT
Breakfast Gravy, 2.^{4} oz	175	6	465	28	1¾ST+1FAT
Hash Browns, 1 ¾ oz	178	13	350	15	1ST+2½FAT
Hotcake, 1	68	3	171	9	½ST+ ½FAT
Sausage, 1 ¾ oz	240	22	240	0	1½MT+3FAT
Cinnamon Roll, 3.^{7} oz	380	14	310	55	3½CHO+3FAT
BET Sandwich	532	30	851	40	2½ST+3MT+3FAT
Lunch:					
Chicken Leg	197	11	428	6	½ST+2MT
Wing	329	22	906	12	½ST+2½MT+2FAT
Thigh	570	43	792	18	1ST+3½MT+5FAT
Breast	538	33	1330	21	1½ST+4½MT+2FAT
Nugget, 1	47	2	107	3	¼ST+ ½MT
Grilled Fillet, 3 oz	149	6	285	1	3MT(lean)
Grilled Fillet Sandwich	396	13	1006	38	2ST+3½MT
Chicken Fried Chicken, 5 oz	318	15	700	18	1ST+3½MT
Roast Chicken, white meat, 9oz	477	28	1667	1	8MT(lean)+½FAT
Dark meat, 7.^{6} oz	429	27	1067	2	6½MT
Country Steak, 4 ½ oz	456	31	1088	27	1½ST+3MT+3FAT
Dinner:					
Steak Finger, 1	100	7	200	6	½ST+½MT+½FAT
Smoked Rib, 3 ½ oz	250	19	385	3	3MT+1FAT
Dinner Roll	109	3	93	18	1ST+½FAT
Mashed Potatoes, 3 ½ oz	130	5	340	17	1ST+1FAT
Brown Gravy, 3 oz	67	4	428	8	½ST+1FAT
White Gravy, 3 oz	49	2	269	6	½ST+½FAT
Baked Beans, 3.^{4} oz	130	1	705	26	1½ST
Cole Slaw, 3 ½ oz	110	7	210	9	1V+ ¼CHO+1½FAT
Green Beans	30	1	372	4	1V
Seasoned Rice, 4 oz	90	1	300	20	1¼ST
Fried Okra, 4 oz	332	19	760	36	2ST+1V+4FAT
Frozen Corn	110	3	140	18	1ST+½FAT
Small Fries	343	17	192	43	2½ST+3½FAT
Peach Cobbler, 5 oz	300	11	200	48	2CHO+1FR+2FAT
Cherry Cobbler, 5 oz	400	15	200	59	3CHO+1FR+3FAT

*Carbs=Carbohydrate, na=not available **Exchanges: ST=Starch, Mlk=Milk (skim)
FR=Fruit, CHO=Other Carbohydrates, V=Vegetable, MT=Meat (medium fat), FAT=Fat

GRANDY'S® (continued)

Salad:	Calories	Fat (g)	Sodium (mg)	Carbs* (g)	Exchanges**
Garden Salad	217	8	400	28	1ST+2V+1MT+½FAT
Dinner Salad	30	0	67	5	1V
SW Salad	280	11	774	10	½ST+1V+4MT(lean)
SW Caesar	394	15	718	31	2ST+3½MT

Source: Grandy's® Nutritional Information. Current as of 12/99.

HARDEE'S® - all items may not be available at all locations

Breakfast:	Calories	Fat (g)	Sodium (mg)	Carbs* (g)	Exchanges**
Made From Scratch™ Biscuit	390	21	1000	44	3ST+4FAT
Jelly Biscuit	440	21	1000	57	3ST+1FR+4FAT
Apple Cinnamon 'N' Raisin™ Biscuit	250	8	350	42	2ST+1FR+1½FAT
Sausage Biscuit	550	36	1310	44	3ST+1MT+6FAT
Sausage & Egg Biscuit	620	41	1370	45	3ST+2MT+6FAT
Bacon, Egg & Cheese Biscuit	520	30	1420	45	3ST+1½MT+4½FAT
Country Ham Biscuit	440	22	1710	44	3ST+1MT+3½FAT
Frisco™ Breakfast Sandwich, Ham	450	22	1290	42	3ST+2½MT+2FAT
Ham Biscuit	410	20	1200	45	3ST+1MT+3FAT
Regular Hash Rounds™, 16	230	14	560	24	1½ST+3FAT
Biscuit 'N' Gravy™	530	30	1550	56	3½ST+6FAT
Omelet™ Biscuit	550	32	1350	45	3ST+2MT+4½FAT
Chicken Biscuit	590	27	1820	62	4ST+2MT+3½FAT
Steak Biscuit	580	32	1580	56	3½ST+1MT+5½FAT

Sandwiches:	Calories	Fat (g)	Sodium (mg)	Carbs* (g)	Exchanges**
Hamburger (varies)	270-330	11-13	480-550	29-34	2ST+2MT
Cheeseburger	320	15	780	30	2ST+2MT+1FAT
Big Deluxe™ Burger	650	44	870	40	2½ST+2½MT+6FAT
Big Deluxe™ Burger with Cheese	710	49	1140	40	2½ST+3MT+7FAT
Famous Star™ Hamburger	580	32	910	49	3½ST+2MT+4FAT
Super Star® Hamburger	790	46	970	50	3½ST+4½MT+4FAT
Double Cheeseburger	480	28	1055	31	2ST+3MT+2½FAT
Monster Burger®	1060	79	1860	37	2½ST+6MT+10FAT
Chicken Fillet Sandwich	480	23	1190	44	3ST+2½MT+2FAT
Grilled Chicken Sandwich	350	16	860	28	1¾ST+3MT
Regular Roast Beef	310	16	800	26	1½ST+2MT+1FAT
Big Roast Beef™ Sandwich	410	24	1140	26	1½ST+3MT+2FAT
Frisco™ Burger	720	49	1180	37	2½ST+3½MT+6FAT
Classic Bacon Cheeseburger	720	48	1200	42	2½ST+3½MT+6FAT
Classic Bacon Double Cheeseburger	1000	70	1575	42	2½ST+6MT+8FAT
Western Bacon Cheeseburger®	650	30	1430	63	4ST+3MT+2FAT
Dble Western Bacon Cheeseburger®	900	49	1770	64	4ST+5½MT+3FAT
Hot Ham 'N' Cheese™	300	12	1390	34	2ST+2MT+½FAT
Fisherman's Fillet™	530	28	1280	45	3ST+2½MT+3FAT

*Carbs=Carbohydrate, na=not available   **Exchanges:** ST=Starch, Mlk=Milk (skim)
FR=Fruit, CHO=Other Carbohydrates, V=Vegetable, MT=Meat (medium fat), FAT=Fat

HARDEE'S® (continued)

	Calories	Fat (g)	Sodium (mg)	Carbs* (g)	Exchanges**
Sandwiches, continued:					
Hot Dog with condiments	450	32	1240	25	1½ST+2MT+4½FAT
Charbroiled BBQ Chicken SW™	280	3	830	37	2½ST+2½MT(very lean)
Charbroiled Chicken Club SW™	460	22	1110	33	2ST+3½MT+½FAT
Crispy Chicken Sandwich	620	29	1220	65	4ST+2MT+3FAT
Bacon Swiss Crispy Chicken SW	720	36	1610	66	4ST+3MT+3½FAT
Chicken & Sides:					
Breast	370	15	1190	29	2ST+3MT
Wing	200	8	740	23	1½ST+1MT+½FAT
Thigh	330	15	1000	30	2ST+2MT+1FAT
Leg	170	7	570	15	1ST+1½MT
Cole Slaw, small	240	20	340	13	1V+½CHO+4FAT
Gravy, 1.^{5} oz	20	<1	260	3	¼ST
Mashed Potatoes, small	70	<1	330	14	1ST
Salads & Fries:					
French Fries, regular	340	16	390	45	3ST+3FAT
French Fries, large	440	21	520	59	4ST+4FAT
French Fries, monster	510	24	590	67	4½ST+5FAT
Crispy Curls™ Potatoes, med	340	18	950	41	2½ST+3½FAT
Crispy Curls™ Potatoes, large	520	28	1450	62	4ST+5½FAT
Crispy Curls™ Potatoes, monster	590	31	1640	70	4½ST+6FAT
Onion Rings	430	21	700	53	3½ST+3½FAT
Chicken Stars, 6 piece	280	19	330	15	1ST+1½MT+2FAT
Shakes & Desserts:					
Shake, Vanilla, 12.^{3} oz	350	5	300	65	3CHO+1½Mlk+1FAT
Shake, Chocolate, 12.^{3} oz	370	5	270	67	3CHO+1½Mlk+1FAT
Cool Twist™ Cone, Vanilla/Choc	180	2	120	34	2CHO+½Mlk+½FAT
Apple Turnover	270	12	250	38	2½CHO+2½FAT
Peach Cobbler, small	310	7	360	60	3CHO+1FR+1½FAT

Source: Hardee's® Nutritional Guide 7/98. Current as of 12/99. All ® in this section are
trademarks of Hardee's®.

HARTZ CHICKEN® INC.

	Calories	Fat (g)	Sodium (mg)	Carbs* (g)	Exchanges**
Meats & Dinners:					
2 Piece White Dinner	970	47	1440	na	na
2 Piece Dark Dinner	770	36	1130	na	na
3 Piece White Dinner	1550	77	2060	na	na
3 Piece Dark Dinner	1000	54	1440	na	na
Roasted Chicken Dinner	910	39	460	na	na
3 Piece Fish Dinner	590	24	450	na	na
Fish Snack	610	20	550	na	na

*Carbs=Carbohydrate, na=not available   ****Exchanges:** ST=Starch, Mlk=Milk (skim)
FR=Fruit, CHO=Other Carbohydrates, V=Vegetable, MT=Meat (medium fat), FAT=Fat

HARTZ CHICKEN® INC. (continued)

	Calories	Fat (g)	Sodium (mg)	Carbs* (g)	Exchanges**
Gizzards, ¾ c	130	4	50	na	3MT(lean)
Livers, ¾ c	100	3	60	na	2MT(lean)
Fish Fillet, 1	240	9	280	na	½ST+4MT(lean)
Fried Chicken, 1 average	380	22	120	na	5MT
Barbecue Chicken, 5 oz	270	12	880	na	1CHO+3MT+½FAT
Meatloaf, 3 oz	160	8	420	na	¼ST+2MT
2 Piece White Dinner	970	47	1440	na	na
2 Piece Dark Dinner	770	36	1130	na	na
3 Piece White Dinner	1550	77	2060	na	na
3 Piece Dark Dinner	1000	54	1440	na	na
Roasted Chicken Dinner	910	39	460	na	na
3 Piece Fish Dinner	590	24	450	na	na
Fish Snack	610	20	550	na	na
Gizzards, ¾ c	130	4	50	na	3MT(lean)
Livers, ¾ c	100	3	60	na	2MT(lean)
Fish Fillet, 1	240	9	280	na	½ST+4MT(lean
Fried Chicken, 1 average	380	22	120	na	5MT
Barbecue Chicken, 5 oz	270	12	880	na	1CHO+3MT+½FAT
Meatloaf, 3 oz	160	8	420	na	¼ST+2MT
Vegetables & Starches (½ c):					
Broccoli, average	35	1.5	25	na	1V+¼FAT
Broccoli & Cauliflower, average	30	1	220	na	1V+¼FAT
Broc, Caul, & Carrots, average	35	1	430	na	1V+¼FAT
Cabbage	40	1	200	na	1V+¼FAT
Candied Carrots, average	70	0.5	155	na	1V+½CHO
Cauliflower, average	30	1.7	175	na	1V+½FAT
Corn, average	85	1.7	175	na	1ST+½FAT
Mexican Corn	100	1.5	180	na	1ST+¼FAT
Beans	130	2	350	na	1ST+½FAT
Green Beans, average	40	1.3	455	na	1V+¼FAT
Corn on Cob, 1	140	1	800	na	1½ST+¼FAT
Green Beans/Potatoes	60	0	350	na	¾ST
Green Beans/Onion Casserole	80	5	330	na	1V+½ST+½FAT
Gr Beans/Mushroom/Cheese Sauce	50	2	440	na	1V+¼ST+½FAT
Green Bean Supreme	140	11	490	na	1V+2FAT
Green Peas	50	1.5	180	na	½ST+¼FAT
Green Peas/Carrots, average	65	1.2	180	na	½ST+¼FAT
Macaroni & Cheese	270	17	470	na	1½ST+½MT+3FAT
Mustard/Turnip Greens, average	68	4.2	450	na	1V+1FAT
Okra & Tomatoes	60	2	600	na	1V+½FAT
Pinto Beans, average	110	1.5	600	na	1ST+½FAT
Golden Ex Rich Potatoes	160	5	65	na	1½ST+1FAT
Whipped Potatoes	100	3	300	na	1St+1FAT
Fry's, 3 oz	190	7	25	na	1½ST+1½FAT
Rice, average	150	1.7	310	na	2ST+½FAT
Squash	30	1	28	na	1V+¼FAT

*Carbs=Carbohydrate, na=not available   **Exchanges:** ST=Starch, Mlk=Milk (skim)
FR=Fruit, CHO=Other Carbohydrates, V=Vegetable, MT=Meat (medium fat), FAT=Fat

HARTZ CHICKEN® INC. (continued)

	Calories	Fat (g)	Sodium (mg)	Carbs* (g)	Exchanges**
Vegetables & Starches, continued (½c):					
Squash & Tomato, average	45	1.^{3}	330	na	1V+¼FAT
Stewed Tomatoes, average	47	1	630	na	1V+¼FAT
Steamed Red Potatoes	110	7	890	na	¾ST+1½FAT
Candied Yams	190	2	65	na	1ST+1½CHO+½FAT
Hot Beets	40	0	320	na	1V
Baked Beans	170	2	560	na	1½ST+½FAT
Carrots & Bacon	100	5	380	na	1V+1FAT
Hominy	80	2	240	na	1ST+½FAT
Casseroles (½ c):					
Broccoli & Rice Casserole	130	5	400	na	1V+1ST+1FAT
Broccoli/Rice/Cheese	120	5	470	na	1ST+1FAT
Cornbread Dressing	270	8	660	na	3ST+1½FAT
Spanish Rice	150	4	510	na	1½ST+1FAT
Squash Casserole	300	29	780	na	1V+6FAT
Derty Rice	150	4	650	na	1½ST+1FAT
Chicken & Rice Casserole	300	15	280	na	2ST+1MT+2FAT
Chicken & Rice Cass, steamer	250	4	650	na	2ST+1MT
Chicken Spaghetti	370	12	970	na	3ST+1½MT+1FAT
Chicken Spaghetti, steamer	210	8	550	na	1½ST+1MT+½FAT
Chicken Enchiladas Casserole	400	22	990	na	2ST+2MT+2FAT
Chicken Creole	240	13	630	na	1ST+2½MT
Chicken Vegetable Stew	230	10	400	na	1ST+1V+2MT
Corn & Rice Casserole, average	160	4.^{3}	335	na	1½ST+1FAT
King Ranch Chicken	350	22	900	na	1ST+3MT+1½FAT
Liver & Onions w/Gravy	170	5	740	na	½ST+2½MT(lean)
Macaroni & Tomato Casserole	130	4	460	na	1ST+1FAT
Green Bean/Onion Casserole	60	2.^{5}	480	na	1V+½FAT
Chicken & Dumplings	280	13	940	na	2ST+1MT+1½FAT
Chicken Cabbage	240	18	430	na	1V+1½MT+2FAT
Paella	350	14	900	na	1ST+1V+3MT
Spicy Shrimp & Rice	230	2.^{5}	860	na	2ST+1MT(lean)
Breads (1):					
Cornbread Muffins	150	5	240	na	1½ST+1FAT
Jalapeño Cornbread Muffin	150	5	290	na	1½ST+1FAT
Yeast Rolls	180	3	260	na	2ST+½FAT
Dinner Rolls	220	3.^{5}	230	na	2½ST+½FAT
Soup (1c):					
Cream of Chicken/Rice Soup	210	10	390	na	1ST+1MT+1FAT
Cream of Chicken Noodle Soup	210	11	430	na	1ST+1½MT+1FAT
Vegetable Soup	80	0	770	na	1V+½ST

*Carbs=Carbohydrate, na=not available **Exchanges: ST=Starch, Mlk=Milk (skim)
FR=Fruit, CHO=Other Carbohydrates, V=Vegetable, MT=Meat (medium fat), FAT=Fat

HARTZ CHICKEN® INC. (continued)

	Calories	Fat (g)	Sodium (mg)	Carbs* (g)	Exchanges**
Salad (½ c):					
Beet Salad	60	0	260	na	1V+½CHO
Broccoli Salad	35	0	115	na	1V
Carrot/Raisin Salad	380	28	330	na	1V+1½CHO+5½FAT
Green Pea & Carrot Salad	110	8	210	na	1½V+1½FAT
Macaroni & Pea Salad	300	23	210	na	1ST+1MT+3FAT
Green Bean Salad	160	13	580	na	1V+2½FAT
Pasta Salad	210	13	210	na	1½ST+2½FAT
Cole Slaw	220	18	115	na	1V+3½FAT
Fruit Salad	110	0.5	5	na	1FR+1CHO
Mexican Salad	90	1	480	na	1ST+¼FAT
Three Bean Salad	130	3.5	80	na	1V+1ST+½FAT
Rice & Egg Salad	480	22	330	na	2ST+2CHO+4½FAT
Garden Salad, 1	130	6	110	na	1V+1MT
Croutons, 3T	25	1.5	60	na	¼ST+¼FAT
Green Pea & Egg Salad	280	23	580	na	1V+1MT+3½FAT
Potato Salad	150	3.5	610	na	1½ST+½FAT
Cool Salad	70	0	0	na	1CHO
Plain Jello	80	0	0	na	1CHO
Fruit Jello Salad	80	0	0	na	1CHO
Cold Spicy Pasta Salad	200	7	310	na	1½ST+1½FAT
Krab Slaw	160	12	380	na	1V+2½FAT
Sauces & Gravy (2T):					
Cocktail Sauce	30	0	350	na	½CHO
Hartz Gravy	10	0	135	na	FREE
Tartar Sauce	220	23	200	na	4½FAT
White Sauce	40	3	115	na	½FAT
Cheese Sauce	80	6	260	na	½MT+1FAT
White Gravy	0	0	30	na	FREE
Desserts:					
Apple Cobbler 4 oz	250	2.5	280	na	1FR+2½CHO+½FAT
Pineapple Cobbler, 4 oz	240	2.5	280	na	1FR+2½CHO+½FAT
Bread Pudding, 4 oz	240	8	170	na	2½CHO+1½FAT
Crunchy Dessert, 4½ oz	330	12	160	na	3½CHO+2½FAT
Peach Cobbler, 4 oz	250	3	290	na	1FR+2½CHO+½FAT
Coffee Cake Dessert, 1 pc	240	2.5	280	na	3CHO+½FAT
Cinnamon Rolls, 1	820	8	520	na	12CHO+1½FAT
Pineapple Dessert, 4 oz	180	2	210	na	1FR+1½CHO+½FAT
Lemon Apple Cobbler, ½ c	320	7	380	na	1FR+3CHO+1½FAT
Chocolate Cake, 1 average piece	260	8	245	na	3CHO+1½FAT
Yellow Cake, 1 average piece	200	7	270	na	2CHO+1½FAT
Banana Flavored Pudding, ½ c	160	3	340	na	2CHO+½FAT

Source: Hartz Chicken® Inc. Current as of 12/99.

*Carbs=Carbohydrate, na=not available **Exchanges: ST=Starch, Mlk=Milk (skim)
FR=Fruit, CHO=Other Carbohydrates, V=Vegetable, MT=Meat (medium fat), FAT=Fat

IHOP®

Pancake, Waffle, and Crepe (per individual piece):	Calories	Fat (g)	Sodium (mg)	Carbs* (g)	Exchanges**
Buttermilk Pancake	110	3	450	17	1ST+½FAT
Buckwheat Pancake	110	4	280	15	1ST+½FAT
Harvest Grain'N Nut Pancake	180	9	410	20	1¼ST+2FAT
Country Griddle Pancake	120	3.⁵	440	19	1¼ST+½FAT
Regular Waffle	310	15	380	37	2½ST+3FAT
Regular Belgian Waffle	390	19	850	48	3ST+4FAT
Other Items:					
Old-Fashioned Syrup, 2 fl oz	230	0	230	58	4CHO
Whipped Butter, 0.⁴ oz	80	9	74	0	2FAT

Source: IHOP® Nutritional Data 12/98

IN-N-OUT BURGER®

	Calories	Fat (g)	Sodium (mg)	Carbs* (g)	Exchanges**
Hamburger	390	19	640	39	2½ST+1½MT+2FAT
w/mustard & ketchup instead of spread	310	10	720	41	2½ST+1½MT+½FAT
Cheeseburger	480	27	1000	39	2½ST+2MT+3½FAT
w/mustard & ketchup instead of spread	400	18	1080	41	2½ST+2MT+1½FAT
Double-Double®	670	41	1430	40	2½ST+4MT+4FAT
w/mustard & ketchup instead of spread	590	32	1510	42	2½ST+4MT+2½FAT
French Fries	400	18	245	54	3½ST+3½FAT
Chocolate Shake, 15 oz	690	36	350	83	1Mlk+4½CHO+7FAT
Vanilla Shake, 15 oz	680	37	390	78	1Mlk+4CHO+7½FAT
Strawberry Shake, 15 oz	690	33	280	91	1Mlk+5CHO+6½FAT

Source: In-N-Out Burger® Nutrition Facts ©1999. Exchanges calculated by J. Lichten, PhD RD

JACK IN THE BOX®

Burgers:	Calories	Fat (g)	Sodium (mg)	Carbs* (g)	Exchanges**
Sourdough Jack™	690	45	1180	37	2½ST+3½MT+5½FAT
Ultimate Cheeseburger	950	66	1370	37	2½ST+6MT+7FAT
Bacon Ultimate Cheeseburger	1020	71	1740	37	2½ST+7MT+6FAT
Jumbo Jack®	590	37	670	39	2½ST+3MT+4½FAT
Jumbo Jack® with Cheese	680	45	1130	39	2½ST+3½MT+5½FAT
Double Cheeseburger	460	27	1090	32	2ST+2½MT+3FAT
Hamburger	280	12	490	30	2ST+1MT+1½FAT
Hamburger with Cheese	320	16	720	30	2ST+1½MT+1½FAT
Sandwiches and Tacos:					
Chicken Supreme	570	37	1440	39	2½ST+2MT+5½FAT
Jack's Spicy Chicken™	570	29	1020	52	3½ST+2MT+4FAT
Chicken Fajita Pita	280	9	840	25	1½ST+2½MT
Chicken Sandwich	420	23	950	39	2½ST+2MT+2½FAT
Grilled Chicken Fillet	480	24	1110	39	2½ST+3MT+2FAT

*Carbs=Carbohydrate, na=not available   **Exchanges: ST=Starch, Mlk=Milk (skim)
FR=Fruit, CHO=Other Carbohydrates, V=Vegetable, MT=Meat (medium fat), FAT=Fat

JACK IN THE BOX® (continued)

	Calories	Fat (g)	Sodium (mg)	Carbs* (g)	Exchanges**
Sandwiches and Tacos, continued:					
Philly Cheesesteak	580	16	1860	56	3½ST+3MT
Taco	170	10	460	12	1ST+½MT+1½FAT
Monster Taco	270	17	670	19	1ST+1½MT+2FAT
American Cheese, 1 slice	45	4	230	1	1FAT
Swiss-style Cheese, 1 slice	40	3	210	1	1FAT
Teriyaki Bowls & Salads:					
Chicken Teriyaki Bowl	670	4	1730	128	7½ST+1V+1MT
Soy Sauce	5	0	480	1	FREE
Garden Chicken Salad	200	9	420	8	2V+2MT
Side Salad	50	3	75	3	½V+½FAT
Bleu Cheese Dressing	210	15	750	11	4¾FAT
Buttermilk House Dressing	290	30	560	6	6½FAT
Low Calorie Italian Dressing	25	1.⁵	670	2	½FAT
Thousand Island Dressing	250	24	570	10	5½FAT
Croutons	50	2	105	8	½ST+½FAT
Finger Foods and More:					
Bacon & Cheddar Potato Wedges	800	58	1470	49	3ST+1½MT+10FAT
Stuffed Jalapeños, 7 piece	530	31	1730	46	3ST+1MT+5FAT
Stuffed Jalapeños, 10 piece	750	44	2470	65	4ST+1MT+8FAT
Egg Rolls, 3 piece	440	24	1020	40	2½ST+1V+1MT+3½FAT
Egg Rolls, 5 piece	730	41	1700	67	4ST+1½V+1½MT+6½FAT
Fish & Chips	780	39	1740	86	5ST+2MT+6FAT
Tartar Sauce	210	22	340	2	4½FAT
Chicken Breast Pieces, 5 pieces	360	17	970	24	1½ST+3MT+½FAT
Chicken (4) & Fries	730	34	1690	79	5ST+1½MT+5FAT
Barbecue Dipping Sauce	45	0	310	11	½ST
Buttermilk House Dipping Sauce	130	13	240	3	2½FAT
Sweet & Sour Dipping Sauce	45	0	160	11	½ST
Salsa	10	0	200	2	FREE
Sour Cream	60	6	30	1	1½FAT
Sides:					
French Fries, Regular	350	16	710	46	3ST+3FAT
Fries, Jumbo	430	20	890	58	3¾ST+4FAT
French Fries, Super Scoop	610	28	1250	82	5½ST+5½FAT
Ketchup Packet	10	0	105	2	FREE
Onion Rings	410	23	1010	45	3ST+4½FAT
Seasoned Curly Fries	410	23	1010	45	3ST+4½FAT
Chili Cheese Curly Fries	650	41	1760	60	4ST+½MT+7½FAT
Desserts:					
Carrot Cake	370	16	340	54	3½CHO+3FAT
Hot Apple Turnover	340	18	510	41	2¼CHO+3½FAT
Cheesecake	320	18	220	32	2CHO+3½FAT
Double Fudge Cake	300	10	320	50	3¼CHO+2FAT

*Carbs=Carbohydrate, na=not available   **Exchanges: ST=Starch, Mlk=Milk (skim)
FR=Fruit, CHO=Other Carbohydrates, V=Vegetable, MT=Meat (medium fat), FAT=Fat

JACK IN THE BOX® (continued)

Breakfast:

	Calories	Fat (g)	Sodium (mg)	Carbs* (g)	Exchanges**
Breakfast Jack®	280	12	750	28	2ST+2MT+½FAT
French Toast Sticks with bacon	470	23	700	53	3½ST+1MT+3½FAT
Syrup	130	0	5	30	2CHO
Sausage Croissant	700	51	1000	38	2½ST+2MT+8FAT
Supreme Croissant	530	32	960	37	2½ST+2MT+4½FAT
Sourdough Breakfast Sandwich	450	24	1040	36	2ST+2MT+2½FAT
Ultimate Breakfast Sandwich	600	34	1470	39	2½ST+4MT+3FAT
Hash Browns	170	12	250	14	¾ST+2½FAT
Country Crock Spread®	25	3	40	0	½FAT
Grape Jelly	40	0	5	10	¾CHO

Ice Cream Shakes (regular):

	Calories	Fat (g)	Sodium (mg)	Carbs* (g)	Exchanges**
Cappuccino Ice Cream Shake	630	29	320	80	4½CHO+1Mlk+5½FAT
Chocolate Ice Cream Shake	630	27	330	85	4½CHO+1Mlk+5½FAT
Strawberry Ice Cream Shake	640	28	300	85	4½CHO+1Mlk+5½FAT
Vanilla Ice Cream Shake	610	31	320	73	4CHO+1Mlk+6FAT
Oreo® Cookie Ice Cream Shake	740	36	490	91	5CHO+1Mlk+7FAT

Source: Jack in the Box® Nutrition Facts © 1999. Jumbo Jack and Breakfast Jack are trademarks of Jack in the Box®

JASON'S DELI®

	Calories	Fat (g)	Sodium (mg)	Carbs* (g)	Exchanges**
Healthy Heart Super Combo - Each sandwich is served with your choice of:					
Pretzels	110	1	na	na	1ST
Baked Lays®	130	2	170	na	1ST+½FAT
Fruit	50	0.[3]	na	na	1FR
German Potato Salad	108	4	na	na	1ST+1FAT
Steamed Vegetables	7	0.[2]	na	na	FREE
Turkey Reuben	335	3	na	na	2ST+4MT(very lean)
"Lite" Tuna Sandwich	324	6	1000	na	na
"Lite" Chicken Salad Sandwich	324	6	1000	na	na
Ham It Down®	386	7	na	na	2ST+6MT(very lean)
Garden Sandwich	374	18	500	na	2ST+3FAT
King Ranch Lite	541	5	na	na	Na
Southwestern Pita	266	4	794	na	2ST+3MT(very lean)
Pita Plus	387	13	1000	na	2ST+3MT
Philly Chick®	524	13	na	na	na
Turkey Wrap	417	15	na	na	na
Spinach Veggie Wrap	426	17	694	na	na
Tuna Wrap	510	5	na	na	na

---

*Carbs=Carbohydrate, na=not available   ****Exchanges:** ST=Starch, Mlk=Milk (skim)
FR=Fruit, CHO=Other Carbohydrates, V=Vegetable, MT=Meat (medium fat), FAT=Fat

JASON'S DELI® (continued)

Healthy Heart Super Spuds:

	Calories	Fat (g)	Sodium (mg)	Carbs* (g)	Exchanges**
Pollo Mexicano Lite	650	5	na	na	na
Spud Lite	499	1.3	na	na	na
Veggie Jane	476	1.6	658	na	na
Chicken Pepper Sauté "Lite"	529	10	1000	na	na

Healthy Heart Soups & Salads:

	Calories	Fat (g)	Sodium (mg)	Carbs* (g)	Exchanges**
Marinated Chicken Breast Salad	257	11	718	na	na
Gazpacho Soup, cup	53	2	434	na	na
bowl	70	3	579	na	na
French Onion Soup, cup	77	5	751	na	na
bowl	128	9	na	na	na
Vegetarian Vegetable Soup, cup	75	2	532	na	na
bowl	100	3	710	na	na
Fruit Plate (no dressing), small	100	1	na	na	na
large	200	2	na	na	na

Source: Jason's Deli® nutritional information. Current as of 12/99.

KFC®

	Calories	Fat (g)	Sodium (mg)	Carbs* (g)	Exchanges**
Tender Roast® Chicken (not available at all restaurants):					
Wing with skin, 1.8 oz	121	7.7	331	1	1½MT
Breast with skin, 4.9 oz	251	10.8	830	1	5MT(lean)
Breast without skin, 4.2 oz	169	4.3	797	1	4½MT(very lean)
Thigh with skin, 3.2 oz	207	12	504	<2	2½MT
Thigh without skin, 2.1 oz	106	5.5	312	<1	2MT(lean)
Drumstick with skin, 1.9 oz	97	4.3	271	<1	2MT(lean)
Drumstick without skin, 1.2 oz	67	2.4	259	<1	1½MT(lean)
Original Recipe® Chicken:					
Whole Wing, 1.6 oz	140	10	414	5	¼ST+1MT+1FAT
Breast, 5.4 oz	400	24	1116	16	1ST+4MT+1FAT
Drumstick, 2.2 oz	140	9	422	4	¼ST+2MT
Thigh, 3.2 oz	250	18	747	6	½ST+2MT+1½FAT
Extra Crispy™ Chicken:					
Whole Wing, 1.9 oz	220	15	415	10	½ST+1½MT+1FAT
Breast, 5.9 oz	470	28	874	17	1ST+4MT+1½FAT
Drumstick, 2.4 oz	195	12	375	7	½ST+1½MT+1FAT
Thigh, 4.2 oz	380	27	625	14	1ST+2½MT+2½FAT
Hot & Spicy Chicken:					
Whole Wing, 1.9 oz	210	15	350	9	½ST+1MT+2FAT
Breast, 6.5 oz	505	29	1170	23	1½ST+4MT+3FAT
Drumstick, 2.3 oz	175	10	360	9	½ST+1½MT+½FAT
Thigh, 3.8 oz	355	26	630	13	1ST+2MT+3½FAT

*Carbs=Carbohydrate, na=not available   **Exchanges: ST=Starch, Mlk=Milk (skim)
FR=Fruit, CHO=Other Carbohydrates, V=Vegetable, MT=Meat (medium fat), FAT=Fat

KFC® (continued)

	Calories	Fat (g)	Sodium (mg)	Carbs* (g)	Exchanges**
Sandwiches:					
Original Recipe® Chicken SW	450	22	940	33	2ST+3MT+1FAT
without sauce	360	13	890	33	2ST+3MT
Triple Crunch® Chicken SW	490	29	710	39	2½ST+3MT+2½FAT
without sauce	390	15	650	29	2ST+3MT
Triple Crunch® Zinger™ Chicken SW	550	32	830	39	2½ST+3MT+3FAT
without sauce	390	15	650	36	2ST+3MT
Tender Roast® Chicken SW	350	15	880	26	1½ST+3½MT
without sauce	270	5	690	23	1½ST+3½MT(lean)
Honey BBQ Flavored Chicken SW	310	6	560	37	2½ST+3MT(lean)
Other Specialty Items:					
Hot Wings™ Pieces, 6	471	33	1230	18	1ST+3½MT+3FAT
Honey BBQ Wings Pieces, 6	607	38	1145	33	2ST+3½MT+4FAT
Colonel's Crispy Strips®, 3	300	16	1165	18	1ST+2½MT+1FAT
Spicy Crispy Strips®, 3	335	15	1140	23	1½ST+2½MT+½FAT
Popcorn Chicken, small	362	23	610	21	1½ST+2MT+2FAT
Popcorn Chicken, large	620	40	1046	36	2ST+3½MT+4FAT
Chunky Chicken Pot Pie	770	42	2160	69	4ST+2MT+6½FAT
Vegetables:					
Mashed Potatoes with Gravy	120	6	440	17	1ST+1FAT
Potato Wedges	280	13	750	28	2ST+2½FAT
Macaroni & Cheese	180	8	860	21	1½ST+½MT+1FAT
Corn on the Cob	150	1.⁵	20	35	2ST+¼FAT
BBQ Baked Beans	190	3	760	33	2ST+½FAT
Salads:					
Coleslaw	232	13.⁵	284	26	1ST+1V+3FAT
Potato Salad	230	14	540	23	1½ST+3FAT
Breads:					
Biscuit, 1	180	10	560	20	1½ST+2FAT
Desserts:					
Double Chocolate Chip Cake	320	16	230	41	2½CHO+3FAT
Little Bucket™ Parfaits, Fudge Brownie	280	10	190	44	3CHO+1½FAT
lemon crème	410	14	290	62	4CHO+2½FAT
chocolate cream	290	15	330	37	2½CHO+2½FAT
strawberry shortcake	200	7	220	33	2CHO+1FAT
Colonel's™ Pies, pecan pie slice	490	23	510	66	4CHO+4FAT
apple pie, slice	310	14	280	44	1FR+2CHO+2½FAT
strawberry crème pie slice	280	15	130	32	2CHO+3FAT

Source: KFC® Nutrition Facts ©1999. Current as of 12/99. All ® in this section are trademarks of KFC®.

---

*Carbs=Carbohydrate, na=not available   ****Exchanges:** ST=Starch, Mlk=Milk (skim)
FR=Fruit, CHO=Other Carbohydrates, V=Vegetable, MT=Meat (medium fat), FAT=Fat

KOO-KOO-ROO®

	Calories	Fat (g)	Sodium (mg)	Carbs* (g)	Exchanges**
Original Skinless Flame Broiled Chicken™:					
Original Leg & Thigh	173	8	364	3	3MT (lean)
Original Breast & Wing (wing portion contains skin)	218	8	495	3	5MT (lean)
1 Original Breast Meat	159	4	400	2	4MT (very lean)
Half Original Chicken (wing portion contains skin)	391	16	859	6	8MT (lean)
Rotisserie Chicken:					
Rotisserie Leg & Thigh	300	18	513	1	4MT
Rotisserie Breast & Wing	355	16	675	1	6½MT(lean)
Half Rotisserie Chicken	655	34	1188	2	11MT
Fresh Roasted Carved Turkey:					
Turkey Breast Sandwich	538	7	800	68	4ST+6MT(very lean)
½ Turkey Breast Sandwich	269	4	400	34	2ST+3MT(very lean)
¼ # Sliced White Meat	153	1	59	0	5MT (very lean)
¼ # Sliced Dark Meat	212	8	89	0	5MT (lean)
Open-Faced Turkey Sandwich	672	21	1394	69	3ST+1FR+5½MT
Hand Carved Turkey Dinner	705	21	1421	76	3½ST+1FR+1V+5½MT
Turkey Pot Pie	905	45	1381	83	5ST+4MT+5FAT
Salads:					
Koo Koo Roo House Salad	164	6	360	21	1ST+2V+1FAT
Caesar Salad	170	8	483	16	½ST+2V+1½FAT
12 Vegetable Chopped Salad	78	1	65	16	3V
Chicken Caesar Salad	310	11	545	16	½ST+2V+4MT (very lean)+1½FAT
Chinese Chicken Salad	296	8	169	23	1ST+1V+3½MT (very lean)+1FAT
BBQ Chicken Salad	466	21	738	30	2ST+5MT(very lean)+3FAT
Soups:					
Ten Vegetable Soup	121	3	620	21	1ST+1V+½FAT
Turkey Dumpling Soup	166	4	890	14	1ST+2MT
Chicken Chili	98	2	334	13	1ST+½MT
Sandwiches:					
Original Chicken Breast SW	752	47	1076	50	3ST+3½MT+6FAT
BBQ Chicken Sandwich	568	14	1542	69	4ST+4MT
Chicken Caesar Sandwich	728	37	2137	49	3ST+6MT+1½FAT
Turkey Breast Sandwich	538	7	800	68	4ST+5½MT(very lean)
Hot Side Dishes:					
Artichokes	33	0	250	8	1½V
Asparagus	24	0	5	4	1V
Baby Carrots	73	0	173	18	1V+½CHO

*Carbs=Carbohydrate, na=not available **Exchanges:** ST=Starch, Mlk=Milk (skim)
FR=Fruit, CHO=Other Carbohydrates, V=Vegetable, MT=Meat (medium fat), FAT=Fat

KOO-KOO-ROO® (continued)

	Calories	Fat (g)	Sodium (mg)	Carbs* (g)	Exchanges**
Hot Side Dishes (continued):					
Baked Yams	362	0	25	86	3ST+2½CHO
BBQ Beans	139	2	505	28	1½ST+½FAT
Black Beans	139	2	567	23	1½ST+½FAT
Brussels Sprouts	49	0	177	10	2V
Butternut Squash	87	0	7	23	1ST+½CHO
Confetti Rice	131	0	166	29	2ST
Cracked Wheat Rice	97	1	140	21	1½ST
Creamed Spinach	141	12	396	9	1V+½MT+2FAT
Green Beans	50	2	130	7	1½V
Hand-Mashed Potatoes	185	5	362	32	2ST
Homemade Stuffing	189	9	613	23	1½ST
Hot Potatoes	115	3	118	21	1½ST
Italian Vegetables	36	2	123	4	1V
Kernel Corn	97	0	200	25	1½ST
Macaroni & Cheese	270	11	243	28	2ST+1MT+1½FAT
Roasted Garlic Potatoes	116	2	163	22	1½ST+½FAT
Steamed Vegetables	33	0	27	7	1½V
Cold Side Dishes:					
Cucumber Salad	30	0	109	7	1V
Koo Koo Roo Slaw	55	2	230	10	2V+½FAT
Lentil Salad	175	5	273	24	1½ST+1MT
Tangy Tomato Salad	56	3	425	7	1½V
Pasta Salads:					
Tomato Basil Pasta	108	2	223	19	1½ST
Pesto Pasta	168	5	251	21	1½ST+1FAT
Santa Fe Pasta	206	6	327	27	2ST+1MT
Extras:					
Balsamic Vinaigrette Dressing	90	9	240	3	2FAT
BBQ Dressing	40	0	280	10	½CHO
Caesar Dressing	160	18	180	1	3½FAT
Chinese Chicken Salad Dressing	110	8	110	8	1½FAT
Chopped Salad Dressing	100	7	350	8	1½FAT
Cranberry Sauce	45	0	14	11	½CHO
Gravy	24	1	312	3	½FAT
Lahvash (flatbread)	94	0	143	20	1½ST
Roll	107	1	191	21	1½ST

Source: Koo-Koo-Roo® Nutrition Information. Current as of 12/99.

Carbs=Carbohydrate, na=not available **Exchanges:** ST=Starch, Mlk=Milk (skim)
FR=Fruit, CHO=Other Carbohydrates, V=Vegetable, MT=Meat (medium fat), FAT=Fat

KRISPY KREME DOUGHNUTS®

	Calories	Fat (g)	Sodium (mg)	Carbs* (g)	Exchanges**
Glazed Yeast Doughnut	180	10	95	17	1CHO+2FAT
Maple Iced Glazed Yeast	200	9	100	28	1¾CHO+2FAT
Cinn Apple Filled Sugar Coated	210	9	150	29	1¾CHO+2FAT
Blueb Filled Pow'd Sugar Coated	200	9	160	26	1½CHO+2FAT
Fudge Iced Custard Filled Yeast	250	9	150	38	2¼CHO+2FAT
Fudge Iced Glazed w/sprinkles	220	10	95	31	2CHO+2FAT
Glazed Lemon *or* Rasp Filled Yeast	210	10	150-160	27-28	1½CHO+2FAT
Traditional Cake Doughnut	200	11	280	22	1½CHO+2FAT
Cinn Bun, Pow'd Sugar Coated Cake	220	11	160-250	26	1½CHO+2FAT
Fudge Iced Cake Doughnut	230	12	280	28	1¾CHO+2½FAT
Old Fashioned Devil's Fd Cake	240	13	180	29	2CHO+2½FAT
Fudge Iced Glazed Yeast	260	14	105	30	2CHO+3FAT
Fudge Iced Crème Filled Yeast	270	14	150	32	2CHO+3FAT
Glazed Crème Filled Yeast	270	14	150	32	2 CHO+3FAT
Glazed Cruller	220	14	150	22	1½CHO+3FAT
Fudge Iced Glazed Cruller	240	14	160	26	1½CHO+3FAT
Glazed Blueberry Old Fashioned	300	15	200	37	2½CHO+3FAT

Source: Krispy Kreme Doughnuts® Nutritional Information.

KRYSTAL®

Breakfast:

	Calories	Fat (g)	Sodium (mg)	Carbs* (g)	Exchanges**
Krystal Sunriser	240	14	460	14	1ST+1MT+2FAT
Biscuit, plain	260	15	570	27	2ST+3FAT
Sausage Biscuit	440	32	850	27	2ST+1MT+5½FAT
Bacon, Egg, Cheese Biscuit	390	25	870	28	2ST+1MT+4FAT
Chik Biscuit	340	17	990	34	2ST+1MT+2½FAT
Hash Browns	190	13	340	17	1ST+2½FAT
Country Breakfast	660	42	1450	46	2½ST+2½MT+6FAT

Sandwiches, Chili, Fries, Shakes and Desserts:

Krystal	160	7	260	17	1ST+1MT+½FAT
Cheese Krystal	180	9	430	16	1ST+1MT+1FAT
Double Krystal	260	13	550	24	1½ST+1½MT+1FAT
Double Cheese Krystal	310	16	800	26	1½ST+2MT+1FAT
Bacon Cheese Krystal	190	10	430	16	1ST+1MT+1FAT
Krystal Chik	240	11	640	24	1½ST+1MT+1FAT
Regular Fries	370	18	85	49	3ST+3½FAT
Chili Cheese Fries	540	28	800	59	3½ST+1MT+4½FAT
Krystal Chili	200	7	1130	22	1ST+1½MT+½FAT
Plain Pup	170	9	500	15	1ST+½MT+1FAT
Chili Cheese Pup	210	12	510	17	1ST+1MT+1½FAT
Corn Pup	260	19	480	19	1ST+½MT+3FAT
Chocolate Shake	380	11	410	58	4CHO+2FAT
Apple Turnover	220	10	300	31	2CHO+2FAT
Lemon Pie	360	10	190	60	4CHO+2FAT

Source: Krystal Company nutrition information.

*Carbs=Carbohydrate, na=not available   **Exchanges: ST=Starch, Mlk=Milk (skim)
FR=Fruit, CHO=Other Carbohydrates, V=Vegetable, MT=Meat (medium fat), FAT=Fat

LA MADELEINE® FRENCH BAKERY & CAFÉ

	Calories	Fat (g)	Sodium (mg)	Carbs* (g)	Exchanges**
Breads (50 g serving, unless indicated):					
Sourdough/Baguette	120	0.^{5}	400	25	1½ST
Country Wheat	120	0.^{5}	400	24	1½ST
Seven Grain	129	2	300	24	1½ST
Rye Caraway	120	0.^{5}	400	24	1½ST
Mediterranean Ciabatta	120	0.^{5}	400	25	1½ST
Focaccia Roll, 1 roll	240	3	na	na	3ST
White Chocolate, 1 roll	160	4	na	na	2ST
Soups (6 oz serving):					
French Onion w/out cheese/croutons	50	1.^{5}	na	na	1V+¼FAT
Salads (small servings) & Dressings (2 Tbsp):					
Fresh Fruit Salad	65	0.^{5}	na	na	1FR
Strawberries Romanoff	141	5	na	na	1½FR+1FAT
Wild Field Salad (w/fat-free Caesar Drsg)	27	0.^{5}	na	na	½V
Entrees & Sandwiches (whole):					
Light Tuna Salad Sandwich	266	4	na	na	na
Smoked Turkey SW, no cheese	330	1	na	na	na
Grilled Chicken SW, no dressing	345	4	na	na	na
Rotisserie Turkey w/rice & veg	628	8	na	na	na
Grilled Chicken Breast and Rice	433	7	na	na	na
Pastries:					
Light Apricot Tart	237	4	na	na	3CHO+½FAT
Light Yogurt Mousse	212	2	na	na	1Mlk+1½CHO
Light Fruit and Cinnamon Muffin	429	7	na	na	3CHO+2½FAT

Source: La Madeleine® Nutritional Information. Current as of 12/99.

LITTLE CAESARS® PIZZA

	Calories	Fat (g)	Sodium (mg)	Carbs* (g)	Exchanges**
Medium Round (one slice):					
Cheese only	170	6	330	22	1½ST+½MT+½FAT
Pepperoni	190	8	410	22	1½ST+½MT+1FAT
PIZZA!PIZZA!® (one slice):					
Medium Cheese	160	6	410	21	1½ST+½MT+½FAT
Medium Pepperoni	170	7	480	21	1½ST+½MT+½FAT
Large Cheese	170	7	430	21	1½ST+½MT+1FAT
Large Pepperoni	190	9	490	21	1½ST+½MT+1FAT
Single Slice:					
Cheese only	350	13	670	45	3ST+1MT+1½FAT
Pepperoni	390	16	830	45	3ST+1½MT+1½FAT

*Carbs=Carbohydrate, na=not available   **Exchanges:** ST=Starch, Mlk=Milk (skim)
FR=Fruit, CHO=Other Carbohydrates, V=Vegetable, MT=Meat (medium fat), FAT=Fat

LITTLE CAESARS® PIZZA (continued)

	Calories	Fat (g)	Sodium (mg)	Carbs* (g)	Exchanges**
Other Menu Items:					
Crazy Bread®, 1 stick	100	3	105	16	1ST+½FAT
Crazy Sauce®, 4 oz	60	0	260	11	1½V
Chicken Wings, 5 wings	250	35	710	0	1MT+6FAT
Italian Cheese Bread, 1 stick	110	5	230	11	¾ST+1FAT
Italian Cheese Bread, lunch order	300	16	750	30	2ST+3FAT
Baby Pan! Pan!®	308	14	770	31	2ST+1MT+2FAT
Cold Deli-Style Sandwiches:					
Italian	690	31	1660	68	4ST+3MT+3FAT
Tuna	820	39	1330	71	4½ST+4½MT+3FAT
Ham & Cheese	600	22	1410	68	4ST+3MT+1½FAT
Turkey	600	21	1570	68	4ST+3½MT+1FAT
Veggie	550	24	940	70	4½ST+2MT+3FAT
Hot Oven-Baked Sandwiches:					
Pepperoni	930	58	2290	75	4½ST+5MT6½FAT
Veggie	760	38	1360	74	4½ST+5MT+2½FAT
Supreme	900	49	2040	74	4½ST+5MT+4½FAT
Cheeser	900	48	2130	73	4½ST+5MT+4½FAT
Meatsa	980	53	2240	72	4½ST+5MT+5½FAT
Side Salads:					
Greek	60	3	330	5	1V+½MT
Caesar	80	3	190	7	1½V+½MT
Antipasto	80	6	340	4	1V+½MT+½FAT
Tossed	50	1	60	9	2V
Salad Dressings (1½oz):					
Golden Italian	210	22	360	2	4½FAT
Buttermilk Ranch	270	29	380	1	6FAT
Honey French	220	18	310	14	3½FAT
Fat Free Italian	25	0	390	5	¼CHO
Thousand Island	220	21	360	7	½CHO+4FAT
Chunky Blue Cheese	230	24	450	2	5FAT
LC Caesar Dressing	230	25	260	1	5FAT
Creamy Caesar	220	23	540	2	4½FAT

Source: Little Caesar's® Nutrition Guide ©1999. Current as of 12/99. All ® in this section are the
trademark of Little Caesars®

LONG JOHN SILVER'S®

	Calories	Fat (g)	Sodium (mg)	Carbs* (g)	Exchanges**
Regular Battered Fish, 1 piece	230	13	700	16	1ST+1½MT+1FAT
Junior Battered Fish, 1 piece	120	8	410	8	½ST+½MT+1FAT
Battered Chicken Plank, 1 piece	140	8	400	9	½ST+1MT+½FAT

*Carbs=Carbohydrate, na=not available   ****Exchanges:** ST=Starch, Mlk=Milk (skim)
FR=Fruit, CHO=Other Carbohydrates, V=Vegetable, MT=Meat (medium fat), FAT=Fat

LONG JOHN SILVER'S®

	Calories	Fat (g)	Sodium (mg)	Carbs* (g)	Exchanges**
Batter Shrimp, 1 piece	45	2.5	125	3	5=1ST+1MT+1½FAT
Breaded Clams, 1 order	250	14	560	26	1½ST+1MT+2FAT
Lemon Crumb Fish, 2 pieces	240	12	790	10	½ST+3MT
Lemon Crumb Fish a-la-carte, 2 fish w/rice	480	17	1490	52	3½ST+3MT+½FAT
Lemon Crumb Fish Add A Piece, 1 fish w/rice	150	7	460	9	½ST+1½MT
Popcorn Shrimp, 1 serving	320	15	1440	33	2ST+1½MT+1½FAT
Country Style Breaded Fish	200	10	300	17	1ST+1MT+1FAT
Side Items:					
Regular Fries	250	15	500	28	1½ST+3FAT
Large Fries	420	24	830	46	2½ST+5FAT
Hushpuppies, 1 pc	60	2.5	25	8	½ST+½FAT`
Cole Slaw, 4 oz	170	7	310	23	1V+1CHO+1½FAT
Corn Cobbette	80	0.5	0	19	1ST
Corn Cobbette w/butter	140	8	0	19	1ST+1½FAT
Rice, 4 oz	180	4	560	34	2ST+1FAT
Cheesesticks, 5 pieces	160	9	360	12	1ST+½MT+1FAT
Broccoli Cheese Soup, 1 bowl	180	12	1240	13	½ST+1V+2½FAT
Sandwiches & Meals:					
Ultimate Fish™ Sandwich	480	25	1400	46	3ST+1½MT+3½FAT
Lemon Crumb Fish Meal	730	29	1720	89	na
Salads:					
Ocean Chef Salad	130	2	540	15	½ST+1V+2MT(very lean)
Grilled Chicken Salad	140	2.5	260	10	¼ST+1V+2½MT(very lean)
Garden Salad	45	0	25	9	1½V
Side Salad	20	0	10	3	1V
Salad Dressings & Condiments (1 packet):					
Ranch	170	18	260	1	3½FAT
Fat-Free Ranch	40	0	290	9	½CHO
Fat-Free French	40	0	240	10	½CHO
Italian	90	9	290	2	2FAT
Thousand Island	120	10	290	5	¼CHO+2FAT
Tartar Sauce	40	3.5	105	2	½FAT
Shrimp Sauce	15	0	180	3	1=FREE
Ketchup	10	0	110	2	1=FREE
Honey Mustard Sauce	20	0	60	5	¼CHO
Sweet'N'Sour Sauce	20	0	45	5	¼CHO
Malt Vinegar	0	0	15	0	FREE
Desserts:					
Pineapple Crème Cheesecake Pie	310	17	105	35	2CHO+3½FAT

Source: Long John Silver® Product Nutritional Database 5/17/99. Current as of 12/99.

*Carbs=Carbohydrate, na=not available   ****Exchanges:** ST=Starch, Mlk=Milk (skim)
FR=Fruit, CHO=Other Carbohydrates, V=Vegetable, MT=Meat (medium fat), FAT=Fat

LUBY'S® CAFETERIAS

	Calories	Fat (g)	Sodium (mg)	Carbs* (g)	Exchanges**
Fruit Salad	172	0	10	44	2FR+1CHO
Cucumbers w/vinegar & oil	80	5	305	9	1½V+1FAT
Shredded Carrots	276	17	84	31	2V+1CHO+3½FAT
Spanish Slaw	54	2	189	8	1V+½FAT
Chopped Steak, 5½oz serving	311	21	596	5	¼ST+3MT+1FAT
Baked Haddock Almondine, 7oz	409	24	317	7	½ST+5½MT
Roast Turkey Breast, 5½oz serving	153	1	59	0	5MT(very lean)
Roast Turkey Breast w/drsg & gravy	352	12	791	19	1ST+5MT
Roast Beef	327	12	93	0	7MT(lean)
Fried Fish (haddock), 7 oz	377	12	625	37	2ST+4MT(lean)
Vegetable Soup Bowl	112	1	2449	19	1ST+1V
Seasoned Leaf Spinach	67	5	484	5	1V+1FAT
Grilled Texaican Chicken Breast, 7oz	305	8	188	2	8MT(very lean)
Seasoned Green Beans, canned	27	1	605	5	1V
Fresh Steamed Broccoli	40	0	38	7	1½V
Mashed Potatoes	204	7	415	32	2ST+1½FAT
Mexicalli Rice	170	5	242	28	2ST+1FAT
Baked Potato, 11 oz	350	5	23	72	4ST+1FAT
Cloverleaf Roll	125	3	179	21	1½ST+½FAT
Whole Wheat Roll	174	8	32	23	1½ST+1½FAT

Source: Luby's®. Info based on company recipe & standard Luby's order size. Current as of 12/99.

MAZZIO'S PIZZA®

	Calories	Fat (g)	Sodium (mg)	Carbs* (g)	Exchanges**
Appetizers:					
Meat Nachos	500	37	1200	21	1½ST+2½MT+5FAT
Garlic Bread w/cheese, appx 2 sl	700	35	1280	74	5ST+1MT+5FAT
Sandwiches:					
Ham and Cheese	790	39	1900	71	4ST+4MT+4FAT
Deluxe Submarine	810	43	2240	68	4ST+4MT+4½FAT
BBQ Beef & Cheddar	580	24	1260	51	3ST+4MT+1FAT
Chicken & Cheddar	570	24	1350	56	3½ST+3MT+2FAT
Pizza (1 slice medium pizza):					
Original Crust Cheese	260	8	450	33	2ST+1MT+½FAT
Thin Crust Cheese	220	9	440	22	1½ST+1MT+1FAT
Deep Pan Cheese	350	13	620	42	2½ST+1½MT+1FAT
Original Crust Pepperoni	280	11	600	30	2ST+1½MT+1FAT
Deep Pan Pepperoni	380	17	740	38	2½ST+1½MT+2FAT
Original Crust Sausage	350	16	890	34	2ST+1½MT+1½FAT
Deep Pan Sausage	430	21	1040	41	2½ST+2MT+2FAT
Original Crust Combo	320	13	780	34	2ST+1½MT+1FAT
Deep Pan Combo	410	18	930	42	2½ST+1½MT+2FAT

*Carbs=Carbohydrate, na=not available   **Exchanges: ST=Starch, Mlk=Milk (skim)
FR=Fruit, CHO=Other Carbohydrates, V=Vegetable, MT=Meat (medium fat), FAT=Fat

MAZZIO'S PIZZA® (continued)

Pasta:	Calories	Fat (g)	Sodium (mg)	Carbs* (g)	Exchanges**
Chicken Parmesan	590	19	1600	68	4ST+4MT
Small Meat Lasagna	460	25	1370	36	2ST+3MT+2FAT
Small Fettuccine Alfredo	440	28	680	34	2ST+1MT+4½FAT
Small Spaghetti	290	10	800	39	2ST+2V+2FAT

Source: Mazzio's Pizza®. Current as of 12/99.

McDONALD'S®

Sandwiches:	Calories	Fat (g)	Sodium (mg)	Carbs* (g)	Exchanges**
Hamburger	270	9	600	35	2ST+1½MT
Cheeseburger	320	13	830	35	2ST+1½MT+1FAT
Quarter Pounder®	430	21	840	37	2½ST+3MT+1FAT
Quarter Pounder® w/Cheese	530	30	1310	38	2½ST+3½MT+2FAT
Big Mac®	570	32	1100	45	3ST+3MT+3FAT
Arch Deluxe®	550	31	1010	39	2½ST+3MT+3FAT
Arch Deluxe® with Bacon	590	34	1150	39	2½ST+4MT+3FAT
Crispy Chicken Deluxe™	500	25	1100	43	3ST+3MT+2FAT
Filet-O-Fish®	470	26	890	45	3ST+1MT+4FAT
Grilled Chicken Deluxe™	440	20	1040	38	2½ST+3MT+1FAT
Grilled Chicken Deluxe™, no mayo	300	5	930	38	2½ST+3MT(lean)
French Fries:					
French Fries, small	210	10	135	26	1½ST+2FAT
French Fries, medium	450	22	290	57	3½ST+4FAT
French Fries, large	540	26	350	68	4½ST+5FAT
French Fries, Super Size®	610	29	390	77	5ST+5FAT
Chicken McNuggets®/Sauces:					
Chicken McNuggets®, 4 piece	190	11	360	13	1ST+1MT+1FAT
Chicken McNuggets®, 6 piece	290	17	540	20	1ST+2MT+1FAT
Chicken McNuggets®, 9 piece	430	25	810	29	2ST+3MT+1FAT
Hot Mustard Sauce, 1 pkg	60	3.^{5}	240	7	½CHO+½FAT
Barbecue Sauce, 1 pkg	45	0	250	10	1CHO
Sweet'N Sour Sauce, 1 pkg	50	0	140	11	1CHO
Honey, 1 pkg	45	0	0	12	1CHO
Honey Mustard, 1 pkg	50	4.^{5}	85	3	1FAT
Light Mayonnaise, 1 pkg	40	4	80	<1	1FAT
Salads & Dressings (1 pkg):					
Garden Salad	35	0	20	7	1V
Grilled Chicken Salad Deluxe	120	1.^{5}	240	7	1V+3MT(lean)
Croutons, 1 pkg	50	1	105	9	½ST
Caesar Dressing	160	14	450	7	3FAT
Fat Free Herb Vinaigrette	50	0	330	11	½CHO
Ranch Dressing	230	21	550	10	½CHO+4FAT
Red French Reduced Calorie Dressing	160	8	490	23	1½CHO+1FAT

*Carbs=Carbohydrate, na=not available   **Exchanges: ST=Starch, Mlk=Milk (skim)
FR=Fruit, CHO=Other Carbohydrates, V=Vegetable, MT=Meat (medium fat), FAT=Fat

McDONALD'S® (continued)

	Calories	Fat (g)	Sodium (mg)	Carbs* (g)	Exchanges**
Breakfast:					
Egg McMuffin®	290	12	790	27	2ST+2MT
Sausage McMuffin®	360	23	740	26	2ST+1MT+3FAT
Sausage McMuffin® w/Egg	440	28	890	27	2ST+2MT+3FAT
English Muffin	140	2	210	25	2ST
Sausage Biscuit	470	31	1080	35	2ST+1MT+4½FAT
Sausage Biscuit w/Egg	550	37	1160	35	2ST+2MT+5FAT
Bacon, Egg & Cheese Biscuit	540	34	1550	36	2ST+2½MT+4FAT
Biscuit	290	15	780	34	2ST+2FAT
Ham, Egg, & Cheese Bagel	550	23	1490	58	4ST+3MT+1FAT
Spanish Omelete Bagel	690	38	1560	59	4ST+3MT+4FAT
Steak, Egg, & Cheese Bagel	660	31	1300	57	4ST+4MT+1FAT
Sausage	170	16	290	0	1MT(high fat)+1½FAT
Scrambled Eggs, 2	160	11	170	1	2MT
Hashbrowns	130	8	330	14	1ST+1FAT
Hotcakes, plain	340	8	630	58	4ST+1FAT
Hotcakes, w/2 pats margarine & syrup	600	17	770	104	4ST+3CHO+3FAT
Breakfast Burrito	320	20	660	21	1½ST+1½MT+2FAT
Muffins/Danish:					
Low Fat Apple Bran Muffin	300	3	380	61	4CHO
Apple Danish	340	15	340	47	3CHO+2½FAT
Cheese Danish	400	21	400	45	3CHO+4FAT
Cinnamon Roll	390	18	310	50	3½CHO+3FAT
Desserts/Shakes:					
Vanilla Red. Fat Ice Cream Cone	150	4.5	75	23	1½CHO+1FAT
Strawberry Sundae	290	7	95	50	3½CHO+1FAT
Hot Caramel Sundae	360	10	180	61	4CHO+2FAT
Hot Fudge Sundae	340	12	170	52	3½CHO+2FAT
Nuts, added to sundaes	40	3.5	55	2	1FAT
Butterfinger® McFlurry™	620	22	260	90	6CHO+3FAT
M&M® McFlurry™	630	23	210	90	6CHO+4FAT
Nestle Crunch® McFlurry™	630	24	230	89	6CHO+4FAT
Oreo® McFlurry™	570	20	280	82	5½CHO+3FAT
Baked Apple Pie	260	13	200	34	2½CHO+2FAT
Chocolate Chip Cookie	170	10	120	22	1½CHO+2FAT
McDonaldland® Cookies, 1 pkg	180	5	190	32	2CHO+1FAT
Vanilla Shake, small	360	9	250	59	4CHO+2FAT
Chocolate Shake, small	360	9	250	60	4CHO+2FAT
Strawberry Shake, small	360	9	180	60	4CHO+2FAT

Source: McDonald's® Today © October 1999. Current as of 12/99. The following trademarks used in this section are owned by McDonald's Corporation: McDonald's, Quarter Pounder, Big Mac, Crispy Chicken Deluxe, Filet-O-Fish, Grilled Chicken Deluxe, Super Size, Chicken McNuggets, Egg McMuffin, Sausage McMuffin, McDonaldland, McFlurry.

*Carbs=Carbohydrate, na=not available   **Exchanges: ST=Starch, Mlk=Milk (skim)
FR=Fruit, CHO=Other Carbohydrates, V=Vegetable, MT=Meat (medium fat), FAT=Fat

MIAMI SUBS®

	Calories	Fat (g)	Sodium (mg)	Carbs* (g)	Exchanges**
Broiled Chicken Club Salad	376	16	505	20	½ST+2V+4MT(lean) +1½FAT
Chicken Pita	392	13	546	34	2ST+4MT(lean)
Gyros Platter w/salad & fries	1041	62	4007	77	4½ST+1V+4MT+8½FAT
12" Cheese Steak Sub	1024	48	1386	63	4ST+10MT
12" Turkey Breast Sub	820	43	2312	69	4ST+1V+4MT+4½FAT
6" Tuna Sub	427	20	758	31	2ST+1MT+3FAT

Source: Miami Subs®. Current as of 12/99.

MR GATTI'S®

	Calories	Fat (g)	Sodium (mg)	Carbs* (g)	Exchanges**
Gourmet Pizza (per slice):					
BBQ Chicken	282	8	411	39	2½ST+1MT
Black Bean	269	9	593	38	2½ST+1½MT
Burgeroni	311	13	586	36	2½ST+2MT
Deluxe	366	9	518	37	2½ST+2MT
Double Cheeseburger	310	13	580	36	2½ST+2MT
Fiesta with Pace Picante	290	10	674	37	2½ST+1½MT
Meat Market	298	12	625	36	2½ST+2MT
Sampler	314	13	602	39	2½ST+2MT
Superoni	286	11	457	36	2½ST+1½MT
Vegetable Sampler	260	8	424	38	2½ST+1MT
Cheese Sticks (per stick)	104	5	142	12	1ST+½FAT
Pizza (per slice):					
Mr. Gatti's® Original (crust, sauce, and cheese	222	5	383	35	2ST+1MT
Mr. Gatti's® Pan Perfect (crust, sauce, and cheese)	250	7	375	37	2ST+1½MT
Pizza with Toppings (per slice add):					
Anchovies	4	0.7	188	0	FREE
Bell Peppers	2	0	0	0	FREE
Black Beans	5	0	7	1	FREE
Burger	58	5	77	0	1MT
Canadian Bacon	9	0.5	92	0	FREE
Cheddar Cheese	27	2	4	0	½MT
Extra Cheese	22	2	60	0	½MT
Italian Sausage	61	5	73	0	1MT
Jalapenos	3	0	0	0	FREE
Onions, red	3	0	0	1	FREE
Onions, white	4	0	0	1	FREE
Olives, black	14	1	54	1	¼ FAT
Olives, green	14	1	48	0	¼ FAT
Mushrooms	2	0	0	0	FREE

*Carbs=Carbohydrate, na=not available   **Exchanges: ST=Starch, Mlk=Milk (skim)
FR=Fruit, CHO=Other Carbohydrates, V=Vegetable, MT=Meat (medium fat), FAT=Fat

MR GATTI'S® (continued)

	Calories	Fat (g)	Sodium (mg)	Carbs* (g)	Exchanges**
Pizza with Toppings (per slice add):					
Pepperoni	27	3	12	0	½MT
Sausage	57	5	70	0	1MT
Spicy Burger	48	4	43	1	1MT
Tomatoes	3	0	1	1	FREE
White Cheddar Cheese	27	2	5	0	½MT
Sandwiches (per sandwich):					
Roll	180	2	420	36	2½ST
Provolone	75	6	186	0	1MT
Salami	111	10	44	0	1MT+1FAT
Ham	48	1	91	1	1MT (lean)
Lettuce	4	0	1	0	FREE
Tomatoes	6	0	2	1	FREE
Smoked Sausage	53	4	25	1	1FAT
Mustard	5	0	71	1	FREE
Mayonnaise	51	6	41	0	1FAT
Pickles	20	1	170	0	FREE
Chips, bag	160	10	150	15	1ST+2FAT
Pasta (per serving):					
Fettuccini Alfredo	373	10	196	58	3½ST+2FAT
Spaghetti Marinara	291	1	157	58	3ST+1V
Spaghetti, meat	304	2	164	59	3ST+1V+½MT
Desserts:					
Very Cherry Pizza, slice	272	6	284	51	3½CHO+1FAT
Dutch Apple Treat, slice	285	8	294	50	3½CHO+1½FAT
Cinnamon Rolls, each	381	29	333	41	2 ½CHO+5FAT
Cinnamon Sticks, per stick	87	2	117	15	1CHO+½FAT

Source: Mr Gatti's® Nutritional Information. Current as of 12/99. All ® in this section are the trademark of Mr Gatti's®

OLIVE GARDEN®

	Calories	Fat (g)	Sodium (mg)	Carbs* (g)	Exchanges**
Garden Fare® Lunch Entrees:					
Capellini Pomodoro	340	11	700	52	3ST+2V+1½FAT
Capellini Primavera	350	7	820	58	3ST+2V+1FAT
Capellini Primavera w/Chicken	510	13	1550	59	3ST+2V+3MT
Chicken Giardino	300	7	910	40	3ST+3MT(lean)
Linguine Alla Marinara	280	5	510	48	3ST+2V+½FAT
Shrimp Primavera	440	9	830	53	3ST+2V+2MT(lean)
Penne Arrabbiata	300	7	530	49	3ST+1FAT

*Carbs=Carbohydrate, na=not available   **Exchanges:** ST=Starch, Mlk=Milk (skim)
FR=Fruit, CHO=Other Carbohydrates, V=Vegetable, MT=Meat (medium fat), FAT=Fat

OLIVE GARDEN® (continued)

	Calories	Fat (g)	Sodium (mg)	Carbs* (g)	Exchanges**
Garden Fare® Dinner Entrees:					
Capellini Pomodoro	550	17	1090	84	5½ST+3V+2½FAT
Capellini Primavera	600	12	1450	99	5½ST+3V+1½FAT
Capellini Primavera w/Chicken	760	18	2190	101	5½ST+3V+4MT
Chicken Giardino	460	8	1180	59	4½ST+5MT(lean)
Grilled Chicken Capri	500	9	640	45	3ST+7MT(lean)
Linguine Alla Marinara	450	9	770	79	5½ST+3V+1FAT
Shrimp Primavera	830	14	1390	103	5½ST+3V+5MT(lean)
Penne Arrabbiata	410	11	800	67	4ST+2FAT
Garden Fare® Breadsticks, Soup, & Dessert:					
Minestrone, 6 fl oz bowl	100	1	610	18	¾ST+1V
Plain Breadstick, 1	140	1.5	270	26	1½ST
Apple Carmellina	570	2.5	260	131	1FR+7CHO

Source: Olive Garden®. Current as of 12/99. All ® in this section are the trademarks of Olive
 Garden®. Note: Recipes and their respective nutritional information are subject to change.
Other tips: You may request alternative food preparation or serving instructions including cheese
 topping omitted, sauce served on the side, or lunch portions at dinner.

PAPA JOHN'S

	Calories	Fat (g)	Sodium (mg)	Carbs* (g)	Exchanges**
One Slice Original Pizza (¹/₈ of a 14" Large Pizza):					
Cheese	270	9	660	37	2¼ST+1MT+½FAT
Pepperoni	305	12	800	37	2¼ST+1MT+1FAT
Sausage	335	14	900	37	2¼ST+1MT+1½FAT
All the Meats	390	19	1110	37	2¼ST+1½MT+2FAT
Garden Special	290	10	720	39	2¼ST+1MT+1FAT
The Works	345	14	920	38	2¼ST+1½MT+1FAT
One Slice Thin Pizza (¹/₈ of a 14" Large Pizza):					
Cheese	225	12	440	22	1½ST+½MT+2FAT
Pepperoni	260	15	580	22	1½ST+1MT+2FAT
Sausage	285	17	680	22	1½ST+1MT+2½FAT
All the Meats	345	22	890	22	1½ST+1½MT+3FAT
Garden Special	240	12	500	24	1½ST+¾MT+1½FAT
The Works	295	17	700	23	1½ST+1¼MT+2FAT
Sides:					
Cheese Sticks, 2, ¹/₇ of an order	180	8	380	20	1¼ST+½MT+1FAT
Bread Sticks, 1, ¹/₈ of an order	140	2	260	26	1½ST+½FAT
Nacho Cheese, 1T	30	2	115	0	½FAT or ½MT
Garlic Sauce, 1 T	75	9	115	0	2FAT
Pizza Sauce, 1T	10	0.5	50	1	FREE

Source: Papa John's® Nutritional Information. Current as of 12/99.

---

*Carbs=Carbohydrate, na=not available   ****Exchanges:** ST=Starch, Mlk=Milk (skim)
FR=Fruit, CHO=Other Carbohydrates, V=Vegetable, MT=Meat (medium fat), FAT=Fat

PETER PIPER™ PIZZA

Based on One Slice (¼ Express Lunch Pizza *or* ELP, ¹/₆ Sm, ¹/₈ Med, ¹/₈ Lg or ¹/₁₂XL):

	Calories	Fat (g)	Sodium (mg)	Carbs* (g)	Exchanges**
Cheese, ELP	152	4	152	21	1½ST+½MT
small	177	4	179	25	1½ST+½MT
medium	203	5	202	29	2ST+½MT
large	270	6	271	39	2½ST+¾MT
extra large	257	6	260	36	2½ST+¾MT
Extra Mozzarella, ELP	174	6	186	21	1½ST+¾MT
small	198	6	213	25	1½ST+¾MT+½FAT
medium	236	7	253	30	2ST+1MT
large	319	10	349	39	2½ST+1¼MT+½FAT
extra large	300	9	327	37	2½ST+1¼MT
Extra Cheddar, ELP	180	6	196	21	1½ST+¾MT
small	196	6	208	25	1½ST+¾MT+½FAT
medium	224	6	235	29	2ST+¾MT+½FAT
large	306	9	327	39	2½ST+1¼MT+½FAT
extra large	290	9	311	37	2½ST+1¼MT
Salami, ELP	164	5	199	21	1½ST+½MT
small	189	5	226	25	1½ST+¾MT+½FAT
medium	216	6	254	29	2ST+¾MT
large	288	8	342	39	2½ST+1MT+½FAT
extra large	273	8	322	37	2½ST+1MT
Pepperoni, ELP	168	6	293	21	1½ST+¾MT
small	198	6	367	25	1½ST+¾MT+½FAT
medium	229	7	431	29	2ST+1MT
large	308	9	555	39	2½ST+1¼MT+½FAT
extra large	284	9	507	36	2½ST+1¼MT
Beef, ELP	165	5	257	21	1½ST+½MT
small	194	5	319	25	1½ST+¾MT+½FAT
medium	222	6	359	29	2ST+¾MT
large	296	8	482	39	2½ST+1MT+½FAT
extra large	280	8	446	36	2½ST+1MT
Green Pepper, ELP	153	4	152	21	1½ST+½MT
small	178	4	179	26	1½ST+½MT+½FAT
medium	204	5	202	30	2ST+½MT+½FAT
large	272	6	272	39	2½ST+¾MT+½FAT
extra large	259	6	260	37	2½ST+¾MT
Onion, ELP	153	4	152	21	1½ST+½MT
small	177	4	179	25	1½ST+½MT+½FAT
medium	204	5	202	30	2ST+½MT
large	271	6	272	39	2½ST+¾MT+½FAT
extra large	258	6	260	37	2½ST+¾MT

Carbs=Carbohydrate, na=not available **Exchanges:** ST=Starch, Mlk=Milk (skim)
FR=Fruit, CHO=Other Carbohydrates, V=Vegetable, MT=Meat (medium fat), FAT=Fat

PETER PIPER™ PIZZA (continued)

Based on One Slice (¼ Express Lunch Pizza *or* ELP, ¹/₆ Sm, ¹/₈ Med, ¹/₈ Lg or ¹/₁₂ L):

	Calories	Fat (g)	Sodium (mg)	Carbs* (g)	Exchanges**
Black Olive, ELP	157	4	198	21	1½ST+½MT
small	182	5	230	36	1½ST+½MT+½FAT
medium	209	5	256	30	2ST+¾MT
large	279	7	349	40	2½ST+1MT
extra large	265	7	331	37	2½ST+¾MT
Sausage, ELP	178	6	362	21	1½ST+¾MT
small	197	6	342	25	1½ST+¾MT+½FAT
medium	224	6	377	29	2ST+¾MT
large	300	8	517	39	2½ST+1MT+½FAT
extra large	284	8	481	36	2½ST+1MT
Mushroom, ELP	153	4	152	21	1½ST+½MT
small	178	4	179	25	1½ST+½MT+½FAT
medium	204	5	202	30	2ST+½MT
large	181	4	182	26	1½ST+½MT+½FAT
extra large	259	6	260	37	2½ST+¾MT
Ham, ELP	156	4	191	21	1½ST+½MT
small	180	4	218	25	1½ST+½MT+½FAT
medium	207	5	245	29	2ST+½MT
large	276	6	330	39	2½ST+¾MT+½FAT
extra large	261	6	311	36	2½ST+¾MT
Tomato, ELP	153	4	152	21	1½ST+½MT
small	177	4	179	25	1½ST+½MT+½FAT
medium	204	5	202	30	2ST+½MT
large	275	6	274	40	2½ST+¾MT+½FAT
extra large	258	6	260	37	2½ST+¾MT
Jalapeno, ELP	153	4	198	21	1½ST+½MT
small	178	4	219	26	1½ST+½MT+½FAT
medium	205	5	247	30	2ST+½MT
large	266	6	336	39	2½ST+¾MT
extra large	259	6	314	37	2½ST+¾MT
Pineapple, ELP	155	4	152	22	1½ST+½MT
small	179	4	179	26	1½ST+½MT+½FAT
medium	206	5	202	30	2ST+½MT
large	274	6	273	40	2½ST+¾MT+½FAT
extra large	260	6	260	37	2½ST+¾MT
Bacon Pizza, ELP	182	7	237	21	1½ST+¾MT
small	217	7	293	25	1½ST+¾MT+½FAT
medium	249	9	330	29	2ST+1MT
large	331	11	442	39	2½ST+1¾MT
extra large	311	11	411	37	2½ST+1½MT

Source: Peter Piper Pizza. Current as of 12/99.

*Carbs=Carbohydrate, na=not available ****Exchanges:** ST=Starch, Mlk=Milk (skim)
FR=Fruit, CHO=Other Carbohydrates, V=Vegetable, MT=Meat (medium fat), FAT=Fat

PICCADILLY CAFETERIA®

Piccadilly Cafeteria is willing to satisfy most special dietary requests. Call ahead to make your request or go to the beginning of the line and ask to speak to the manager. All weights listed below refer to uncooked weights.

Fresh fruits and many salads without dressing are offered. Low fat Ranch salad dressing and fat-free Italian and Ranch salad dressings can be requested. Sugar Free Jello is often available.

The "Dilly Dish" offers a choice of a selected entree, two vegetables, and bread. The leanest Dilly Dish entrees include: Baked Cod, Roast Beef, Quartered Chicken (remove the skin), and Carved Turkey Breast. Each are approximately 4 oz uncooked servings. Another lean entree is the boneless, skinless chicken breast (6 oz) or the baked catfish (6 oz). The leanest steak is the 6 oz choice filet (remove the bacon). The fish is kept on the food line in a sauce that contains mostly chicken broth and is thickened with an oleo/flour roux.

Many vegetables such as broccoli and squash are steamed. The fats are added just before being brought out to the line so you may be able to ask for your portion to be served without fat. Baked potatoes are served dry.

Yeast rolls are 2 oz in weight. Often you can request a roll to be served before it has been brushed with butter. Sugar-free desserts are often served. Lowfat or skim milk is also available.

Source: Picadilly Cafeteria®.   Current as of 12/99.

PIZZA HUT®

	Calories	Fat (g)	Sodium (mg)	Carbs* (g)	Exchanges**
Pan Pizza (1 med slice):					
Cheese	361	15	678	44	2¾ST+¾MT+2FAT
Beef Topping	399	18	773	45	2¾ST+¾MT+2½FAT
Ham	331	12	687	44	2¾ST+¾MT+1½FAT
Pepperoni	353	14	697	44	2¾ST+¾MT+1½FAT
Italian Sausage	415	20	805	45	2¾ST+¾MT+3FAT
Pork Topping	394	18	820	45	2¾ST+¾MT+2½FAT
Meat Lover's®	428	21	607	45	2¾ST+1MT+2½FAT
Veggie Lover's®	333	12	601	46	2¾ST+½MT+1½FAT
Pepperoni Lover's®	370	16	767	44	2¾ST+¾MT+2FAT
Supreme	385	17	757	45	2¾ST+1MT+1½FAT
Super Supreme	401	18	854	46	2¾ST+1MT+1FAT
Chicken Supreme	343	12	671	45	2¾ST+1MT+1FAT
Chicken Taco	320	15	830	36	2ST+1MT+2FAT
Taco	310	13	800	36	2ST+1MT+1FAT
Meatless Taco	290	12	680	36	2ST+½MT+1½FAT
Beef Taco	300	12	770	36	2ST+1MT+1FAT
Hand Tossed Style (1 med slice):					
Cheese	309	9	848	43	2¾ST+1MT+½FAT
Beef Topping	347	12	943	44	2¾ST+1MT+1FAT
Ham	279	6	857	43	2¾ST+½MT

*Carbs=Carbohydrate, na=not available   **Exchanges: ST=Starch, Mlk=Milk (skim)
FR=Fruit, CHO=Other Carbohydrates, V=Vegetable, MT=Meat (medium fat), FAT=Fat

PIZZA HUT® (continued)

	Calories	Fat (g)	Sodium (mg)	Carbs* (g)	Exchanges**
Hand Tossed Style, continued (1 med slice):					
Pepperoni	301	8	867	43	2¾ST+½MT+1FAT
Italian Sausage	363	14	975	44	2¾ST+1MT+1½FAT
Pork Topping	342	12	990	44	2¾ST+1MT+1FAT
Meat Lover's®	376	15	1077	44	2¾ST+1½MT
Veggie Lover's®	281	6	771	45	2¾ST+½MT+½FAT
Pepperoni Lover's®	372	14	1123	43	2¾ST+1½MT+½FAT
Supreme	333	11	927	44	2¾ST+1MT+½FAT
Super Supreme	359	12	1024	45	2¾ST+1MT+1FAT
Chicken Supreme	291	6	841	44	2¾ST+1MT
Taco	280	11	870	34	2ST+1MT+1FAT
Meatless Taco	250	8	790	35	2ST+1MT+½FAT
Beef Taco	270	8	870	35	2ST+1MT+½FAT
Chicken Taco	290	11	940	35	2ST+1MT+1FAT
Thin 'n Crispy® Pizza (1 med slice):					
Cheese	243	10	653	27	1¾ST+¾MT+1FAT
Beef Topping	305	15	814	28	1¾ST+1MT+1½FAT
Ham	212	7	662	27	1¾ST+½MT+1FAT
Pepperoni	235	10	672	27	1¾ST+½MT+1½FAT
Italian Sausage	325	18	865	28	1¾ST+1MT+2FAT
Pork Topping	298	15	875	28	1¾ST+1MT+2FAT
Meat Lover's®	339	19	970	28	1¾ST+1¼MT+2½FAT
Veggie Lover's®	222	8	621	30	1¾ST+½MT+1FAT
Pepperoni Lover's®	289	14	859	28	1¾ST+1MT+2FAT
Supreme	284	13	784	29	1¾ST+1MT+1½FAT
Super Supreme	304	15	902	29	1¾ST+1MT+2FAT
Chicken Supreme	232	7	681	29	1¾ST+1MT
Taco	260	11	860	27	1¾ST+1MT+1FAT
Meatless Taco	230	8	700	27	1¾ST+½MT+1FAT
Beef Taco	260	10	850	29	1¾ST +1MT+1FAT
Chicken Taco	260	12	850	26	1¾ST+¾MT+1½FAT
Stuffed Crust Pizza (1 med slice):					
Cheese	445	19	1090	46	3ST+2MT+1½FAT
Beef Topping	466	22	1137	46	3ST+2MT+2FAT
Ham	404	22	1190	45	2ST+2MT+2FAT
Pepperoni	438	19	1116	45	3ST+1¾MT+1½FAT
Italian Sausage	478	23	1164	46	3ST+2MT+2FAT
Pork Topping	461	21	1176	46	3ST+2MT+2FAT
Meat Lover's®	543	29	1427	46	3ST+2½MT+3FAT
Veggie Lover's®	421	17	1039	48	3ST+1½MT+1½FAT
Pepperoni Lover's®	525	26	1413	46	3ST+2½MT+2FAT
Supreme	487	23	1227	47	3ST+2MT+2FAT
Super Supreme	505	25	1371	46	3ST+2MT+2½FAT
Chicken Supreme	432	17	1111	47	3ST+2MT+1FAT

*Carbs=Carbohydrate, na=not available   **Exchanges: ST=Starch, Mlk=Milk (skim)
FR=Fruit, CHO=Other Carbohydrates, V=Vegetable, MT=Meat (medium fat), FAT=Fat

PIZZA HUT® (continued)

Sicilian Pizza:	Calories	Fat (g)	Sodium (mg)	Carbs* (g)	Exchanges**
Cheese	295	13	815	32	2ST+1MT+1½FAT
Beef	282	12	824	31	2ST+1MT+1FAT
Ham	257	10	745	30	2ST+¾MT+1FAT
Pepperoni	277	13	754	31	2ST+¾MT+1FAT
Italian Sausage	333	18	855	31	2ST+1MT+2FAT
Pork Topping	314	16	868	31	2ST+1MT+2FAT
Meat Lover's®	344	18	948	31	2ST+1MT+2½FAT
Veggie's Lover's®	252	10	627	32	2ST+½MT+1FAT
Pepperoni Lover's®	321	16	899	31	2ST+1MT+2FAT
Supreme	307	15	815	32	2ST+1MT+1½FAT
Super Supreme	323	16	911	32	2ST+1MT+2FAT
Chicken Supreme	269	10	732	32	2ST+1MT+½FAT
Personal Pan Pizza®:					
Cheese	813	27	1581	110	6ST+1V+2MT+3FAT
Pepperoni	810	28	1661	111	6ST+1V+2MT+3FAT
Supreme	808	27	1579	111	6ST+1V+2MT+3FAT
Taco Pizza	780	35	1900	90	5½ST+1V+1½MT+5FAT
The Big New Yorker Pizza:					
Cheese	393	17	1099	42	2½ST+1¾MT+1FAT
Pepperoni	380	16	1116	42	2½ST+1½MT+1½FAT
Supreme	459	22	1310	44	2½ST+1¾MT+2FAT
The Edge™:					
The Works	140	5	390	16	1ST+½MT+½FAT
Veggie	110	2.5	250	16	1ST+½MT
Meaty	150	7	430	15	1ST+½MT+½FAT
Chicken Veggie	120	3	310	16	1ST+½MT
Taco Pizza	140	6	450	17	1ST+½MT+½FAT
Other Menu Items:					
Mild Buffalo Wings, 5 pieces	200	12	510	<1	3MT
Hot Buffalo Wings, 5 pieces	210	12	900	4	3MT
Garlic Bread, 1 piece	150	8	240	16	1ST+1½FAT
Bread Stick, 1	130	4	170	20	1¼ST+½FAT
Bread Stick Dipping Sauce, 1 serv	30	0.5	170	5	1V
Spaghetti w/Marinara	490	6	730	91	5ST+2V+1FAT
Spaghetti w/Meat Sauce	600	13	910	98	5½ST+2V+1MT+1FAT
Spaghetti w/Meatballs	850	24	1120	120	7ST+2V+2MT+½FAT
Cavatini® Pasta	480	14	1170	66	3ST+2V+1½MT+1FAT
Cavatini Supreme® Pasta	560	19	1400	73	3½ST+2V+2MT+1FAT
Ham & Cheese Sandwich	550	21	2150	57	3½ST+3MT+1FAT
Supreme Sandwich	640	28	2150	62	4ST+3MT+1FAT

Source: infomration obtained from Pizza Hut and current as of 12/17/99. The ® in this section
designates the registered trademarks of PizzaHut®, Inc.

---

*Carbs=Carbohydrate, na=not available   ****Exchanges:** ST=Starch, Mlk=Milk (skim)
FR=Fruit, CHO=Other Carbohydrates, V=Vegetable, MT=Meat (medium fat), FAT=Fat

QUIZNO'S® SUBS

	Calories	Fat (g)	Sodium (mg)	Carbs* (g)	Exchanges**
Small Beefeater	324	8	na	na	na
Small Chicken Teriyaki	373	5	na	na	na
Regular Chicken Teriyaki	635	8	na	na	na
Small Turkey Lite	310	2	na	na	na
Regular Turkey Lite	524	4	na	na	na
Large Turkey Lite	818	6	na	na	na
Small Turkey Guacamole	337	6	na	na	na

Source: Quizno's® Subs. Current as of 12/99.

ROUND TABLE® PIZZA

	Calories	Fat (g)	Sodium (mg)	Carbs* (g)	Exchanges**
Thin Crust Pizzas ($^1/_{16}$ of large):					
Cheese	160	$6.^2$	240	16	1ST+½MT+½FAT
Pepperoni	170	8	240	17	1ST+1MT+½FAT
King Arthur's Supreme	200	$10.^1$	340	18	1ST+1 MT+1FAT
Guinever's Garden Delight	150	$5.^6$	250	18	1ST+½ MT+½FAT
Gourmet Veggie	160	$6.^5$	200	18	1ST+½ MT+½FAT
Chicken & Garlic Gourmet	170	$7.^2$	280	17	1ST+1 MT+½FAT
Italian Garlic Supreme	200	$10.^4$	220	17	1ST+1 MT+1FAT
Garden Pesto	170	$7.^7$	200	18	1ST+1 MT+½FAT
Saluté Chicken & Garlic	150	$5.^4$	250	18	1ST+1 MT
Saluté Veggie	140	$4.^7$	170	19	1ST+1V+½MT+¼FAT
Classic Pesto	170	$7.^9$	210	18	1ST+½ MT+1FAT
Bacon Super Deli	200	$12.^6$	360	16	1ST+1 MT+1½FAT
Maui Zaui (Red Pizza Sauce)	170	$6.^5$	350	18	1ST+1MT+¼FAT
Roastin Toastin Garlic	190	9	310	18	1ST+1MT+1FAT
Pan Pizza ($^1/_{16}$ of large):					
Cheese	210	$7.^2$	250	26	1½ST+1MT+½FAT
Pepperoni	220	$8.^1$	240	26	1½ST+1MT+½FAT
King Arthur's Supreme	240	$9.^8$	320	27	2ST+½MT+1FAT
Guinever's Garden Delight	200	$6.^2$	250	27	2ST+½MT+½FAT
Gourmet Veggie	220	$7.^4$	230	28	2ST+½MT+½FAT
Chicken & Garlic Gourmet	230	$8.^1$	310	27	2ST+1MT+½FAT
Italian Garlic Supreme	250	$10.^5$	240	27	2ST+½MT+1½FAT
Garden Pesto	230	$8.^6$	230	28	2ST+½MT+1FAT
Saluté Chicken & Garlic	200	$5.^8$	270	28	2ST+½MT+½FAT
Saluté Veggie	190	$5.^1$	190	28	1½ST+1V+½MT+½FAT
Classic Pesto	230	$8.^8$	240	27	2ST+½MT+1FAT
Bacon Super Deli	260	$13.^5$	380	26	1½ST+1MT+1½FAT
Maui Zaui (Red Pizza Sauce)	310	10	490	37	2½ST+1MT+1FAT
Roastin Toastin Garlic	255	11	353	28	2ST+1MT+1FAT

Source: Round Table Pizza® Nutritional information. Current as of 12/99.

*Carbs=Carbohydrate, na=not available ****Exchanges:** ST=Starch, Mlk=Milk (skim)
FR=Fruit, CHO=Other Carbohydrates, V=Vegetable, MT=Meat (medium fat), FAT=Fat

RUBY TUESDAY

Fit N Trim Menu Items:	Calories	Fat (g)	Sodium (mg)	Carbs* (g)	Exchanges**
Lowfat Baked Potato	587	4	71	94	6ST+1FAT
Teriyaki Chicken	516	3	1650	20	1ST+3MT(very lean)
Chicken Stir-fry	834	1	1980	40	2ST+7MT(very lean)
Herb Grill Chicken Sandwich	538	7	1320	na	na
Fat Free Strawberry Sundae	646	0	25	118	8CHO
Fat Free Fudge Sundae	675	0	37	132	9CHO
Tilapia, 3 ½ oz fillet only	98	2	52	0	2½MT(very lean)
Marinara Sauce, 3 oz	51	2	59	7	½V+½FAT
Clam Chowder, 3 oz	80	5	130	6	½ST+1FAT
Potato Cheese Soup, 3 oz	96	6	410	6	½ST+1FAT
French Onion Soup, 3 oz	26	1	220	4	¼ST
Broccoli Cheese Soup, 3 oz	74	6	220	3	¼ST+1FAT
Italian Vegetable Soup, 3 oz	90	6	300	5	1V+1FAT

Source: Ruby Tuesday®

SCHLOTZSKY'S® DELI

Light & Flavorful Sandwiches (on sourdough bun unless noted):	Calories	Fat (g)	Sodium (mg)	Carbs* (g)	Exchanges**
Chicken Breast, small	360	7	1617	50	3ST+2MT(lean)
medium	536	10	2490	76	4½ST+3½MT(lean)
large	791	14	4204	103	6½ST+6MT(lean)
Smoked Turkey Breast, small	334	5	1403	50	3ST+2MT(lean)
medium	500	7	2104	76	4½ST+3½MT(lean)
large	772	12	3613	106	6ST+6MT(lean)
The Vegetarian on wheat, small	322	10	805	48	2½ST+1V+½MT+1½FAT
medium on wheat	515	16	1232	72	4ST+1V+1MT+2FAT
large on sourdough	743	25	1708	103	5½ST+2V+2MT+3FAT
Albacore Tuna on wheat, sm	370	11	1208	47	3ST+2MT
medium on wheat	566	17	1795	70	4½ST+3½MT
large on sourdough	852	28	2853	99	5½ST+6MT
Dijon Chicken on wheat, sm	305	3	1206	47	3ST+2MT(lean)
medium on wheat	475	4	1814	70	4½ST+3½MT(lean)
large on sourdough	726	7	3067	102	5½ST+6MT(lean)
Santa Fe Chick on jalapeno cheese, sm	445	14	1756	52	3ST+3MT
medium on jalapeno cheese	645	19	2578	79	4½ST+4MT
large on jalapeno cheese	976	28	4361	107	5½ST+7MT
Pesto Chicken, sm	344	6	1269	49	3ST+2MT(lean)
medium	513	9	1902	73	4½ST+3½MT(lean)
large	779	14	3172	100	5½ST+6MT(lean)

*Carbs=Carbohydrate, na=not available **Exchanges: ST=Starch, Mlk=Milk (skim) FR=Fruit, CHO=Other Carbohydrates, V=Vegetable, MT=Meat (medium fat), FAT=Fat

SCHLOTZSKY'S® DELI (continued)

	Calories	Fat (g)	Sodium (mg)	Carbs* (g)	Exchanges**
Original Sandwiches (all on sourdough bun):					
The Original, small	581	30	1566	49	3ST+2½MT+3½FAT
regular	795	39	2314	75	5ST+3MT+4½FAT
large	1403	78	3983	103	7ST+7MT+8FAT
Deluxe Original, small	786	43	2897	52	3ST+5MT+3½FAT
regular	1030	53	3968	79	5ST+6MT+4½FAT
large	1876	106	7291	111	7ST+13MT+8FAT
Ham & Cheese Original, small	534	22	2278	52	3ST+3MT+1½FAT
regular	773	32	3348	78	5ST+4MT+2½FAT
large	1366	65	6051	110	7ST+9MT+4FAT
Turkey Original, small	636	32	2167	52	3ST+4MT+2½FAT
regular	894	42	3073	78	5ST+5MT+3½FAT
large	1558	81	5498	109	7ST+12MT+4FAT
Cheese Original, small	584	31	1350	49	3ST+2½MT+3½FAT
regular	833	43	2005	75	5ST+3MT+5FAT
large	1580	95	3550	103	7ST+7MT+11FAT
Specialty Deli Sandwiches (on sourdough bun unless otherwise noted):					
Roast Beef & Cheese, small	606	27	1731	49	3ST+4MT+1½FAT
regular	870	37	2512	75	5ST+6MT+1½FAT
large	1524	71	4235	103	7ST+12MT+2FAT
Turkey & Bacon Club on wheat, small	679	37	2107	49	3ST+4MT+3½FAT
regular on wheat	1006	53	3079	73	5ST+6MT+4½FAT
large on sourdough	1749	97	5502	108	7ST+12MT+7½FAT
Pastrami & Swiss on dark rye, small	618	27	2804	54	3ST+4MT+1½FAT
regular on dark rye	918	40	4053	79	5ST+5½MT+2½FAT
large on sourdough	1556	75	7114	108	7ST+11MT+4FAT
Chicken Club, small	552	24	1621	49	3ST+4MT+1FAT
regular	864	37	2479	78	5ST+5½MT+2FAT
large	1492	73	4340	109	7ST+11MT+3½FAT
The Philly, small	560	21	1684	52	3ST+4MT
regular	817	29	2525	80	5ST+6MT
large	1452	61	4151	110	7ST+12MT
Corned Beef Reuben on dark rye, sm	536	23	2272	52	3ST+3MT+1½FAT
regular on dark rye	842	37	3560	77	5ST+4½MT+3FAT
large on sourdough	1403	66	6559	105	7ST+9MT+4FAT
Corned Beef on dark rye, small	390	11	2004	50	3ST+2½MT
regular on dark rye	576	16	2853	73	5ST+3MT
large on sour dough	872	26	4714	98	7ST+5MT
Pastrami Reuben on dark rye, sm	655	31	2622	55	3ST+4MT+2FAT
regular on dark rye	966	45	3860	80	5ST+5½MT+3½FAT
large on sourdough	1651	84	7159	113	7½ST+11MT+4FAT
Roast Beef, small	439	14	1203	48	3ST+3MT
regular	654	20	1795	73	5ST+4MT
large	1005	31	2845	98	7ST+7MT

*Carbs=Carbohydrate, na=not available **Exchanges: ST=Starch, Mlk=Milk (skim)
FR=Fruit, CHO=Other Carbohydrates, V=Vegetable, MT=Meat (medium fat), FAT=Fat

SCHLOTZSKY'S® DELI (continued)

	Calories	Fat (g)	Sodium (mg)	Carbs* (g)	Exchanges**
Turkey Reuben on dark rye, sm	615	27	2582	55	3ST+4MT+1½FAT
regular on dark rye	906	39	3800	80	5ST+5½MT+2½FAT
large on sourdough	1531	72	7039	113	7½ST+11MT+3½FAT
Albacore Tuna Melt, wheat, sm	576	29	1633	48	3ST+4MT+2FAT
regular on wheat	860	42	2428	72	5ST+5½MT+3FAT
large on sourdough	1494	80	4219	104	7ST+11MT+5FAT
Western Vegetarian, small	449	23	790	51	3ST+1V+½MT+3FAT
regular	651	33	1161	75	5ST+2V+1MT+4FAT
large	1261	61	2235	150	8ST+3V+1½MT+9½FAT
Vegetable Club, small	414	18	982	49	2½ST+1V+½MT+3FAT
regular	616	28	1473	74	4ST+1V+½MT+5FAT
large	916	44	2158	101	6ST+2V+1½MT+7FAT
BLT, small	558	31	1166	47	3ST+½MT+5½FAT
regular	861	48	1786	72	5ST+2MT+7½FAT
large	1400	86	2792	98	6½ST+4MT+13FAT
Turkey Guacamole, small	493	19	1862	55	3½ST+2½MT+1FAT
regular	761	31	2872	86	5½ST+3MT+3FAT
large	1215	52	4987	124	8ST+6MT+4½FAT
TX Schlotzsky's® jalapeno cheese, sm	604	30	2235	51	3ST+3MT+3FAT
regular on jalapeno cheese	856	41	3287	78	5ST+4½MT+4FAT
large on sourdough	1491	78	6048	108	7ST+9MT+6½FAT

8" Pizzas:

	Calories	Fat (g)	Sodium (mg)	Carbs* (g)	Exchanges**
Double Cheese & Pepperoni	680	32	1057	67	4ST+2½MT+4FAT
Barbeque Chicken	618	18	1274	76	4½ST+3½MT
Thai Chicken	642	18	1292	83	5ST+3½MT
Chicken & Pesto	579	16	828	69	4ST+3½MT
The Original Combination	602	25	844	70	4ST+2MT+3FAT
Vegetarian Special	504	15	569	68	4ST+2MT+1FAT
Smoked Turkey & Jalapeno	582	17	1463	71	4ST+3½MT
Double Cheese	534	19	591	67	4ST+2MT+2FAT
Southwestern	601	19	3410	72	4ST+3½MT
New Orleans	581	17	2837	70	4ST+3½MT
Bacon, Tomato & Mushroom	639	28	725	69	4ST+2½MT+3FAT
Fresh Tomatoes & Pesto	528	19	454	67	4ST+1½MT+2½FAT
Mediterranean	513	19	815	67	4ST+1MT+3FAT

Soups (8 oz cup):

	Calories	Fat (g)	Sodium (mg)	Carbs* (g)	Exchanges**
7 Bean Medley	145	2	1260	25	1½ST+½MT
New England Clam Chowder	148	7	1062	16	1ST+1½FAT
Broccoli Cheese	252	17	1104	23	1½ST+1MT+1½FAT
Cauliflower Cheese	167	10	993	16	1ST+2FAT
Chicken Noodle (Old Fashioned)	122	1	810	8	1ST+1MT(very lean)
Chicken Tortilla	167	3	1026	24	1½ST+½MT
Chicken with Wild Rice	378	28	1201	25	1½ST+1MT+4FAT
Corn Chowder	140	4	1209	22	1½ST+½FAT
Cream of Broccoli	121	5	1152	16	1ST+1FAT

Carbs=Carbohydrate, na=not available   **Exchanges:** ST=Starch, Mlk=Milk (skim) FR=Fruit, CHO=Other Carbohydrates, V=Vegetable, MT=Meat (medium fat), FAT=Fat

SCHLOTZSKY'S® DELI (continued)

	Calories	Fat (g)	Sodium (mg)	Carbs* (g)	Exchanges**
Soups, continued (8 oz cup):					
Cream of Potato with Bacon	226	13	1209	31	2ST+2FAT
Creamy Turkey Vegetable	219	14	871	21	1ST+1V+1MT+1FAT
French Onion	78	3	1715	9	½ST+½FAT
Minestrone	89	1	1048	17	1ST
Ravioli Tomato	111	2	1115	21	1½ST+½MT
Red Beans and Rice	166	1	934	32	2ST
Timberline Chili	210	7	814	24	1½ST+1½MT
Tomato Florentine	100	1	855	25	1ST+1V
Tomato Milano	89	0	437	19	1ST
Tortellini	122	3	1360	19	1ST+½MT
Vegetable Beef Barley	100	3	1160	12	1ST+1V
Vegetable Cheese	289	19	1338	24	1½ST+½MT+3FAT
Vegetable Lumberjack	133	6	1482	6	1V+1FAT
Vegetable Vegetarian	138	6	1536	20	¾ST+1V+1FAT
Wisconsin Cheese	319	25	1104	26	1½ST+5FAT
Heartland Chicken Noodle	96	1	867	14	1ST
Salads (does not include dressing):					
Chicken Caesar	146	5	437	4	1V+2½MT(lean)
Caesar	66	4	177	2	1V+1MT
Smoked Turkey Chef's	233	10	1342	14	½ST+1V+3MT(lean)
Garden	110	3	120	14	½ST+1V+½FAT
Small Garden	70	3	55	8	1½V+½FAT
Chinese Chicken	181	4	267	14	½ST+1V+2MT(lean)
Greek	190	12	595	14	½ST+1V+½MT+2FAT
Ham & Turkey Chef's	253	12	1490	14	½ST+1V+3MT
Deli Salads:					
Potato Salad, Choice, 2/3 cup	270	19	560	19	1ST+4FAT
Potato Salad, Mustard/egg, 2/3 c	240	16	570	18	1ST+4FAT
Potato Salad, Diced w/egg, 2/3 c	230	14	640	19	1ST+3FAT
Cole Slaw, Country-style, ½ cup	180	13	230	13	½CHO+1V+2½FAT
Cole Slaw, Shredded, ½ cup	180	13	310	13	½CHO+1V+2½FAT
Macaroni Salad, 2/3 cup	360	25	660	25	1½ST+5FAT
Schlotzsky's® Deli Style Potato Chips (1½ oz bag):					
Reg, Jalapeno, & Sour Cream & Onion	210	10	190-220	25	1½ST+2FAT
Barbeque and Salt & Vinegar	210	10	270-310	25	1½ST+2FAT
Kid's Deals (nutritional information doesn't include cookie or soft drink):					
Kid's Cheese Pizza	452	13	396	66	4ST+1MT+1½FAT
Kid's Pepperoni Pizza	492	17	517	66	4ST+1MT+2½FAT
Kid's Cheese Sandwich	412	17	971	46	3ST+1MT+2½FAT
Kid's PBJ Sandwich	494	15	748	78	3ST+2CHO+1MT+2FAT
Kid's Ham & Cheese Sandwich	442	18	1341	47	3ST+2MT+1½FAT

*Carbs=Carbohydrate, na=not available   **Exchanges: ST=Starch, Mlk=Milk (skim)
FR=Fruit, CHO=Other Carbohydrates, V=Vegetable, MT=Meat (medium fat), FAT=Fat

SCHLOTZSKY'S® DELI (continued)

Cookies:

	Calories	Fat (g)	Sodium (mg)	Carbs* (g)	Exchanges**
Chocolate Chip	160	7	140	24	1½CHO+1½FAT
Oatmeal Raisin	150	5	140	24	1½CHO+1½FAT
Peanut Butter	170	8	190	21	1½CHO+1½FAT
Sugar	160	6	180	23	1½CHO+1½FAT
Chocolate Chunk	160	7	150	23	1½CHO+1½FAT
White Macadamia Nut	170	8	140	22	1½CHO+1½FAT
Chocolate Pecan Chunk	170	8	140	23	1½CHO+1½FAT
Fudge Chocolate Chunk	170	8	170	22	1½CHO+1½FAT
Peanut Butter Chocolate Chunk	170	8	160	22	1½CHO+1½FAT

Other Desserts:

	Calories	Fat (g)	Sodium (mg)	Carbs* (g)	Exchanges**
New York-style Cheesecake	310	18	230	31	2CHO+3½FAT
Fudge Brownie Cake	410	25	135	46	3CHO+5FAT
Strawberry Swirl Cheesecake	300	17	230	30	2CHO+3½FAT

Source: Scholtzsky's® Inc. Current as of 12/99. All ® in this section are the trademarks of Scholtzsky's® Inc.

SMOOTHIE KING®

Smoothies, 20 oz (each is custom-made to your order & nutritional content may vary slightly):

	Calories	Fat (g)	Sodium (mg)	Carbs* (g)	Exchanges**
Activator® - vanilla, choc, or banana	429	1	260	90	na
Activator® - strawberry	559	1	260	123	na
Angel Food™	330	0.5	71	79	na
Blackberry Dream™	343	0.3	39	86	na
Caribbean Way®	392	0.4	18	96	na
Celestial Cherry High™	285	0.4	22	69	na
Coconut Surprise™	457	5.9	126	99	na
Cranberry Cooler™	538	0.1	95	132	na
Cranberry Supreme™	577	0.6	120	139	na
High Protein - almond mocha	402	12.9	245	45	na
High Protein – banana	412	13.8	315	44	na
High Protein – chocolate	401	12.9	244	45	na
High Protein – lemon	390	12.8	177	41	na
High Protein – pineapple	380	12.9	206	41	na
Grape Expectations™	399	0.4	24	96	na
Grape ExpectationsII™	529	0.4	24	129	na
GoGuava™	300	0	50	72	na
Hawaiian Café Au Lei™	286	0.3	170	62	na
Hulk™ - chocolate	846	29	626	129	na
Hulk – strawberry	953	29	645	156	na
Hulk™ - vanilla	846	29	646	129	na
Immune Builder™	333	1	47	80	na
Instant Vigor™	359	1.2	38	87	na
Island Treat®	334	0.8	29	81	na

*Carbs=Carbohydrate, na=not available   **Exchanges: ST=Starch, Mlk=Milk (skim)
FR=Fruit, CHO=Other Carbohydrates, V=Vegetable, MT=Meat (medium fat), FAT=Fat

SMOOTHIE KING® (continued)

	Calories	Fat (g)	Sodium (mg)	Carbs* (g)	Exchanges**
Smoothies, 20 oz (each is custom-made to your order & nutritional content may vary slightly):					
Lemon Twist® - Banana	339	0.4	24	82	na
Lemon Twist® - Strawberry	399	0.3	23	97	na
Light & Fluffy®	389	0.4	12	98	na
Malt	887	41.4	370	119	na
MangoFest™	320	0	50	78	na
Mo'cuccino™	420	12	190	71	na
Muscle Punch®	339	1.3	75	80	na
Muscle Plus Punch™	340	1.2	65	80	na
Peach Slice™	341	0.2	93	80	na
Peach Slice Plus®	471	0.2	93	113	na
Peanut Power®	502	20.8	88	72	na
Peanut Power Plus™ - grape	703	20.8	87	119	na
Peanut Power Plus™ - strawberry	632	20.8	87	104	na
Pep Upper®	334	0.8	39	80	na
Pineapple Pleasure®	313	0.4	29	76	na
Power Punch®	430	1.3	91	102	na
Power Punch Plus®	499	2	91	113	na
Raspberry Surprise™	335	0.7	39	85	na
Shake	875	41.4	359	117	na
Slim & Trim™ - chocolate	270	1.6	261	55	na
Slim & Trim™ - strawberry	357	1	149	79	na
Slim & Trim™ - vanilla	227	1	150	51	na
Slim & Trim™ - orange-vanilla	199	0.5	150	43	na
Super Punch™	425	0.4	179	95	na
Super Punch™ Plus	516	0.4	195	118	na
Yogurt D-Lite™	341	3.9	183	65	na
Youth Fountain™	267	0.4	40	65	na
Kid's Kups:					
Gimme-Grape™	170	0	5	42	na
Choc-A-Laka	210	2	200	44	na
Berry Interesting™	150	0	5	37	na
Smarti Tarti™	150	0	5	36	na

Source: Smoothie King® Nutritional Guide. Current as of 12/99. All ® in this section are trademarks of Smoothie King®.

Carbs=Carbohydrate, na=not available   **Exchanges:** ST=Starch, Mlk=Milk (skim)
FR=Fruit, CHO=Other Carbohydrates, V=Vegetable, MT=Meat (medium fat), FAT=Fat

SOUPLANTATION & SWEET TOMATOES™

	Calories	Fat (g)	Sodium (mg)	Carbs* (g)	Exchanges**
Fat-Free Signature Prepared Salads (½ c):					
Aunt Doris' Red Pepper Slaw	70	0	480	18	½CHO+1V
Cucumber Tomato w/chile lime	20	0	20	4	1V
Marinated Summer Vegetables	80	0	210	19	3V
Low-Free Signature Prepared Salads (½ c):					
Baja Bean & Cilantro Salad	180	3	190	29	1¼ST+1V+1MT(lean)
Carrot Raisin Salad	90	3	80	17	1FR+1V+½FAT
Gemelli Pasta w/chicken/citrus vinaigr	130	3	380	20	1ST+½MT
German Potato Salad	120	3	260	18	1ST+½FAT
Mandarin Krab Salad	150	3	280	26	1½FR+½FAT
Mandarin Noodles Salad w/broccoli	120	3	380	19	1ST+1V+½FAT
Mandarin Shells Salad w/almonds	120	3	360	19	1ST+½FAT
Mediterranean Harvest Salad	120	3	180	17	1ST+½FAT
Moroccan Marinated Vegetables	90	3	230	9	2V+½FAT
Oriental Ginger Slaw w/krab	70	3	80	8	1V+½FAT
Southern Dill Potato Salad	120	3	300	20	1½ST+½FAT
Spicy Southwestern Pasta Salad	130	3	350	21	1½ST+½FAT
Summer Barley Salad w/black beans	110	3	280	19	1ST+½FAT
Signature Prepared Salads (½ c):					
Artichoke Rice Salad	160	8	780	21	1ST+1V+1½FAT
BBQ Potato Salad	160	8	270	20	1½ST+1½FAT
Carrot Ginger Salad w/herb vinaigrette	150	12	40	9	1V+2½FAT
Chinese Krab Salad	160	8	260	19	1ST+½MT+1FAT
Confetti Pasta w/cheddar & dill	150	12	40	9	½ST+½MT+2FAT
Dijon Potato w/garlic dill vinaigr.	150	12	40	9	½ST+1½FAT
Greek Couscous w/feta cheese	170	9	480	19	1ST+½MT+1FAT
Italian White Bean Salad	140	5	480	19	1ST+1FAT
Jalapeño Potato Salad	140	5	490	20	1ST+1FAT
Joan's Broccoli Madness Salad	180	14	250	11	1½V+3FAT
Lemon Orzo Salad w/feta & mint	130	5	270	18	1ST+1FAT
Old Fashioned Macaroni w/ham	180	11	360	15	1ST+2FAT
Pesto Pasta Salad	160	7	320	18	1ST+1½FAT
Picnic Potato Salad	150	7	320	19	1ST+1½FAT
Pineapple Coconut Slaw	150	10	190	14	1FR+2FAT
Poppyseed Coleslaw	120	9	130	9	2V+2FAT
R'sted Potato Salad w/Chipotle Chile V	140	6	250	18	1ST+1FAT
Thai Noodle Salad w/Peanut Sauce	170	8	310	17	1ST+1½FAT
Three Bean Marinade Salad	170	6	320	27	1½ST+1FAT
Tortellini Salad with Basil	170	10	260	14	1ST+2FAT
Tumbleweed Tortelli Salad	140	9	330	11	½ST+2FAT
Tuna Tarragon Salad	240	14	480	21	1½ST+½MT+2FAT
Turkey Chutney Pasta Salad	230	9	310	21	1½ST+1MT+1FAT
Zesty Tortellini Salad	190	15	460	18	1ST+3FAT

*Carbs=Carbohydrate, na=not available   **Exchanges: ST=Starch, Mlk=Milk (skim)
FR=Fruit, CHO=Other Carbohydrates, V=Vegetable, MT=Meat (medium fat), FAT=Fat

SOUPLANTATION & SWEET TOMATOES™ (continued)

	Calories	Fat (g)	Sodium (mg)	Carbs* (g)	Exchanges**
Fresh Tossed Salads (1 c):					
Antipasto Salad	140	10	370	6	1V+½MT+1½FAT
Antipasto Salad w/peppered salami	150	11	390	6	1V+ ½MT+2FAT
Bartlett Pear & Walnut Salad	180	12	220	13	1FR+½MT+2FAT
BBQ Chopped Salad	130	9	190	7	1V+1MT+½FAT
California Cobb Salad	180	8	190	4	1V+1MT+½FAT
Caribbean Krab Salad	120	7	180	10	2V+1½FAT
Classic Caesar Salad	190	14	280	10	2V+3FAT
Country French Salad w/bacon	210	18	420	7	1V+1MT+2½FAT
Ensalada Azteca	130	9	230	7	1½V+2FAT
Garden Fresh Pasta w/ripe avocado	240	12	360	27	1½ST+2½FAT
Ginger Lime Shrimp Salad	120	5	130	12	½ST+1MT
Greek Salad	120	9	320	4	1V+2FAT
Lox & Bagels Salad	130	9	250	8	½ST+½MT+1FAT
Mandarin Spinach w/carmel'd walnuts	170	11	150	14	1V+½FR+2FAT
Ranch House BLT Salad w/turkey	180	11	390	10	2V+ ½MT+2FAT
Roasted Vegetables w/feta & olives	140	11	340	5	1V+2FAT
Roma Tomato, Mozzarella & Basil	120	9	180	7	1V+½MT+1FAT
Shrimp & Krab Louis Salad	180	12	340	6	1V+1MT+1½FAT
Traditional Spinach Salad w/bacon	160	11	310	7	2V+2FAT
Won Ton Chicken Salad	150	8	220	12	¾ST+1MT+½FAT
Fat-Free Salad Dressings (2T):					
Honey Mustard Dressing	45	0	160	10	½CHO
Italian Dressing	20	0	340	5	FREE
Ranch Dressing	50	0	180	2	½CHO
Low-Fat & Reduced Calorie Salad Dressings (2T):					
Garden Fresh French Tomato	40	1.5	270	7	½CHO+½FAT
Creamy Cucumber Dressing	80	7	290	4	1½FAT
Parmesan & Garlic Croutons, 10 pieces	40	3	160	2	½FAT
Salad Dressings (2T):					
Balsamic House Vinaigrette	180	19	190	1	4FAT
Basil House Vinaigrette	160	17	160	1	3½FAT
Blue Cheese Dressing	140	14	230	3	3FAT
Blush Vinaigrette	120	12	320	3	2½FAT
Honey Ginger Dressing	150	15	200	5	¼CHO+3FAT
Honey Mustard Dressing	150	13	230	8	½CHO+2½FAT
Parmesan Pepper Cream Dressing	160	17	330	2	3½FAT
Ranch House Dressing	130	13	180	1	2½FAT
Raspberry Vinaigrette	120	13	150	3	2½FAT
Roasted Garlic Dressing	140	14	300	2	3FAT
Thousand Island Dressing	110	11	250	3	2FAT
Zesty Italian Dressing	160	18	280	1	3½FAT

*Carbs=Carbohydrate, na=not available   **Exchanges: ST=Starch, Mlk=Milk (skim)
FR=Fruit, CHO=Other Carbohydrates, V=Vegetable, MT=Meat (medium fat), FAT=Fat

SOUPLANTATION & SWEET TOMATOES™ (continued)

	Calories	Fat (g)	Sodium (mg)	Carbs* (g)	Exchanges**
Low-Fat Soups & Chilies (1 c):					
Chicken Tortilla Soup with Jalapeño Chilies & Tomatoes	100	3	990	5	1V+1½MT(lean)
Classic Chicken Noodle Soup	160	3	480	17	1ST+1½MT(lean)
French Onion Soup	80	3	990	11	½ST+½FAT
Garden Fresh Vegetable Soup	110	1	890	22	1ST+1V
House Chili	230	3	560	26	1½ST+1½MT(lean)
Pasta Fagioli	100	3	940	14	1ST+½FAT
Santa Fe Black Bean Chili	190	3	580	26	1½ST+1MT(lean)
Spicy 4-Bean Minestrone	140	3	980	23	1ST+1V+½FAT
Sweet Tomato Onion Soup	110	3	450	12	2V+½FAT
Turkey Noodle Soup	170	3	550	16	1ST+2MT(lean)
Vegetable Medley Soup	90	1	520	14	½ST+1V
Soups & Chilies (1 c):					
Albondigas Buenas (meatball soup)	190	9	720	17	1ST+1MT+1FAT
Arizona Chili	220	8	690	25	1ST+2MT
Butternut Squash Soup	140	6	670	15	1ST+1FAT
Chesapeake Corn Chowder	310	13	720	43	2½ST+2½FAT
Chicken Fajitas & Black Bean	280	7	980	33	1¾ST+2½MT(lean)
Chicken Jambalaya	160	7	980	13	1ST+1½MT
Chunky Potato Cheese w/Thyme	210	10	480	19	1ST+1MT+1FAT
Cream of Broccoli Soup	210	15	960	14	2V+3FAT
Cream of Chicken Soup	250	15	350	21	1½ST+1MT+1½FAT
Cream of Mushroom Soup	290	21	820	15	½ST+1V+1MT+3FAT
Green Chile Stew	150	6	980	14	1V+½ST+1MT
Irish Potato Leek Soup	260	16	680	23	1ST+1V+3FAT
Longhorn Beef Chili	190	6	790	25	1ST+1V+1MT
Minestrone with Italian Sausage	210	11	890	14	½ST+1V+1MT+1FAT
Navy Bean Soup with Ham	340	10	980	30	1½ST+4MT(lean)
New England Clam Chowder	330	20	630	21	1ST+2MT+2FAT
New Orleans Style Jambalaya	160	8	900	14	½ST+1V+½MT+1FAT
Posole	150	6	980	8	½ST+1½MT
Shrimp Bisque	300	19	880	20	1ST+1MT+3FAT
Split Pea Soup with Ham	350	10	980	32	1½ST+4MT(lean)
Southwest Tomato Cream Soup	120	6	720	14	1ST+1FAT
Texas Red Chili	240	8	680	30	1½ST+1V+1½MT
Turkey Cassoulet	360	12	890	32	2ST+4MT(lean)
Turkey Vegetable Soup	270	12	990	16	½ST+1V+2½MT
Vegetable Beef Stew	250	14	780	21	1V+1ST+1MT+1½FAT
Vegetarian Harvest Soup	190	8	990	23	½ST+2V+1½FAT
Yucatan Chili	280	10	890	31	1ST+1V+3MT(lean)

---

*Carbs=Carbohydrate, na=not available   **Exchanges: ST=Starch, Mlk=Milk (skim)
FR=Fruit, CHO=Other Carbohydrates, V=Vegetable, MT=Meat (medium fat), FAT=Fat

SOUPLANTATION & SWEET TOMATOES™ (continued)

	Calories	Fat (g)	Sodium (mg)	Carbs* (g)	Exchanges**
Hot Tossed Pasta (1 c):					
Bruschetta	260	4	450	41	2ST+2V+1FAT
Chipotle Chicken w/cilantro	390	16	560	42	2½ST+2½MT+½FAT
Creamy Pesto w/sundried tomatoes	430	21	410	44	2½ST+1V+1MT+3FAT
Creamy Bruschetta	360	16	510	43	2ST+1V+1MT+2FAT
Fettucine Alfredo	390	18	580	41	2½ST+1½MT+2FAT
Garden Vegetable w/meatballs	270	7	460	42	2ST+1V+1MT
Garden Vegetable w/Italian saus.	300	10	540	42	2ST+1V+1MT+1FAT
Italian Vegetable Beef	270	6	470	43	2ST+1V+1MT
Jalapeño Salsa	240	4	430	41	2ST+1V+1MT
Linguini with Clam Sauce	380	10	890	56	3½ST+1MT+1FAT
Nutty Mushroom	390	20	410	42	2ST+1V+1MT+2½FAT
Pasta Florentine	360	10	920	54	3ST+1V+1MT+1FAT
Pasta Primavera	350	8	630	60	3ST+2V+1½FAT
Sicilian with Capers & Olives	220	6	570	28	2ST+½MT+½FAT
Smoked Salmon & Dill	360	16	390	41	2ST+1V+1MT+2FAT
Tuscany Sausage w/Capers & Olives	240	10	920	29	2ST+½MT+1FAT
Vegetarian Marinara w/basil	260	4	750	44	2ST+2V+1FAT
Vermouth Cream Pasta	360	17	490	30	2ST+1MT+2½FAT
Walnut Pesto	310	9	610	42	3ST+1MT+½FAT
Low-Fat Fresh Baked Muffins & Breads (1 piece):					
Bran Muffins: Apple Cinn, Cranb Orange or Fruit Medley, 96% fat-free	80	0.5	110	17	1CHO
Buttermilk Corn Bread	140	2	270	27	1½ST+½FAT
Chile Corn Muffin	140	3	320	27	1½ST+½FAT
Garlic Parmesan Focaccia	100	3	170	15	1ST+½FAT
Indian Grain Bread	200	1.5	260	35	2½ST+½FAT
Sourdough Bread	150	0.5	240	27	1½ST
Fresh Baked Muffins & Breads (1 piece):					
Muffins: Apple Raisin, Apricot Nut, Banana Nut, or Cherry Nut	150	7	190	22	1½CHO+1½FAT
Carrot Pineapple Muffin w/Oat Bran	150	6	230	23	1½CHO+1FAT
Choc. Brownie, Choc. Chip, or Choc. Chip Mandarin Muffin	170	8	190	22	1½CHO+1½FAT
Georgia Peach Poppyseed Muffin	150	6	210	20	1½CHO+1FAT
Lemon Muffin	140	4	190	24	1½CHO+1FAT
Mandarin Alm. Muffin w/Oat Bran	140	7	210	20	1CHO+1½FAT
Maple Walnut Muffin	230	10	230	33	2CHO+2FAT
Nutty Peanut Butter Muffin	170	8	210	21	1½CHO+1½FAT
Pauline's Apple Walnut Cake	180	7	180	28	1½CHO+1½FAT
Peanut Butter Choc. Chip Muffin	190	9	230	23	1½CHO+2FAT
Pizza Focaccia	140	6	220	16	1ST+1FAT
Pumpkin Raisin Muffin	150	6	210	25	1½CHO+1FAT
Roasted Potato Focaccia	150	6	220	17	1ST+1FAT

*Carbs=Carbohydrate, na=not available   **Exchanges: ST=Starch, Mlk=Milk (skim)
FR=Fruit, CHO=Other Carbohydrates, V=Vegetable, MT=Meat (medium fat), FAT=Fat

SOUPLANTATION & SWEET TOMATOES™ (continued)

	Calories	Fat (g)	Sodium (mg)	Carbs* (g)	Exchanges**
Fresh Baked Muffins & Breads (1 piece):					
Strawberry Buttermilk Muffin	140	6	210	21	1½ST+1FAT
Sweet Orange & Cranberry Muffin	200	7	220	33	2CHO+1½FAT
Tomatillo Focaccia	140	6	270	16	1ST+1FAT
Tropical Papaya Coconut Muffin	180	7	210	28	1½CHO+1½FAT
Wild Maine Blueberry Muffin	140	5	180	22	1CHO+½FR+1FAT
Wild Maine Blueberry Muffin, lg	310	12	380	46	2CHO+1FR+2½FAT
Zucchini Nut Muffin	150	7	190	22	1½CHO+1½FAT
Fat-Free Desserts (½ c unless specified):					
Apple Medley	70	0	5	18	1CHO
Banana Royale	80	0	5	20	1CHO
Ghiradelli Choc. Frozen Yogurt	95	0	80	21	1½CHO
Jello, flavored	80	0	40	20	1CHO
Tropical Fruit Salad	75	0	5	19	1FR
Low-Fat *or* Reduced Fat Desserts (½ c):					
Chocolate Pudding	140	3	220	23	1½CHO+½FAT
Nutty Waldorf Salad	80	3	80	12	1FR+½FAT
Rice Pudding	110	2	50	20	1ST+½FAT
Tapioca Pudding	140	3	160	24	1½CHO+½FAT
Vanilla Soft Serve	140	4	70	22	1½CHO+1FAT
Yogurt Bar Toppings:					
Chocolate Syrup, 2T	70	0	15	18	1CHO
Candy Sprinkles, 1T	70	2	0	11	½CHO+½FAT
Granola Topping, 2T	110	4	14	16	1CHO+1FAT
Desserts:					
Banana Pudding, ½ c	160	4	220	27	1½CHO+1FAT
Chocolate Chip Cookie, 1 small	70	3	90	10	½CHO+½FAT
Vanilla Pudding, ½ c	140	4	160	24	1Mlk+½CHO+½FAT

Source: Souplantation & Sweet Tomatoes™. Current as of 12/99.

STARBUCKS COFFEE

	Calories	Fat (g)	Sodium (mg)	Carbs* (g)	Exchanges**
Drip Coffee:					
Short	5	0	5	1	FREE
Tall	10	0	10	1	FREE
Grande	10	0	15	2	FREE
Blended Coffee Frappuccino® (coffee, ice, & milk):					
Tall	180	2	180	38	½Mlk+2CHO
Grande	240	2.5	230	50	½Mlk+3CHO+½FAT
Venti	300	3	290	63	¾Mlk+3½CHO+½FAT

*Carbs=Carbohydrate, na=not available   **Exchanges: ST=Starch, Mlk=Milk (skim)
FR=Fruit, CHO=Other Carbohydrates, V=Vegetable, MT=Meat (medium fat), FAT=Fat

STARBUCKS COFFEE (continued)

	Calories	Fat (g)	Sodium (mg)	Carbs* (g)	Exchanges**
Blended Mocha Frappuccino® (coffee, ice, milk, chocolate syrup & flavoring):					
Tall	210	2	190	43	½Mlk+2½CHO+½FAT
Grande	280	3	250	58	½Mlk+3½CHO+½FAT
Venti	350	3.⁵	310	72	¾Mlk+4CHO+½FAT
Blended Rhumba Frappuccino® (coffee, ice, milk, chocolate syrup & flavoring):					
Tall	220	4	210	42	½Mlk+2½CHO+1FAT
Grande	290	5	290	56	½Mlk+3½CHO+1FAT
Venti	360	7	360	70	¾Mlk+4CHO+1½FAT
Espresso:					
Solo	5	0	0	1	FREE
Doppio	10	0	0	2	FREE
Espresso Con Panna (espresso w/whipped cream on top):					
Solo	35	3	0	1	½FAT
Dopio	40	3	5	2	1FAT
Espresso Macchiato (espresso dotted w/foamed milk):					
Solo, nonfat milk	10	0	10	2	FREE
Solo, lowfat milk	15	0	10	2	FREE
Solo, whole milk	15	0.⁵	10	2	FREE
Solo, soy milk	10	0	0	1	FREE
Doppio, nonfat milk	15	0	10	3	FREE
Doppio, lowfat milk*	20	0	10	3	FREE
Doppio, whole milk	20	0.⁵	10	3	FREE
Doppio, soy milk	15	0	0	2	FREE
Cappuccino:					
Short, nonfat milk	60	0	80	8	¾Mlk
Short, lowfat milk	80	2.⁵	80	8	¾Mlk+½FAT
Short, whole milk	100	5	75	8	¾Mlk+1FAT
Short, soy milk	60	3	20	4	½CHO+½MT
Tall, nonfat milk	80	0	110	11	1Mlk
Tall, lowfat milk	110	3.⁵	110	11	1Mlk+½FAT
Tall, whole milk	140	7	105	11	1Mlk+1½FAT
Tall, soy milk	70	4	25	5	¾CHO+¾MT
Grande, nonfat milk	110	0	140	15	1¼Mlk
Grande, lowfat milk	140	5	140	15	1¼Mlk+1FAT
Grande, whole milk	180	9	135	15	1¼Mlk+2FAT
Grande, soy milk	100	5	35	7	¾CHO+1MT
Venti, nonfat milk	120	0.⁵	160	17	1½Mlk
Venti, lowfat milk	160	5	160	17	1½Mlk+1FAT
Venti, whole milk	200	10	150	16	1¼Mlk+2FAT
Venti, soy milk	110	6	40	8	¾CHO+1MT

Carbs=Carbohydrate, na=not available   **Exchanges:** ST=Starch, Mlk=Milk (skim)
FR=Fruit, CHO=Other Carbohydrates, V=Vegetable, MT=Meat (medium fat), FAT=Fat

STARBUCKS COFFEE (continued)

	Calories	Fat (g)	Sodium (mg)	Carbs* (g)	Exchanges**
Caffè Americano (espresso & water):					
Short	5	0	5	1	FREE
Tall	10	0	10	2	FREE
Grande	15	0	15	3	FREE
Venti	15	0	20	3	FREE
Latte:					
Short, nonfat milk	80	0	110	11	1Mlk
Short, lowfat milk	110	3.5	110	11	1Mlk +½FAT
Short, whole milk	140	7	105	11	1Mlk +1FAT
Short, soy milk	70	4	25	5	¼CHO+¾MT
Tall, nonfat milk	120	0.5	170	17	1½Mlk
Tall, lowfat milk	170	6	170	17	1½Mlk+1FAT
Tall, whole milk	210	11	170	17	1½Mlk+2FAT
Tall, soy milk	110	6	40	7	½CHO+1MT
Grande, nonfat milk	160	1	220	23	2Mlk
Grande, lowfat milk	220	7	220	22	2Mlk+1½FAT
Grande, whole milk	270	14	210	22	2Mlk+3FAT
Grande, soy milk	150	8	55	10	½CHO+1½MT
Venti, nonfat milk	200	1	290	29	2½Mlk
Venti, lowfat milk	280	10	280	28	2½Mlk+2FAT
Venti, whole milk	350	18	270	28	2½Mlk+3FAT
Venti, soy milk	190	10	65	12	1CHO+2MT
Iced Latte:					
Short, nonfat milk	60	0	85	8	¾Mlk
Short, lowfat milk	80	2.5	80	8	¾Mlk+½FAT
Short, whole milk	100	5	80	5	¾Mlk+1FAT
Short, soy milk	60	3	25	4	¼CHO+½MT
Tall, nonfat milk	70	0	100	10	1Mlk
Tall, lowfat milk	90	3	100	10	1Mlk +½FAT
Tall, whole milk	120	6	95	10	1Mlk +1FAT
Tall, soy milk	70	3.5	30	4	¼CHO+¾MT
Grande, nonfat milk	100	0	135	14	1¼Mlk
Grande, lowfat milk	130	4.5	130	14	1¼Mlk+1FAT
Grande, whole milk	160	8	130	13	1¼Mlk+1½FAT
Grande, soy milk	90	4.5	35	6	½CHO+1MT
Venti, nonfat milk	110	0	150	15	1¼Mlk
Venti, lowfat milk	140	5	150	15	1¼Mlk+1FAT
Venti, whole milk	180	9	140	15	1¼Mlk+2FAT
Venti, soy milk	100	5	40	7	½CHO+1MT
Whipped Cream Topping:					
0.8 fl oz	80	9	10	1	2FAT

*Carbs=Carbohydrate, na=not available   **Exchanges: ST=Starch, Mlk=Milk (skim)
FR=Fruit, CHO=Other Carbohydrates, V=Vegetable, MT=Meat (medium fat), FAT=Fat

STARBUCKS COFFEE (continued)

	Calories	Fat (g)	Sodium (mg)	Carbs* (g)	Exchanges**
Cocoa (w/whipping cream unless specified):					
Short, nonfat milk	230	10	150	26	1Mlk+1CHO+2FAT
Short, lowfat milk	260	14	150	26	1Mlk+1CHO+2½FAT
Short, whole milk	290	17	140	25	1Mlk+1CHO+3½FAT
Short, soy milk w/out cream	140	5	55	19	1CHO+1MT
Tall, nonfat milk	300	11	220	38	1½Mlk+1½CHO+2FAT
Tall, lowfat milk	350	16	220	38	1½Mlk+1½CHO+3FAT
Tall, whole milk	390	21	210	38	1½Mlk+1½CHO+4FAT
Tall, soy milk w/out cream	210	8	85	28	1½CHO+1½MT
Grande, nonfat milk	380	12	290	51	2Mlk+2CHO+2½FAT
Grande, lowfat milk	430	18	280	51	2Mlk+2CHO+3FAT
Grande, whole milk	490	25	280	50	2Mlk+2CHO+5FAT
Grande, soy milk w/out cream	290	10	110	37	2CHO+2MT
Venti, nonfat milk	450	12	360	64	2¾Mlk+2CHO+2½FAT
Venti, lowfat milk	520	21	350	63	2¾Mlk+2CHO+4FAT
Venti, whole milk	590	29	350	62	2¾Mlk+2CHO+6FAT
Venti, soy milk w/out cream	360	13	140	47	3CHO+2½MT
Carmel Macchiato:					
Short, nonfat milk	90	0.⁵	75	17	½Mlk+¾CHO
Short, lowfat milk	110	2.⁵	70	17	½Mlk+¾CHO+½FAT
Short, whole milk	130	4.⁵	70	17	½Mlk+¾CHO+1FAT
Tall, nonfat milk	140	1	110	27	1Mlk+1CHO+¼FAT
Tall, lowfat milk	170	3.⁵	105	27	1Mlk+1CHO+½FAT
Tall, whole milk	190	7	105	27	1Mlk+1CHO+1½FAT
Grande nonfat milk	190	1	140	36	1¼Mlk+1¼CHO
Grande, lowfat milk	225	5	140	36	1¼Mlk+1¼CHO+1FAT
Grande, whole milk	250	9	135	36	1¼Mlk+1¼CHO+2FAT
Venti, nonfat milk	230	1	170	44	1½Mlk+1½CHO
Venti, lowfat milk	270	6	170	44	1½Mlk+1½CHO+1FAT
Venti, whole milk	310	11	170	44	1½Mlk+1½CHO+2FAT
Mocha (w/whipping cream unless specified):					
Short, nonfat milk w/out cream	120	1.⁵	95	22	¾Mlk+1CHO+½FAT
Short, lowfat milk	230	13	105	22	¾Mlk+1CHO+2½FAT
Short, whole milk	250	16	100	22	¾Mlk+1CHO+3FAT
Short, soy milk w/out cream	120	4.⁵	25	16	1CHO+½MT
Tall, nonfat milk w/out cream	180	2	150	33	1Mlk+1½CHO+½FAT
Tall, lowfat milk	300	15	160	33	1Mlk+1½CHO+3FAT
Tall, whole milk	340	20	150	33	1Mlk+1½CHO+4FAT
Tall, soy milk w/out cream	180	7	40	24	1½CHO+1MT
Grande, nonfat milk w/out cream	240	3	190	44	1¼Mlk+2CHO+½FAT
Grande, lowfat milk	370	17	200	44	1¼Mlk+2CHO+3FAT
Grande, whole milk	420	23	190	44	1¼Mlk+2CHO+4FAT
Grande, soy milk w/out cream	230	9	50	33	2CHO+1MT+½FAT

*Carbs=Carbohydrate, na=not available **Exchanges: ST=Starch, Mlk=Milk (skim)
FR=Fruit, CHO=Other Carbohydrates, V=Vegetable, MT=Meat (medium fat), FAT=Fat

STARBUCKS COFFEE (continued)

	Calories	Fat (g)	Sodium (mg)	Carbs* (g)	Exchanges**
Mocha, continued (w/whipping cream unless specified):					
Venti, nonfat milk w/out cream	300	3.^{5}	250	55	1½Mlk+2½CHO+1FAT
Venti, lowfat milk	450	20	250	55	1½Mlk+2½CHO+1FAT
Venti, whole milk	510	27	250	55	1½Mlk+2½CHO+1FAT
Venti, soy milk w/out cream	290	12	60	41	2½CHO+1½MT+1FAT
Iced Mocha (without whipping cream)					
Short, nonfat milk	100	1.^{5}	70	19	¼Mlk+1CHO
Short, lowfat milk	110	3	65	19	¼Mlk+1CHO+½FAT
Short, whole milk	130	5	65	19	¼Mlk+1CHO+1FAT
Short, soy milk	100	3.^{5}	20	15	1CHO+¼MT+½FAT
Tall, nonfat milk	130	2	80	26	¾Mlk+1CHO+¼FAT
Tall, lowfat milk	150	4	75	26	¾Mlk+1CHO+½FAT
Tall, whole milk	160	6	75	26	¾Mlk+1CHO+1FAT
Tall, soy milk	130	4	25	21	1½CHO+¼MT+½FAT
Grande, nonfat milk	170	2.^{5}	105	35	1Mlk+1½CHO+½FAT
Grande, lowfat milk	200	5	105	35	1Mlk+1½CHO+1FAT
Grande, whole milk	220	8	100	35	1Mlk+1½CHO+1½FAT
Grande, soy milk	170	6	35	29	1½CHO+½MT+½FAT
Venti, nonfat milk	210	3	115	42	1Mlk+2CHO+½FAT
Venti, lowfat milk	230	6	115	41	1Mlk+2CHO+1FAT
Venti, whole milk	260	9	110	41	1Mlk+2CHO+1½FAT
Venti, soy milk	200	6	35	36	2½CHO+½MT+1FAT
Steamed Milk:					
Short, nonfat milk	90	0	125	12	1Mlk
Short, lowfat milk	120	4.^{5}	125	12	1Mlk+1FAT
Short, whole milk	150	8	120	11	1Mlk+1½FAT
Short, soy milk	80	4.^{5}	30	4	¼CHO+1MT
Tall, nonfat milk	130	0.^{5}	190	18	1½Mlk
Tall, lowfat milk	180	6	180	17	1½Mlk+1FAT
Tall, whole milk	220	12	180	17	1½Mlk+1½FAT
Tall, soy milk	120	7	45	7	½CHO+1¼MT
Grande, nonfat milk	170	1	250	24	2Mlk
Grande, lowfat milk	240	9	250	23	2Mlk+2FAT
Grande, whole milk	300	16	240	23	2Mlk+3FAT
Grande, soy milk	160	9	60	9	½CHO+1½MT
Venti, nonfat milk	210	1	320	30	2½Mlk
Venti, lowfat milk	290	11	310	29	2½Mlk+2FAT
Venti, whole milk	370	20	300	28	2½Mlk+4FAT
Venti, soy milk	200	12	75	11	½CHO+2MT

---

*Carbs=Carbohydrate, na=not available   **Exchanges:** ST=Starch, Mlk=Milk (skim)
FR=Fruit, CHO=Other Carbohydrates, V=Vegetable, MT=Meat (medium fat), FAT=Fat

STARBUCKS COFFEE (continued)

	Calories	Fat (g)	Sodium (mg)	Carbs* (g)	Exchanges**
Bar Mocha Syrup:					
Short, 1 oz	50	1	0	12	¾CHO
Tall, 1.⁵ oz	70	1.⁵	0	18	1CHO
Grande, 2 oz	100	2	0	24	1½CHO+¼FAT
Venti, 2.⁵ oz	120	2.⁵	0	30	2CHO+½FAT
Frappucino® Mocha Syrup:					
Tall, 1.⁵ oz	25	0	10	5	¼CHO
Grande, 2 oz	35	0	15	7	½CHO
Venti, 2.⁵ oz	45	0.⁵	20	9	½CHO
Vanilla, Hazelnut, Almond, Raspberry, or Irish Creme Syrup:					
Short, 1 oz	40	0	0	10	¾CHO
Tall, 1.⁵ oz	60	0	0	15	1CHO
Grande, 2 oz	80	0	0	21	1½CHO
Venti, 2.⁵ oz	100	0	0	25	2CHO
Crème De Menthe (mint) Syrup:					
Short, 1 oz	45	0	0	11	¾CHO
Tall, 1.⁵ oz	70	0	0	16	1CHO
Grande, 2 oz	90	0	0	21	1½CHO
Venti, 2.⁵ oz	220	0	0	28	2CHO
Egg Nog Latte (whole milk)					
Short	320	14	160	39	¾Mlk+2CHO+2½FAT
Tall	490	22	260	60	1Mlk+3CHO+4FAT
Grande	630	28	330	78	1¼Mlk+4CHO+5FAT
Venti	810	36	420	99	1½Mlk+5CHO+6FAT
Mocha Valencia (with whipping cream unless specified):					
Short, nonfat milk w/out cream	140	1.⁵	80	30	¾Mlk+1½CHO
Short, lowfat milk	240	12	85	30	¾Mlk+1½CHO+2½FAT
Short, whole milk	260	14	85	30	¾Mlk+1½CHO+3FAT
Short, soy milk w/out cream	140	3.⁵	25	25	1½CHO+½MT
Tall, nonfat milk w/out cream	220	2	135	45	1¼Mlk+2CHO+½FAT
Tall, lowfat milk	330	15	140	45	1¼Mlk+2CHO+3FAT
Tall, whole milk	370	18	135	45	1¼Mlk+2CHO+3½FAT
Tall, soy milk w/out cream	220	6	40	38	2½CHO+1MT
Grande, nonfat milk w/out cream	290	2.⁵	170	60	1¾Mlk+2½CHO+½FAT
Grande, lowfat milk	420	16	180	60	1¾Mlk+2½CHO+3FAT
Grande, whole milk	460	21	170	60	1¾Mlk+2½CHO+4FAT
Grande, soy milk w/out cream	290	8	55	51	3½CHO+1½MT
Venti, nonfat milk w/out cream	370	3.⁵	230	75	2¼Mlk+3CHO+½FAT
Venti, lowfat milk	510	19	230	75	2¼Mlk+3CHO+4FAT
Venti, whole milk	560	25	230	75	2¼Mlk+3CHO+5FAT
Venti, soy milk w/out cream	360	10	70	63	2½CHO+2MT

*Carbs=Carbohydrate, na=not available   **Exchanges:** ST=Starch, Mlk=Milk (skim)
FR=Fruit, CHO=Other Carbohydrates, V=Vegetable, MT=Meat (medium fat), FAT=Fat

STARBUCKS COFFEE (continued)

	Calories	Fat (g)	Sodium (mg)	Carbs* (g)	Exchanges**
Iced Chai Latte:					
Tall, nonfat milk	110	0	95	21	¼Mlk+1CHO
Tall, lowfat milk	130	2.⁵	90	21	¼Mlk+1CHO+¼FAT
Tall, whole milk	150	5	90	21	¼Mlk+1CHO+½FAT
Tall, soy milk	100	3	35	16	1CHO+½MT
Grande, nonfat milk	160	0	140	30	½Mlk+1½CHO
Grande, lowfat milk	190	4.⁵	140	30	½Mlk+1½CHO+½FAT
Grande, whole milk	220	8	140	29	½Mlk+1½CHO+1FAT
Grande, soy milk	150	4.⁵	50	22	1½CHO+1MT
Venti, nonfat milk	190	0.⁵	170	36	¾Mlk+2CHO
Venti, lowfat milk	230	5	170	36	¾Mlk+2CHO+½FAT
Venti, whole milk	270	10	160	36	¾Mlk+2CHO+1½FAT
Venti, soy milk	190	6	55	28	2CHO+1MT
Wild Berry Tiazzi Blended Juiced Tea:					
Tall	230	0	40	53	3½CHO
Grande	290	0	55	68	4½CHO
Venti	340	0	65	80	5CHO
Berries & Cream Tiazzi Blended Juiced Tea:					
Tall	320	13	120	45	½Mlk+2½CHO+2FAT
Grande	400	14	150	59	½Mlk+3½CHO+2FAT
Venti	530	18	190	79	½Mlk+5CHO+3FAT
Mango Citrus Tiazzi Blended Juiced Tea:					
Tall	160	0	40	37	2½CHO
Grande	220	0	50	51	3½CHO
Venti	290	0	70	66	4½CHO
Orange & Cream Tiazzi Blended Juiced Tea:					
Tall	340	13	105	47	½Mlk+3CHO+2FAT
Grande	420	14	125	61	½Mlk+3½CHO+2FAT
Venti	550	18	160	82	½Mlk+5CHO+3FAT

Source: Starbucks Beverages Nutritional Information 1/11/99. Current as of 12/99. All ® in this section are trademarks of Starbucks.

*Carbs=Carbohydrate, na=not available   **Exchanges: ST=Starch, Mlk=Milk (skim) FR=Fruit, CHO=Other Carbohydrates, V=Vegetable, MT=Meat (medium fat), FAT=Fat

SUBWAY®

Nutritional information on regular 6" subs and salads includes the standard vegetables of onions, lettuce, tomatoes, pickles, green peppers, & olives. They do not include cheese (unless noted w/▲) or condiments. These are listed separately below.

	Calories	Fat (g)	Sodium (mg)	Carbs* (g)	Exchanges**
6" Cold Subs:					
Veggie Delite®	232	3	582	43	2½ST+1V
Turkey Breast	282	4	1170	45	2½ST+1V+1½MT(lean)
Turkey Breast & Ham	288	4	1256	45	2½ST+1V+1½MT(lean)
Ham	293	5	1342	45	2½ST+1V+1½MT(lean)
Roast Beef	296	5	928	45	2½ST+1V+1½MT(lean)
Subway Club®	304	5	1239	46	2½ST+1V+1½MT(lean)
Subway Seafood & Crab® a processed seafood & crab blend, made w/light mayo	338	9	1034	51	2½ST+1V+½MT+1FAT
Cold Cut Trio™	374	14	1435	45	2½ST+1V+1½MT+1½FAT
Tuna, made w/light mayo	378	14	942	45	3ST+1V+1½MT+1½FAT
Classic Italian B.M.T.®	450	21	1579	45	2½ST+1V+2MT+2FAT
6" Hot Subs:					
Roasted Chicken Breast	342	6	966	46	2½ST+1V+2½MT(lean)
Steak & Cheese▲	363	10	1160	47	2½ST+1V+2MT
Subway Melt®▲	370	11	1619	46	2½ST+1V+2MT
Meatball	413	15	1025	50	3ST+1V+1½MT+1½FAT
Wraps:					
Chicken Parmesan Ranch▲	333	5	1393	56	3½ST+1V+1MT(lean)
Steak & Cheese▲	353	9	1450	53	3ST+1V+1MT+1FAT
Turkey Breast & Bacon▲	355	10	1823	52	3ST+1V+½MT+1½FAT
Super Subs:					
Classic Italian B.M.T.®	668	39	2576	47	3ST+1V+3MT+4FAT
Subway Club®	377	7	1895	48	3ST+1V+3MT(lean)
Cold Cut Trio™	517	24	2289	47	3ST+1V+2½MT+1½FAT
Deli Style Sandwiches:					
Turkey Breast	227	3	839	37	2½ST+½V+½MT(lean)
Ham	224	3	827	37	2½ST+½V+½MT(lean)
Roast Beef	236	4	678	37	2½ST+½V+½MT)lean)
Tuna, made w/light mayo	267	8	627	37	2½ST+½V+½MT+½FAT
Bologna	283	10	785	37	2½ST+½V+½MT+1FAT
Condiments & Extras:					
Vinegar, 1 tsp	1	0	0	0	FREE
Mustard, 2 tsp	8	0	57	1	FREE
Light Mayonnaise, 1 tsp	15	2	33	0	FREE, 3 tsp=1FAT
Bacon, 2 slices	42	3	160	0	½MT or 1FAT
Cheese, 2 triangles	41	3	204	0	½MT
Mayonnaise, 1 tsp	37	4	27	0	1FAT
Olive Oil Blend, 1 tsp	45	5	0	0	1FAT

*Carbs=Carbohydrate, na=not available   ****Exchanges:** ST=Starch, Mlk=Milk (skim) FR=Fruit, CHO=Other Carbohydrates, V=Vegetable, MT=Meat (medium fat), FAT=Fat

SUBWAY® (continued)

	Calories	Fat (g)	Sodium (mg)	Carbs* (g)	Exchanges**
Salads (without salad dressings):					
Veggie Delite®	51	1	308	10	2V
Turkey Breast	101	2	896	12	2V+1½MT(very lean)
Subway Club®	123	3	965	12	2V+2MT(very lean)
Roast Beef	115	3	654	11	2V+1½MT(lean)
Ham	112	3	1068	11	2V+1½MT(lean)
Turkey Breast & Ham	107	2	982	11	2V+1½MT(lean)
Roasted Chicken Breast	162	4	693	13	2V+2½MT(lean)
Subway Seafood & Crab® a processed seafood & crab blend, made w/light mayo	157	7	761	17	½ST+2V+½MT+1FAT
Steak & Cheese▲	182	8	887	13	2V+2MT
Subway Melt®▲	190	9	1346	12	2V+2MT
Cold Cut Trio™	193	12	1162	12	2V+1½MT+1FAT
Tuna, made w/light mayo	198	12	669	11	2V+1MT+1½FAT
Meatball	232	13	751	17	½ST+2V+1MT+1½FAT
Classic Italian B.M.T.®	269	19	1305	11	2V+1MT+3FAT
Salad Dressing, per Tbsp (each packet has approximately 4 Tbsp):					
Creamy Italian	65	7	133	3	1½FAT
Fat Free Italian	5	0	153	1	FREE
French	70	6	100	5	½ST+1FAT
Fat Free French	18	0	98	4	FREE
Thousand Island	65	7	155	3	1½FAT
Ranch	88	10	118	2	2FAT
Fat Free Ranch	15	0	178	4	FREE
Cookies (1):					
Oatmeal Raisin	199	8	159	29	2ST+1½FAT
Low Fat Oatmeal Raisin	168	3	171	33	2ST+½FAT
Chocolate Chunk	215	10	144	29	2ST+2FAT
Chocolate Chip	214	10	144	29	2ST+2FAT
Chocolate Chip M&M®	212	10	144	29	2ST+2FAT
Peanut Butter	223	12	214	27	2ST+2FAT
Sugar	225	12	180	28	2ST+2FAT
Macadamia Nut	222	11	144	28	2ST+2FAT
Brazil Nut	215	10	153	29	2ST+2FAT

Source: Subway® Nutrition Guide ©5/99. Current as of 12/99. All ® in this section are trademarks of Subway®

---

*Carbs=Carbohydrate, na=not available   **Exchanges:** ST=Starch, Mlk=Milk (skim) FR=Fruit, CHO=Other Carbohydrates, V=Vegetable, MT=Meat (medium fat), FAT=Fat

TACO BELL®

	Calories	Fat (g)	Sodium (mg)	Carbs* (g)	Exchanges**
Breakfast:					
Fiesta Breakfast Burrito	280	16	580	25	1½ST+1MT+2FAT
Country Breakfast Burrito	270	14	690	26	1½ST+1MT+2FAT
Grande Breakfast Burrito	420	22	1050	43	3ST+1MT+2½FAT
Double Bacon & Egg Burrito	480	27	1240	39	2½ST+1MT+4½FAT
Breakfast Cheese Quesadilla	380	21	1010	33	2ST+1MT+3FAT
Breakfast Quesadilla with Bacon	450	27	1200	33	2ST+2MT+3FAT
Breakfast Quesadilla w/sausage	430	25	1090	33	2ST+2MT+3FAT
Hash Brown Nuggets	280	18	570	29	2ST+3FAT
Gorditas:					
Gordita Supreme™ - Beef	300	14	550	27	2ST+1MT+1½FAT
Gordita Supreme™ - Chicken	300	13	530	28	2ST+1MT+1½FAT
Gordita Supreme™ - Steak	300	14	550	27	2ST+1MT+1½FAT
Gordita Santa Fe™ - Beef	380	23	700	31	2ST+1MT+3FAT
Gordita Santa Fe™ - Chicken	370	20	610	30	2ST+1MT+3FAT
Gordita Santa Fe™ - Steak	370	20	620	29	2ST+1MT+3FAT
Gordita Baja™ - Beef	360	21	810	29	2ST+1MT+2½FAT
Gordita Baja™ - Chicken	340	18	710	28	2ST+1MT+2FAT
Gordita Baja™ - Steak	340	18	730	27	2ST+1MT+2FAT
Tacos:					
Taco	170	10	340	12	½ST+1MT+1FAT
Soft Taco	210	10	570	20	1ST+1MT+1FAT
Taco Supreme®	210	14	350	14	1ST+1MT+1½FAT
Soft Taco Supreme®	260	13	590	22	1½ST+1MT+1½FAT
Double Decker® Taco	330	15	740	37	2ST+1MT+2½FAT
Double Decker®Taco Supreme®	380	18	760	39	2½ST+1MT+2½FAT
Grilled Steak Soft Taco	200	7	570	19	1ST+1MT+1FAT
Grilled Steak Soft Taco Supreme®	240	11	580	21	1½ST+1MT+1FAT
Grilled Chicken Soft Taco	200	7	530	20	1½ST+1MT
Burritos:					
Bean Burrito	370	12	1080	54	3ST+1MT+1½FAT
Burrito Supreme®	430	18	1210	50	3ST+1MT+3FAT
Big Beef Burrito	400	17	1320	43	3ST+2MT+3FAT
Big Beef Burrito Supreme®	510	23	1500	52	3ST+2MT+3FAT
7-Layer Burrito	520	22	1270	65	4ST+1MT+3FAT
Grilled Chicken Burrito	390	13	1240	49	3ST+1MT+1½FAT
Big Chicken Burrito Supreme®	460	17	1200	50	3ST+2MT+2FAT
Chili Cheese Burrito	330	13	900	40	2½ST+1MT+1FAT

*Carbs=Carbohydrate, na=not available   **Exchanges:** ST=Starch, Mlk=Milk (skim)
FR=Fruit, CHO=Other Carbohydrates, V=Vegetable, MT=Meat (medium fat), FAT=Fat

TACO BELL® (continued)

	Calories	Fat (g)	Sodium (mg)	Carbs* (g)	Exchanges**
Specialty Items:					
Mexican Pizza	540	35	1030	42	2½ST+2MT+5FAT
Mexican Pizza, Chicken	520	32	940	41	2½ST+2MT+4½FAT
Mexican Pizza, Beef	530	33	950	39	2½ST+2MT+4½FAT
Tostada	250	12	640	27	2ST+1MT+1½FAT
Big Beef MexiMelt®	290	15	830	22	1½ST+2MT+1FAT
Taco Salad with Salsa	850	52	2250	69	3½ST+1V+3MT+7FAT
Taco Salad w/Salsa, w/out Shell	430	22	1990	36	1½ST+1V+3MT+1FAT
Cheese Quesadilla	350	18	860	31	2ST+2MT+1½FAT
Chicken Quesadilla	400	19	1050	33	2ST+3MT+1FAT
Chalupas:					
Chalupa Supreme™ - Beef	380	23	580	29	2ST+1MT+3FAT
Chalupa Supreme™ - Chicken	360	20	490	28	2ST+1MT+3FAT
Chalupa Supreme™ - Steak	360	20	500	27	2ST+1MT+3FAT
Chalupa Santa Fe™ - Beef	440	29	660	31	2ST+1MT+4½FAT
Chalupa Santa Fe™ - Chicken	420	26	560	30	2ST+1MT+4FAT
Chalupa Santa Fe™ - Steak	430	27	580	29	2ST+1MT+4½FAT
Chalupa Baja™ - Beef	420	27	760	30	2ST+1MT+4½FAT
Chalupa Baja™ - Chicken	400	24	660	28	2ST+1MT+4FAT
Chalupa Baja™ - Steak	400	24	680	27	2ST+1MT+4FAT
Nachos and Sides:					
Nachos	320	18	560	34	2ST+3½FAT
Big Beef Nachos Supreme	440	24	800	44	3ST+1MT+3½FAT
Nachos BellGrande®	760	39	1300	83	5½ST+1MT+6FAT
Nachos BellGrande® - Chicken	740	36	1200	82	5½ST+1MT+5½FAT
Nachos BellGrande® - Steak	740	37	1220	81	5½ST+1MT+5½FAT
Pintos'N Cheese	180	8	640	18	1ST+1MT+½FAT
Mexican Rice	190	9	750	23	1½ST+1½FAT
Cinnamon Twists	180	8	190	25	1½CHO+1FAT
Choco Taco® Ice Cream Dessert	310	17	100	37	2½CHO+3½FAT

Source: Taco Bell® Nutritional Information 11/30/99. Current as of 12/99. All ® in this section are trademarks of Taco Bell®.

TACO JOHN'S®

	Calories	Fat (g)	Sodium (mg)	Carbs* (g)	Exchanges**
Tacos:					
El Grande Taco	481	29	765	30	2ST+2½MT+3FAT
El Grande Chicken Taco	327	18	736	24	1½ST+2MT+1½FAT
Taco Bravo®	357	15	653	39	2½ST+1½MT+1FAT
Crispy Taco	194	12	253	13	1ST+1MT+1FAT
Softshell Taco	227	10	504	23	1½ST+1MT+1FAT
Softshell Chicken Taco	177	5	615	22	1½ST+1MT
Taco Burger	280	11	580	29	2ST+1½MT+½FAT
Burritos:					
Super Burrito	456	19	907	51	3ST+1½MT+2FAT
Meat & Potato Burrito	507	23	1236	58	4ST+1MT+3FAT
Chicken & Potato Burrito	455	19	1345	56	3½ST+1MT+2FAT
Bean Burrito	382	12	808	54	3½ST+1MT+1 FAT
Beefy Burrito	440	20	859	44	3ST+2MT+1½FAT
Special Features:					
Chicken Festive Burrito	544	28	1148	56	4ST+1MT+3½FAT
Chicken Festiva Salad	685	50	1424	39	2ST+1V+2MT+7½FAT
without dressing	359	19	660	27	1½ST+1V+2MT+2FAT
Taco Salad	716	45	1797	55	3ST+1V+2MT+6FAT
Taco Salad, w/o dressing	544	28	881	50	2½ST+1V+2MT+3FAT
Super Nachos	926	62	1451	69	4ST+2MT+9FAT
Super Potato Oles®	989	63	3023	83	5ST+11FAT
Potato Oles Bravo®	585	36	1807	55	3½ST+7FAT
Sierra Chicken Sandwich	511	28	931	40	2½ST+3MT+3FAT
Platter:					
Beef Enchilada Platter	848	43	2256	80	4½ST+4MT+4FAT
Chicken Enchilada Platter	708	33	2311	72	4ST+3MT+3FAT
Beef & Bean ChimiPlatter	747	34	1769	82	4½ST+2MT+4½FAT
Cheese & Chiles ChimiPlatter	799	43	1915	74	4½ST+2MT+6FAT
Sides:					
Potato Olés®	414	24	1195	45	2½ST+4FAT
Large Potato Olés®	545	32	1572	59	3½ST+5½FAT
Nachos	456	32	851	36	2½ST+6FAT
Texas Style Chili	376	22	945	23	1ST+1V+2MT+2½FAT
Green Chili	223	12	1236	19	1ST+1V+1MT+1½FAT
Refried Beans	377	13	991	46	2ST+2MT+1½FAT
Potato Olés®, small (Kid's meal)	305	18	880	33	2ST+3½FAT
Side Salad	292	24	556	15	½ST+1V+4½FAT
Mexican Rice	250	5	855	44	3ST+½FAT

---

*Carbs=Carbohydrate, na=not available **Exchanges:** ST=Starch, Mlk=Milk (skim)
FR=Fruit, CHO=Other Carbohydrates, V=Vegetable, MT=Meat (medium fat), FAT=Fat

TACO JOHN'S® (continued)

Desserts:

	Calories	Fat (g)	Sodium (mg)	Carbs* (g)	Exchanges**
Churro	158	11	115	13	1ST+2FAT
Choco Taco	311	17	100	37	2CHO+3FAT
Apple Grande	258	9	240	40	2½ST+2FAT
Dichos Cookies, 2 (Kid's meal)	68	4	12	2	¼ST+1FAT
Teddy Graham® Cubs (Kid's Meal)	60	2	80	11	½ST+½FAT
Taco John's Cinnamon Mint Swirl	60	0	5	14	1CHO

Local Favorites (not available in all locations):

	Calories	Fat (g)	Sodium (mg)	Carbs* (g)	Exchanges**
Smothered Burrito	577	27	1126	57	2½ST+3MT+2FAT
Chicken Fajita Burrito	320	10	889	41	2½ST+1½MT
Ranch Burrito	435	22	829	43	2½ST+1MT+2FAT
Chimichanga	589	29	1139	57	3½ST+1½MT+4FAT
Double Enchilada	545	32	857	34	2½ST+3MT+3½FAT
Taco John's Mexican Pizza	583	32	718	14	1ST+3MT+3FAT
Mexi Rolls®	696	41	1346	53	3½ST+3MT+4½FAT
Chicken Fajita Salad	646	39	1943	53	3ST+1V+2MT+5FAT
Combination Burrito	411	16	833	49	2½ST+1½MT+1FAT
Potato Oles® with Nacho Cheese	549	35	2045	51	3½ST+6FAT
Tostada	195	12	254	13	¾ST+1MT+1FAT
Bean Tostada	166	8	228	18	1ST+½MT+1FAT
Cheese Crisp	222	16	252	10	¾ST+1½MT+1½FAT
Chicken Quesadilla	438	20	1138	42	2½ST+2MT+1½FAT
Chilito	445	22	1063	41	2½ST+2½MT+1½FAT
Quesadilla	464	24	942	41	2½ST+1½MT+3FAT

Source: Taco John's® Nutritional Information 11/10/99. Current as of 12/99.

TACO TIME®

Burritos:

	Calories	Fat (g)	Sodium (mg)	Carbs* (g)	Exchanges**
Casita Burrito®, meat	647	31	1233	54	3½ST+5MT+1FAT
Crisp Burrito, bean	427	18	453	53	3ST+1MT+2½FAT
Crisp Burrito, chicken	422	25	795	32	2ST+1½MT+2½FAT
Crisp Burrito, meat	552	30	1000	39	2½ST+3½MT+2½FAT
Double Soft Bean Burrito	506	12	860	77	4½ST+1½MT+1FAT
Value Soft Bean Burrito, single	380	10	715	58	3½ST+1MT+1FAT
Double Soft Combination Burrito	617	23	1343	66	4ST+4MT+½FAT
Double Soft Meat Burrito	726	33	1809	55	3½ST+6½MT
Value Soft Meat Burrito, single	491	21	1197	48	3ST+3 MT+1FAT
Veggie Burrito	491	16	643	70	4ST+1V+1½MT+1½FAT

Carbs=Carbohydrate, na=not available   **Exchanges:** ST=Starch, Mlk=Milk (skim)
FR=Fruit, CHO=Other Carbohydrates, V=Vegetable, MT=Meat (medium fat), FAT=Fat

TACO TIME® (continued)

Tacos:	Calories	Fat (g)	Sodium (mg)	Carbs* (g)	Exchanges**
Chicken Soft Taco	387	16	933	41	2½ST+2MT+1FAT
Crisp Taco	295	17	609	16	1ST+2½MT+1FAT
Natural Super Taco, meat	627	27	915	60	4ST+4MT+1½FAT
Rolled Soft Flour Taco	512	23	1111	46	3ST+3½MT+1FAT
Super Shredded Beef Soft Taco	368	11	556	38	2½ST+1MT+1FAT
Taco Cheeseburger, meat	633	36	1291	48	3ST+3MT+4FAT
Value Soft Taco	316	15	599	23	1½ST+3MT
Salads, Dressing & Sauces:					
Chicken Taco Salad w/o dressing	370	21	861	27	1½ST+2MT+2FAT
Taco Salad w/out dressing, reg.	479	28	895	30	2ST+3½ MT+2FAT
Tostado Delight® Salad, meat	628	33	1004	48	3ST+4MT+2½FAT
Enchilada Sauce	12	0	133	3	FREE
Ranchero Salsa	21	1	192	3	FREE
Sour Cream Dressing	137	14	207	2	3FAT
Thousand Island Dressing	160	16	220	4	3FAT
Other Food Items:					
Crustos®	373	15	86	47	3ST+3FAT
Empanada, cherry	250	9	46	37	2½ST+2FAT
Mexi Fries®. regular	266	17	799	27	1½ST+3½FAT
Mexi Fries®, large	532	34	1598	54	3½ST+7FAT
Mexican Rice	159	2	530	30	2ST+½FAT
Nachos	680	38	1250	61	4ST+2MT+5½FAT
Nachos Deluxe	1048	57	2252	91	6ST+4MT+7½FAT
Quesadilla, cheese	205	11	255	17	1ST+1MT+1FAT
Refritos	326	10	525	44	3ST+1½MT+½FAT

Source: Taco Time International 12/99. Current as of 12/99. All ® in this section are trademarks of
Taco Time®

TCBY® TREATS

Soft-Serve (½ c):	Calories	Fat (g)	Sodium (mg)	Carbs* (g)	Exchanges**
Nonfat (NF) Frozen Yogurt	110	0	60	23	1½CHO
No Sugar Added NF Yogurt w/aspartame	80	0	35	20	1¼CHO
96% Fat Free Frozen Yogurt	130	3	60	23	1½CHO+½FAT
Nonfat & Nondairy Sorbet	100	0	30	24	1½CHO
Hand-Dipped (½ c):					
Lowfat Ice Cream	120	2.5	75	22	1½CHO
No Sugar Added Lowfat Ice Cream w/aspartame	100	2.5	55	20	1¼CHO

(Calorie content will vary with flavors)

Source: TCBY Systems Inc. Current as of 12/99. All ® in this section are trademarks of TCBY®

*Carbs=Carbohydrate, na=not available   **Exchanges: ST=Starch, Mlk=Milk (skim)
FR=Fruit, CHO=Other Carbohydrates, V=Vegetable, MT=Meat (medium fat), FAT=Fat

WENDY'S®

	Calories	Fat (g)	Sodium (mg)	Carbs* (g)	Exchanges**
Sandwiches:					
Plain Single	360	16	580	31	2ST+2MT+1FAT
Single with Everything	420	20	920	37	2ST+1V+2MT+2FAT
Big Bacon Classic	580	30	1460	46	3ST+4MT+1FAT
Jr. Hamburger	270	10	610	34	2ST+1MT(high fat)
Jr. Cheeseburger	320	13	830	34	2ST+2MT
Jr. Bacon Cheeseburger	380	19	850	34	2ST+1V+2MT+1FAT
Jr. Cheeseburger Deluxe	360	17	890	36	2ST+1V+2MT+1FAT
Hamburger, Kid's Meal	270	10	610	33	2ST+1MT(high fat)
Cheeseburger, Kid's Meal	320	13	830	33	2ST+2MT
Grilled Chicken Sandwich	310	8	790	35	2ST+1V+3MT(lean)
Breaded Chicken Sandwich	440	18	840	44	3ST+3MT
Chicken Club Sandwich	470	20	970	44	3ST+3MT(lean)+1FAT
Spicy Chicken Sandwich	410	15	1280	43	3ST+3MT(lean)
Sandwich Components:					
¼ lb Hamburger Patty	200	14	290	0	3MT
2 oz Hamburger Patty	100	7	150	0	1½MT
Grilled Chicken Fillet	110	3	450	0	3MT(very lean)
Breaded Chicken Fillet	230	12	490	10	½ST+2½MT
Spicy Chicken Fillet	210	9	920	10	½ST+3MT(lean)
Kaiser Bun	190	3	340	36	2½ST+½FAT
Sandwich Bun	160	2.5	280	29	2ST+½FAT
American Cheese, 1 sl	70	5	320	1	½MT+½FAT
American Cheese, Jr., 1 sl	45	3.5	220	0	½MT
Bacon, 1 pc	20	1.5	65	0	½FAT
Honey Mustard Red. Cal., 1 t	25	1.5	45	2	½FAT
Ketchup, 1 t	10	0	75	2	1t=FREE, 3t=½CHO
Mayonnaise, 1½ t	30	3	60	1	½FAT
Fresh Stuffed Pitas™ (with dressing):					
Chicken Caesar	490	18	1320	48	3ST+1V+3MT(lean) +1FAT
Classic Greek	440	20	1050	50	3ST+1V+1MT+2FAT
Garden Ranch Chicken	480	18	1180	51	3ST+1V+3MT(lean) + 1FAT
Garden Veggie	400	17	760	52	3ST+1V+3FAT
Pita Dressings (1T):					
Caesar Vinaigrette, Red. Fat, Red. Cal.	70	7	170	1	1½FAT
Garden Ranch Sauce, Red. Fat, Red. Cal	50	4.5	125	1	1FAT

---

*Carbs=Carbohydrate, na=not available   **Exchanges:** ST=Starch, Mlk=Milk (skim)
FR=Fruit, CHO=Other Carbohydrates, V=Vegetable, MT=Meat (medium fat), FAT=Fat

WENDY'S® (continued)

	Calories	Fat (g)	Sodium (mg)	Carbs* (g)	Exchanges**
Garden Spot® Salad Bar (for other items, see *Salads* chapter):					
Bananas & Strawberry Glaze, ¼ c	30	0	0	8	½ FR
Chicken Salad, 2T	70	5	135	2	½MT+½FAT
Pasta Salad, 2T	35	1.⁵	180	4	¼ST+¼FAT
Potato Salad, 2T	80	7	180	5	½ST+1FAT
Fresh-Salads-to-Go (w/out dressing):					
Caesar Side Salad	110	5	650	7	1V+1MT
Deluxe Garden Salad	110	6	350	9	1V+1FAT
Grilled Chicken Salad, no dressing	200	8	720	9	2V+3MT(lean)
Grilled Chicken Caesar Salad, no dressing	260	9		17	3V+3MT(lean)
Side Salad, no dressing	60	3	180	5	1V+1FAT
Taco Salad	380	19	1040	28	3V+1Mlk(whole)+2MT
Taco chips, 15	210	11	180	24	1½ST+2FAT
Soft Breadstick, 1 ea	130	3	250	23	1½ST
Salad Dressings: 2T (1 oz) =1 ladle, Packets = 2 oz except Italian Caesar=1.⁵ oz					
Blue Cheese, 2T	180	19	180	0	4FAT
French, 2T	120	10	330	6	½CHO+2FAT
French Fat Free, 2T	35	0	150	8	½CHO
Italian Caesar, 2T	150	16	240	1	3FAT
Italian, Red. Fat, Red. Cal., 2T	40	3	340	2	½FAT
Hidden Valley Ranch™, 2T	100	10	220	1	2FAT
Hidden Valley Ranch™, Red. Fat Red. Cal., 2T	60	5	240	2	1FAT
Thousand Island, 2T	90	8	125	2	2½FAT
French Fries:					
Small	270	13	85	35	2ST+2FAT
Medium	390	19	120	50	3ST+3FAT
Biggie	470	23	150	61	3½ST+4FAT
Great Biggie	570	27	180	73	4½ST+5FAT
Baked Potato:					
Plain	310	0	25	71	4ST
Bacon & Cheese	530	18	1390	78	5ST+3FAT
Broccoli & Cheese	470	14	470	80	5ST+2FAT
Cheese	570	23	640	78	5ST+4FAT
Chili & Cheese	630	24	770	83	5ST+1MT+3FAT
Sour Cream & Chives	380	6	40	74	4ST+1FAT
Sour Cream, 1 packet	60	6	15	1	1FAT
Whipped Margarine, 1 packet	60	7	115	0	1½FAT

*Carbs=Carbohydrate, na=not available   **Exchanges: ST=Starch, Mlk=Milk (skim)
FR=Fruit, CHO=Other Carbohydrates, V=Vegetable, MT=Meat (medium fat), FAT=Fat

WENDY'S® (continued)

	Calories	Fat (g)	Sodium (mg)	Carbs* (g)	Exchanges**
Chili:					
Small, 8 oz	210	7	800	21	1ST+1V+1MT(high fat)
Large, 12 oz	310	10	1190	32	1½ST+1V+1½MT
Cheddar Cheese, shredded, 2T	70	6	110	1	½MT
Saltine Crackers, 2 ea	25	0.5	80	4	4 crackers=1ST+½FAT
Chicken Nuggets:					
5 pc Nuggets	230	16	470	11	½ST+1½MT+1½FAT
4 pc Kids'Meal	190	13	380	9	½ST+1MT+1½FAT
Barbecue Sauce, 1 pkt	45	0	160	10	½CHO
Honey Mustard Sauce, 1 pkt	130	12	220	6	½CHO+2FAT
Sweet & Sour Sauce, 1 pkt	50	0	120	12	1CHO
Desserts:					
Chocolate Chip Cookie, 1 ea	270	13	120	36	2CHO+2FAT
Frosty Dairy Dessert, sm, 12 oz	330	8	200	56	3CHO+1Mlk(lowfat)
medium, 16 oz	440	11	260	73	4CHO+1½Mlk(lowfat)
large, 20 oz	540	14	320	91	4½CHO+2Mlk(lowfat)

Source: Wendy's® Nutrition/Ingredient Guide ©1998 & Diabetic Exchange List. Current as of 12/99. All ® in this section are trademarks of Wendy's®.

WHATABURGER®

	Calories	Fat (g)	Sodium (mg)	Carbs* (g)	Exchanges**
Breakfast Items:					
Taquito, Potato & Egg	446	22	883	48	2½ST+1MT+3½FAT
Taquito, Sausage & Egg	443	26	790	32	2ST+2MT+3FAT
Taquito, Bacon & Egg	335	16	761	32	2ST+1½MT+1½FAT
Egg Omlette Sandwich	288	13	602	29	2ST+1MT+1½FAT
Breakfast on a Bun™ w/sausage	455	28	886	30	2ST+2MT+3½FAT
Breakfast on a Bun™ w/bacon	365	19	815	29	2ST+1½MT+2½FAT
Pancakes, order of 3	259	6	842	40	2½ST+1FAT
Pancakes, order of 3 w/sausage	426	21	1127	40	2½ST+1½MT+2½FAT
Pancakes, order of 3 w/2 bacon	335	12	1074	40	2½ST+1MT+1½FAT
Biscuit, Plain	280	13	509	37	2½ST+2½FAT
Biscuit w/bacon	359	20	730	37	2½ST+4FAT
Biscuit w/sausage	446	29	794	37	2½ST+1MT+5FAT
Biscuit w/sausage gravy	479	27	1253	48	3½ST+5½FAT
Biscuit w/egg and cheese	434	26	797	38	2½ST+1MT+4FAT
Biscuit w/bacon, egg, & cheese	511	33	1010	38	2½ST+1½MT+5FAT
Biscuit w/sausage, egg, & cheese	601	42	1081	38	2½ST+2MT+6½FAT
Breakfast Platter w/sausage	785	53	1234	54	3½ST+2MT+8½FAT
Breakfast Platter w/bacon	695	44	1162	54	3½ST+1½MT+7FAT
Cinnamon Roll	320	16	190	39	2½CHO+3FAT
Blueberry Muffin	239	8	538	36	2½CHO+1½FAT

Carbs=Carbohydrate, na=not available   **Exchanges:** ST=Starch, Mlk=Milk (skim)
FR=Fruit, CHO=Other Carbohydrates, V=Vegetable, MT=Meat (medium fat), FAT=Fat

WHATABURGER®

	Calories	Fat (g)	Sodium (mg)	Carbs* (g)	Exchanges**
Burgers:					
Whataburger®	598	26	1096	61	4ST+2½MT+2½FAT
on small bun & w/out bun oil	407	19	839	34	2ST+2½MT+1½FAT
Double Meat Whataburger®	823	42	1298	62	4ST+5MT+3½FAT
Whataburger, Jr®	322	13	603	35	2ST+1½MT+1FAT
Justaburger®	298	13	598	30	2ST+1½MT+1FAT
Fajitas:					
Chicken Fajita	272	7	691	35	2ST+1V+1½MT
Beef Fajita	326	12	670	34	2ST+1V+2½MT
Chicken & Fish:					
Grilled Chicken Sandwich	442	14	1103	48	3ST+3½MT
w/out salad dressing	385	9	989	46	3ST+3½MT(lean)
w/out bun oil & w/out dressing	358	6	989	46	3ST+3½MT(lean)
on small bun w/out bun oil & w/mustard instead of dressing	300	3	994	35	2ST+3½MT(very lean)
Whatachick'n® Sandwich	501	23	1122	51	3ST+3MT+1½FAT
Chicken Strips, 2 strips	300	20	630	15	1ST+2MT+2FAT
Whatacatch®	467	25	636	43	3ST+1½MT+3½FAT
Salad and Salad Dressings:					
Garden Salad	56	0.6	32	11	½ST+1V
Grilled Chicken Salad	150	1	434	14	1ST+3MT(very lean)
Fries and Onion Rings:					
French Fries, junior	221	12	139	25	1½ST+2½FAT
French Fries, regular	332	18	208	37	2½ST+3½FAT
French Fries, large	442	24	227	49	3ST+5FAT
Onion Rings, regular	329	19	596	34	2ST+4FAT
Onion Rings, large	493	29	893	51	3½ST+6FAT
Desserts and Shakes:					
Vanilla Shake, junior	325	10	172	51	3½CHO+2FAT
Strawberry Shake, junior	352	9	168	60	4CHO+2FAT
Chocolate Shake, junior	364	9	172	61	4CHO+2FAT
Chocolate Chunk Cookie	247	16	75	28	2CHO+3FAT
Macadamia Nut Cookie	269	16	80	31	2CHO+3FAT
Fried Apple Turnover	215	11	241	27	1FR+1CHO+2FAT

Source: WHATABURGER, Inc. Current as of 12/99. All ® in this section are the trademarks of WHATABURGER, Inc.

---

*Carbs=Carbohydrate, na=not available   **Exchanges:** ST=Starch, Mlk=Milk (skim)
FR=Fruit, CHO=Other Carbohydrates, V=Vegetable, MT=Meat (medium fat), FAT=Fat

WHITE CASTLE®

Menu Items (not all items available in every restaurant):	Calories	Fat (g)	Sodium (mg)	Carbs* (g)	Exchanges**
Hamburger	135	7	135	11	½ST+¾MT+¾FAT
Cheeseburger	160	9	250	11	½ST+1MT+1FAT
Double Hamburger	235	14	200	16	1ST+1MT+1½FAT
Double Cheeseburger	285	18	430	16	1ST+1½MT+2FAT
Bacon Cheeseburger	200	13	400	12	½ST+1½MT+1FAT
Fish Sandwich	160	6	220	18	1ST+¾MT+½FAT
Fish with Cheese	190	8	357	19	1ST+1MT+½FAT
Chicken Sandwich	190	8	360	21	1½ST+¾MT+½FAT
Breakfast Sandwich	340	25	900	17	1ST+1½MT+3FAT
Chicken Rings*	310	21	600-620	14	1ST+1½MT+2½FAT
Onion Rings*	460-540	26-27	550-1300	56-69	4ST+5FAT
French Fries, small	115	6	15	15	1ST+1FAT
Cheese Sticks, 3	290	17	730	19	1ST+1¾MT+1½FAT
Cheese Sticks, 5	491	28	1216	32	2ST+3MT+2½FAT
Vanilla Shake, 14 oz	230	7	150	35	2CHO+1½FAT
Chocolate Shake, 14 oz	220	7	140	32	2CHO+1½FAT
Chili, 12 oz	375	15	1635	45	3ST+3½MT
Chicken Ring Sandwich	170	7	210	15	1ST+½MT+½FAT
Onion Chips, small	180	9	580	25	1½ST+1½FAT

* **Varies among restaurants.**
Source: White Castle Systems. Current as of 12/99. For more information, call 1-800-THE-CRAVE.

---

*Carbs=Carbohydrate, na=not available   **Exchanges:** ST=Starch, Mlk=Milk (skim)
FR=Fruit, CHO=Other Carbohydrates, V=Vegetable, MT=Meat (medium fat), FAT=Fat

Index

Joanne V. Lichten, PhD, RD

helping busy people stay healthy & sane

Get your "ticket" to staying healthy & sane in this whirlwind world. The ticket includes Dr. Lichten's speaking topics. She's available to speak to your company, group, or association.

Call today: 1-888-431-LEAN

Topics include:

How to Stay Healthy & Fit (for Travelers or Busy People)

Defensive Dining (based on Dining Lean)

Keeping Your Energy Up All Day Long

Swimming in a Sea of Priorities (Gettting Your Life in Balance)

How to Defuse Anger & Calm People Down

How to Fix an Attitude (Dealing with Negativity)

Dealing with Difficult People

Stay Calm, State Your Case, & Be Listened To

How to Enjoy the Ride of Your Life (Managing Change)

Order Form

**For credit card orders (Visa, MC, Discover)
or to inquire about quantity discounts
call 1-888-431-LEAN
or email dininglean@aol.com**

_____ copies of Dining Lean @ $14.95 each _____

If shipping to Texas add 7¼% ($1.08 ea)_____

Shipping cost $3 for 1st book, $1 for each add'l _____

_____ Dining Lean Wallet Card @ $3.00 each _____
Price for wallet card includes applicable tax & shipping
(Wallet card is 8 part accordian-folded & laminated)

Total _____

Name:_____

Address:_____

City:_____ State:_____ Zip:_____

Phone: _____ Email: _____

Send check or money order to:
Nutrifit Publishing
PO Box 690452
Houston, TX 77269-0452

Joanne V. Lichten, PhD, RD

helping busy people stay healthy & sane

Get your "ticket" to staying healthy & sane in this whirlwind world. The ticket includes Dr. Lichten's speaking topics. She's available to speak to your company, group, or association.

Call today: 1-888-431-LEAN

Topics include:

How to Stay Healthy & Fit (for Travelers or Busy People)

Defensive Dining (based on Dining Lean)

Keeping Your Energy Up All Day Long

Swimming in a Sea of Priorities (Gettting Your Life in Balance)

How to Defuse Anger & Calm People Down

How to Fix an Attitude (Dealing with Negativity)

Dealing with Difficult People

Stay Calm, State Your Case, & Be Listened To

How to Enjoy the Ride of Your Life

Order Form

**For credit card orders (Visa, MC, Discover)
or to inquire about quantity discounts
call 1-888-431-LEAN
or email dininglean@aol.com**

_____ copies of Dining Lean @ $14.95 each _____

If shipping to Texas add 7¼% ($1.08 ea)_____

Shipping cost $3 for 1st book, $1 for each add'l _____

_____ Dining Lean Wallet Card @ $3.00 each _____

Price for wallet card includes applicable tax & shipping
(Wallet card is 8 part accordian-folded & laminated)

Total _____

Name:_____

Address:_____

City:_____ State:_____ Zip:_____

Phone: _____ Email: _____

Send check or money order to:
Nutrifit Publishing
PO Box 690452
Houston, TX 77269-0452